Sexuality, Health and Human Rights

This new work surveys how rapid changes taking place at the start of the twenty-first century in social, cultural, political and economic domains impact on sexuality, health and human rights. The relationships between men, women and children are changing quickly, as are traditional family structures and gender norms. What were once viewed as private matters have become public, and an array of new social movements – transgender, intersex, sex worker, people living with HIV – have come into the open.

The book is split into three parts:

- Global 'sex' wars – discusses the notion of sexualities, its political landscapes internationally, and the return of religious fervour and extremism.
- Epistemological challenges and research agendas – examines modern 'scientific' understandings of sexuality, its history and the way in which HIV and AIDS have drawn attention to sexuality.
- The promises and limits of sexual rights – discusses human rights approaches to sexuality, its strengths and limitations and new ways of imagining erotic justice.

Offering a unique framework for understanding this new world, set in the context of the major theoretical debates of recent decades, this book will be of interest to professionals, advocates and policy researchers, and is suitable for a wide range of courses covering areas such as gender studies, human sexuality, public health and social policy.

Sonia Corrêa coordinates Sexuality Policy Watch at the Brazilian Interdisciplinary AIDS Association (ABIA), Brazil. **Rosalind Petchesky** is Distinguished Professor of Political Science at Hunter College, City University of New York, USA. **Richard Parker** is Professor of Sociomedical Sciences at Columbia University, USA.

Sexuality, Culture and Health series

Edited by Peter Aggleton, Institute of Education, University of London, UK
Richard Parker, Columbia University, New York, USA
Sonia Corrêa, ABIA, Rio de Janeiro, Brazil
Gary Dowsett, La Trobe University, Melbourne, Australia
Shirley Lindenbaum, City University of New York, USA

This new series of books offers cutting-edge analysis, current theoretical perspectives and up-to-the-minute ideas concerning the interface between sexuality, public health, human rights, culture and social development. It adopts a global and interdisciplinary perspective in which the needs of poorer countries are given equal status to those of richer nations. The books are written with a broad range of readers in mind, and will be invaluable to students, academics and those working in policy and practice. The series also aims to serve as a spur to practical action in an increasingly globalized world.

Also available in the series:

Culture, Society and Sexuality
A reader, 2nd edn
Edited by Richard Parker and Peter Aggleton

Dying to be Men
Youth masculinity and social exclusion
Gary T. Barker

Sex, Drugs and Young People
International perspectives
Edited by Peter Aggleton, Andrew Ball and Purnima Mane

Promoting Young People's Sexual Health
International perspectives
Edited by Roger Ingham and Peter Aggleton

Dangerous Liaisons?
Mobility, sexuality and AIDs
Edited by Felicity Thomas, Mary Haour-Knipe and Peter Aggleton

Sexuality, Health and Human Rights

Sonia Corrêa, Rosalind Petchesky
and Richard Parker

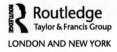
Routledge
Taylor & Francis Group

LONDON AND NEW YORK

First published 2008
by Routledge
2 Park Square, Milton Park, Abingdon, Oxon OX14 4RN

Simultaneously published in the USA and Canada
by Routledge
270 Madison Ave, New York, NY 10016

Routledge is an imprint of the Taylor & Francis Group, an informa business

Transferred to Digital Printing 2010

© 2008 Sonia Corrêa, Rosalind Petchesky and Richard Parker

Typeset in Sabon by Wearset Ltd, Boldon, Tyne and Wear

British Library Cataloguing in Publication Data
A catalogue record for this book is available from the British
Library

Library of Congress Cataloging in Publication Data
Corrêa, S. (Sonia)
Sexuality, health and human rights / Sonia Corrêa, Rosalind
Petchesky and Richard Parker.
p. cm. – (Sexuality, culture and health)
1. Sex–Social aspects. 2. Sex–Political aspects. 3. Sex–Health
aspects. 4. Human rights. I. Petchesky, Rosalind P. II. Parker,
Richard. III. Title.
HQ23.C6473 2008
306.7–dc22   2008002205

ISBN10: 0-415-35117-0 (hbk)
ISBN10: 0-415-35118-9 (pbk)
ISBN10: 0-203-89417-0 (ebk)

ISBN13: 978-0-415-35117-1 (hbk)
ISBN13: 978-0-415-35118-8 (pbk)
ISBN13: 978-0-203-89417-0 (ebk)

Contents

Acknowledgements

All books are constructed through complex processes, and their authors acquire many debts along the way. As three co-authors drawing on work conducted over many years and with broad networks of colleagues, friends, and loved ones who have contributed in myriad ways to the ideas we have tried to develop here, we have many debts – far more than we can do justice to in these brief acknowledgements.

First and foremost, we thank Peter Aggleton for encouraging us to take on this project, for waiting patiently in the face of many delays, and for convincing us that it was worth the wait. We are also deeply grateful to Grace McInnes, our editor at Routledge, whose ongoing support has been essential to the conclusion of this project.

Sonia Corrêa and Richard Parker acknowledge the support of a John D. and Catherine T. MacArthur Foundation Research and Writing Grant on Peace and Security Studies, from 1999 to 2001, which made it possible for them to begin to explore many of the issues examined in this volume. Rosalind Petchesky would like to thank Sexuality Policy Watch (SPW) and the Dean of Arts and Sciences at Hunter College for making it possible for her to take time off in 2005 to 2006 to dedicate to this project.

This effort has evolved from our ongoing work with SPW, with primary support from the Ford Foundation. We particularly thank the programme officers at Ford, Sarah Costa and Barbara Klugman, for the many contributions they have made to our thinking. We also thank our colleagues in the Steering Committee and the Advisory Group for SPW, Amal Abd El-Hadi Abou Halika, Sunila Abeysekera, Dorothy Aken'Ova, Codou Bop, Gloria Careaga, Radhika Chandiramani, Adenike O. Esiet, Maria Luiza Heilborn, Gilbert Herdt, Jodi Jacobson, Rhoda Reddock, Ignacio Saiz, David Satcher, and Michael Tan, whose ideas have helped to shape our thinking in various ways over the past six years.

We acknowledge the influence of the remarkable group of researchers who collaborated with us on the 2007 SPW volume, *SexPolitics: Reports from the Front Lines*, which is, in many ways, the companion volume to the current book: Wesal Afifi, Hossam Bahgat, Belinda Beresford, Carlos

Cáceres, Kenneth de Camargo, Sergio Carrara, Marcos Cueto, Le Minh Giang, Françoise Girard, Nguyen Thi Mai Huong, Pinar Ilkkaracan, Ruben Mattos, Constance A. Nathanson, Wanda Nowicka, Nancy Palomino, Radhika Ramasubban, Helen Schneider, Robert Sember, and Adriana R.B. Vianna.

We owe a huge debt to our colleagues in the SPW Secretariats in New York City, in the Center for Gender, Sexuality and Health and the Department of Sociomedical Sciences of the Mailman School of Public Health at Columbia University, and in Rio de Janeiro, at ABIA (Associação Brasileira Interdisciplinar de AIDS). We particularly thank Vagner de Almeida, Angela Collet, Kirk Fiereck, Jonathan Garcia, Miguel Muñoz-Laboy, Maria Dulce F. Natividad, Mayra Pabon, Robert Sember, and Nancy Worthington from the SPW Secretariats and Lindsay Ryan from Hunter College. Without their help and support, and their intellectual collaboration and partnership, this book would never have been finished.

We acknowledge a wide range of friends and colleagues who have provided comments, offered information, and given us advice, especially Carmen Barroso, Ronald Bayer, Suki Beavers, Alan Berkman, Mauro Cabral, Rhonda Copelon, Andrea Cornwall, Philip Dayle, Diane Di Mauro, Zillah Eisenstein, Amy Fairchild, John Fisher, Jennifer Hirsch, Paul Hunt, Susan Jolly, Scott Long, Elevarti Manohar, Katherine McDonald, Pramada Menon, Alice Miller, Geeta Misra, Vanita Mukherjee, Vera Paiva, Magaly Pazello, Cristina Pimenta, Allan Rosenfield, Alejandra Sardá, Gita Sen, Fatou Sow, Yvonne Szasz, Veriano Terto Jr., Carole S. Vance, Kim Vance, Miriam Ventura, and members of the seminar on Geopolitics and Insecurity at the CUNY Graduate Center.

We thank Joan Ross Frankson for her help in editing the text, smoothing out our very different writing styles and making sense out of our frequent confusions, and for the good spirits, solidarity, and intelligence she brings to her work.

Finally, in memoriam, we record a special acknowledgement to our dear friend José Barzelatto, who did so much in the early 1990s to create the context in which the various threads that unite our work could come together and intertwine. José may never have fully realized how great his legacy would be, or how much his work did to bridge the divides that existed between a number of intellectual fields (and social movements). As he showed, such divides can only be truly overcome through mutual dialogue and deeply rooted coalitions. We owe José a profound debt of gratitude.

All the colleagues mentioned here have made this text much stronger than it would otherwise have been. The limitations that remain are entirely our responsibility.

Introduction

> I have felt the necessity for a chorus, for a choreographic text with poly-sexual signatures.... [W]hat if we were to reach ... the area of a relationship to the other where the code of sexual marks would no longer be discriminating? The relationship would not be a-sexual, far from it, but would be sexual otherwise: beyond the binary difference that governs the decorum of all codes, beyond the opposition feminine–masculine, beyond bi-sexuality as well, beyond homosexuality and heterosexuality, which come to the same thing. As I dream of saving the chance that this question offers I would like to believe in the multiplicity of sexually marked voices. I would like to believe in the masses, this indeterminable number of blended voices, this mobile of non-identified sexual marks whose choreography can carry, divide, multiply the body of each 'individual'.
>
> (Derrida 1982, p. 76)

We write at a time when 'sex' (understood not simply as an empirical reality, but as a complex construct of multiple discursive framings and political struggles) seems to be everywhere around us – in popular culture, media, the Internet, and the rise and resurgence of religion, but also in the tragic march to war and the most remarkable (and often horrifying) actions of governments and states.

In the midst of this sexualized cacophony, complex global transformations and crises intersect with the equally complex dynamics of personal and intimate relations, marking out and defining 'sex', or sexuality, as one of the most charged battlegrounds of the twenty-first century. While sexuality has long been a highly controversial subject – deeply politicized in ways that we will analyse in this book – for many years, research and analysis focusing on the social, cultural, and political dimensions of sexuality languished, and financial support for such work was almost non-existent. Particularly in the wake of the emerging HIV epidemic in the 1980s, the consequences of this long-term neglect became quickly apparent – as did the limitations of existing conceptual frameworks and methodologies. As both researchers and practitioners have struggled to address these issues in recent decades, a new wave of research, intervention, and activism has emerged, more often than not from the ground up, in response to the needs and demands of local communities struggling to react constructively to a range of challenges to both sexuality and health and sexuality and rights in the contemporary world (Parker 2007).

One of the key aspects of research, action, and intervention in relation to these issues – a quality that links this area of work to many others, such as gender studies and postcolonial studies – is the extent to which it has been shaped by an evolving set of highly active and engaged social movements. It is impossible to imagine the recent explosion of work on sexuality, for example, independent of the development of the feminist and women's health movements. Since the 1970s, the analysis of gender and gender power differentials as central to any full understanding of sexual relations and interactions has been a crucial contribution of feminist analysis. It has shaped our understanding of the most pressing issues that must be addressed in seeking to promote sexual well-being and freedom.

But just as the feminist and women's health movements have shaped our understandings of the sexual field, so too have the lesbian, gay, bisexual, transgender, and, in some renderings, queer, movements. Emerging before AIDS in many of the most highly industrialized countries of the world, and often in the wake of AIDS in many developing nations, 'LGBTQI'[1] scholarship and activism have played a central role in calling attention to sexual diversity. In so doing, they have caused us to rethink the understanding of binary categories and classifications previously taken for granted – woman–man; male–female; heterosexual–homosexual; normal–abnormal – that had hitherto been used to map out the sexual field. Like feminism, lesbian, gay, transgender, and queer thinking drew attention to the intimate relations between sexuality and power, and has highlighted the need for new conceptual frameworks and innovative methodological approaches to the study of sexual communities and sexual life, and for strategies that account for the wide spatial, temporal, and cultural variability of sexual practices and meanings.

Drawing strength and inspiration from feminist and lesbian, gay, and transgender rights movements, AIDS activists – first in the industrialized West and subsequently across the global South – have also played a role in advocating for more effective research and programmes related to sexuality, health, and rights. They have been at the forefront in building political alliances around both HIV prevention and treatment access issues – alliances that have remade the way in which public health policy, research agendas, and programmes are designed and implemented, whether at the level of local communities, countries, or international and intergovernmental agencies. Like the feminist and lesbian, gay, and transgender movements, AIDS activism has played a key role in teaching sexual dissidents around the world that silence equals death, and that sexual rights and capabilities – like health, and even a liveable life – are never simply given, but must be achieved and constructed as part of an ongoing, daily struggle.

While these key social movements of the late twentieth and early twenty-first centuries have been quicker to address these issues than have older social and political movements forged in the history of modernity, nevertheless, as time evolved, even the more traditional human rights groups (at first, and still for some, reluctantly in relation to such new claims and recognition), public health and social justice movements have gradually taken up the challenges posed by issues of sexuality. This engagement has been slow and not without tensions for reasons that we analyse in this book, but it has none the less grown rapidly in recent years, shaped by the velocity of social change, economic restructuring, and information exchange that are taken for granted as central to early twenty-first-century globalization. Growing numbers of human rights and social justice activists now fully recognize, as evidenced in slogans on placards and T-shirts, that sexual rights are human rights and that something fundamental is in the process of change, not only within the discursive universe, but also in the shape and structure of human rights practice, as a result of this realization.

One of the key insights to emerge from these social movements and their diverse encounters with sexual controversies, as well as from the work of researchers whose thinking has been influenced by them, is the conviction that sexuality cannot be understood in isolation from the social, political, and economic structures within which it is embedded – or without reference to cultural and ideological discourses that give it meaning. Problems related to both sexual health and sexual rights are never evenly distributed across territories, countries, and population groups. On the contrary, they are systematically shaped by multiple forms of structural violence – social inequalities, poverty and economic exploitation, racism and ethnically based exclusion, gender and sexual oppression, discrimination and stigma, age differentials, disabilities, and other manifestations of disempowerment – in ways that have typically meant that their greatest negative impact has been felt by groups and populations that are *already* marginalized and/or oppressed within society, often in manifold ways. We are only beginning to understand the concrete mechanisms through which various forms of structural violence work in synergy to shape key challenges in specific locations within societies, and how these problems then reinforce the very forms of oppression that helped to create them.

One of the key consequences of the important role played by social movements engaged with sexuality – in relation to both health and rights – has thus been in calling attention to the need to approach both research and intervention in relation to sexuality as extensions of broader struggles for human rights and social justice. Whether the focus is HIV and AIDS, abortion, sexual abuse and violence, genital mutilation, the discrimination and exclusion imposed on sexual minorities, or any other major issue related to sexuality, work being developed in local communities everywhere has emphasized the profound importance of empowerment, or what might be described as socially engaged agency. This is a key precondition for reducing risk and vulnerability and for promoting erotic justice and sexual freedoms. We are convinced, therefore, that human rights approaches offer one of the key theoretical and methodological underpinnings for effective advocacy and programme development aimed at guaranteeing human dignity and worth, and ensuring the realization of health, human development, and freedom for all people. At the same time we are mindful of the serious problems and limitations that encumber human rights – and, by extension, sexual rights – as a normative tradition, and attempt to subject this framework to a rigorous critique while still preserving its liberatory potential.

While sexual rights is the 'the new kid on the block' in the articulation of human rights principles as part of international debates (Petchesky 2000), it is already clear that sexual rights embrace those human rights already recognized in national laws, international human rights documents, and other similar consensus documents developed in processes coordinated by the United Nations and its various agencies. As recently articulated by researchers, activists, and practitioners brought together by the World Health Organization, these sexual rights include the right of all persons, free of coercion, discrimination, and violence, to attain the highest possible standard of health in relation to sexuality, including access to sexual and reproductive health services (WHO 2002). They also include the right to seek, receive, and pass on information in relation to sexuality, and the right to sexuality education. They are based, above all, on respect and choice: respect for bodily integrity; the right to decide whether or not to be sexually active, to choose one's sexual partners, and to enter into consensual sexual relations and relationships; and the right to decide whether or not, and when, to have children. Using a similar approach, in 2006, a group of human rights specialists and 'LGBTQI' activists developed the Yogyakarta Principles for the Application of International Human Rights Law (Yogyakarta Principles 2007) in relation to sexual orientation and gender identity, one key dimension of sexual rights that, since the mid-1990s, has provoked major bottlenecks in intergovernmental negotiations.

Ultimately, what might be described as true sexual citizenship (a concept that we will seek to explore, and also to problematize, below) is possible only when all people in society have the right to pursue a satisfying, safe, and pleasurable sexual life. But importantly, the full realization of sexual citizenship depends not only on rights that are protected by the state. The idea of sexual pleasure, its definitions, its language, and its expression, all typically come from below rather than from above. Social, cultural, religious, biomedical, scientific, and other non-state actors are primarily responsible for respecting (or not) the right to sexual pleasure by adhering (or not) to fundamental principles of social inclusion, freedom, and human dignity (Garcia and Parker 2006). Here we need a whole new language, a cultural revolution.

Given the unequal access to information and cultural capital, which continues to characterize the contemporary world even in the information age (Castells 1996), it is not surprising that access to, and incorporation of, much cutting-edge thinking about sexuality, sexual movements, and erotic justice has remained uneven and fragmented at best. Among the most urgent priorities in seeking to move forward in this field is the challenge of integrating and synthesizing the important insights that have been emerging from recent theorizing, empirical research, and political activism. Without pretending to offer any new theory of sexuality or strategy for sexual politics, this book aims to synthesize perspectives that have surfaced in recent years from different disciplinary and epistemological standpoints as well as different subject positions. In the process, we have tried not to oversimplify the wide range of works and ideas we draw from or to ignore the unresolved challenges that still exist in building broader multidisciplinary and multicultural perspectives and coalitions.

To make greater sense of the complex interconnections and often counter-intuitive convergences of twenty-first-century sexualities and how they connect to both health and human rights is probably unthinkable as an individual intellectual project. While a more collaborative undertaking may not succeed either, there is no question that none of the co-authors of this volume could have attempted such a project on her/his own. Our paths and thinking have come together through a common commitment to a particular kind of intellectual perspective – one that views sexuality as a complex social, cultural, economic, and political construction – and to a very clear political project. That project seeks to build alliances and coalitions across the divisions of identity politics, based on the conviction that only through such common cause can we hope to challenge the forces that are aligned against us.

While each of us brings a perspective to this work that has been shaped by our respective disciplinary training and frameworks, we have shared a deep involvement, over a number of decades, in work on sexuality in relation to women's health and reproductive rights, HIV and AIDS, and sexual health and rights more broadly. Our perspectives have also been shaped, in very important ways, by our ongoing collaborations over some 15 years. Corrêa and Petchesky have worked together within the context of the international feminist and women's reproductive health and rights movements since 1992, collaborating extensively as part of the mobilization and preparation leading up to the United Nations conferences on population and development (Cairo, 1994) and on women (Beijing, 1995). They co-authored an article that has been widely translated and anthologized (Corrêa and Petchesky 1994). They also worked together in projects such as the International Reproductive Rights Research Action Group (IRRRAG) that have provided an important foundation for the analyses developed here, as well as with a range of intertwining networks focusing on issues related to women, development, and the politics of social justice and human rights, including, for example, events at the annual World Social Forum.

Corrêa and Parker began collaborating in the early 1990s, initially in an attempt to build a bridge between the feminist and the HIV and AIDS activist movements in Brazil in response to the growth of the epidemic among women in that country. They have continued to collaborate on a range of related issues in forums such as the Brazilian Commission on Citizenship and Reproduction, through their common engagement with ABIA (the Brazilian Interdisciplinary AIDS Association) in the ongoing response to HIV and AIDS in Brazil, and in a series of collaborative research and writing projects that helped to give rise to this book. Especially important in this regard was an initial project that Corrêa and Parker began to develop in 1999, taking up Petchesky's challenge (Petchesky 2000) to 'map' the changing terrain of emerging sexual rights debates across different countries and regions, as well as in diverse conceptual frameworks (see, e.g., Corrêa and Parker 2004, CREA et al. 2005, Parker and Corrêa 2003, Rojas 2001).

Since 2002, inspired by both local and international initiatives, the three of us have worked together to found and develop Sexuality Policy Watch (SPW), a global forum of researchers and activists from a wide range of countries and regions. SPW aims at contributing to sexuality-related global policy debates through strategic research and analysis, and at promoting more effective linkages between local, regional, and global efforts to change prevailing unjust policies. Within this context, we have worked to develop a cross-national/cross-institutional study of the politics of sexuality within the broader context of global social and economic restructuring taking place in the late twentieth and early twenty-first centuries. Published in late 2007 as *SexPolitics: Reports from the Front Lines* (Parker *et al.* 2007), and including detailed analytic case studies of the politics of sexuality in Brazil, Egypt, India, Peru, Poland, South Africa, Turkey, and Vietnam, and in the United Nations and the World Bank, this project has provided a crucial foundation for many of the comparative and transnational analyses that are developed in the current volume.

In many ways, this book is the companion volume to *SexPolitics*. In it, we try to flesh out some of the conceptual issues underlying much of the thinking behind that more empirically focused project – even as we recognize the magnitude of such a task and its (and our) limitations. Although gender and sexuality are clearly located at the core of current 'real politics', contemporary theories of sexuality have taught us to be cautious about grand historical and political narratives. Sexuality research and thinking have barely started to explore ways of articulating the knowledge accumulated about the microphysics and the political economy of sex. As always, and everywhere, 'sex' is not only about bodies and desires but also the economies, systems of governance, cultural and religious norms, kinship structures, and power dynamics of all of these issues. The vast diversity of how bodies and desires are located in space and time, and across the intersections of gender, race, class, age, and geography, makes us feel more like cartographers than bold theorists of sexual landscapes.

In charting the way forward, it may be useful to clarify a few concepts and terms that appear throughout this book. The first of these concerns the ambiguous conceptualization of 'sex', 'gender', and 'sexuality' and their interrelations. As we shall discuss more fully in Chapter 5, our analysis draws from the work of writers such as Judith Butler and Anne Fausto-Sterling, who call into question the dualism, long taken for granted by feminists, of 'sex' (as a biological given, hence fixed) and 'gender' (as the cultural and social imprints inscribed on sexed bodies, hence malleable). Like Butler and Fausto-Sterling, we subscribe to 'a nondualistic account of the body' and thus understand 'sex' – or the material body – as saturated with, and inseparable from, social and cultural meanings from the start (Fausto-Sterling 2000, pp. 22–23, Butler 1993). Sexuality – as the domain of bodily and social experience produced through ever-changing discourses, norms, and regulatory practices that operate where desire, behaviour, identity, and institutional power meet – is thus a matter of bodies, pleasures, and power all at once. It is, as Michel Foucault revealed, a domain of power, but one where gender norms are always part of the stakes, albeit differently in different contexts. It would seem that researchers in the field of sexuality have been zigzagging between a view that uncritically collapses gender and sexuality studies (as many feminist writers in the 1970s and 1980s tended to do) or envisions an undifferentiated 'sex-gender system' (Rubin 1975), to an insistence on seeing sexuality as its own, separate domain (Foucault 1978, Rubin 1984, Sedgwick 1990), and now back to a more synthetic understanding of sexuality and gender as both distinct and complexly interrelated (Butler 2004b, Halperin 2002, Jackson 2007). In this regard, we strongly sympathize with Peter Jackson's call to reconnect sexuality or queer studies and gender studies, after a long and confining separation (Jackson 2007) and with Judith Butler's observation 'that sexual and gender relations, although in no sense causally linked, are structurally linked in important ways' (Butler 2004b, p. 259, n. 13). One major aim of this book is to examine those structural links.

A second area of terminological confusion concerns the naming of contemporary social movements. The habit of throwing together a wide

range of sexual and gender identity categories into one alphabet soup –
LGBT, LGBTI, or LGBTQ – seems highly unsatisfactory, especially in a
period when the disparate character and political agendas of lesbian, gay,
bisexual, transgender, intersex, queer, and gender/queer groups are rapidly
evolving and sometimes in tension rather than unified in any practical or
ideological sense. We will try to name these distinct movements as much as
possible, and when we feel the need to resort to the questionable acronym,
we ask readers to keep in mind our discomfort with this catch-all category.
But the discomfort is with the collapsing of differences not with the exu-
berant explosion of sexual and gender identities – a cause, we think, for
celebration. In general, we find helpful the definitions offered by Minter,
who refers to

> *transgender* as an umbrella term including transsexuals, transvestites,
> cross-dressers, drag queens and drag kings, butch and femme lesbians,
> feminine gay men, intersex people, bigendered people, and others who
> ... 'challenge the boundaries of sex and gender'. This is distinct from
> 'gay,' 'lesbian' and 'heterosexual,' terms defined exclusively by sexual
> object choice.
>
> (Minter 2006, p. 159, n. 1; see also Currah *et al.* 2006,
> Feinberg 1996)

Also troubling with regard to social movements is the tendency to universalize feminisms and singularize women's movements, when two
decades of working transnationally in this field have made their 'polyver-
sality' (to borrow Zillah Eisenstein's term (2004, ch. 8)) palpably clear.
There is no one strain of feminism any more than there is one expression
of aspirations for sexual freedom. We are profoundly indebted to feminist
research that has uncovered the multiplicity of women's movements as
well as the intersection, everywhere, of gendered power relations with
those of race, class, caste, and empire – however differently those intersections may operate in different spatial and temporal contexts (Crenshaw
1991, Eisenstein 2004, Lorde 1984, Mohanty 2003, Zinn and Dill 1996).

Finally, we have deliberately opted to avoid the term 'fundamentalism'
to describe all manifestations of religious dogmatism, extremism, or other
ideological operations through which contemporary religions are being
remade. While the arguments explaining this choice are fully examined in
Chapter 3, readers should be aware from the start that, in line with many
other authors (Armstrong 2000, Imam 2000), we see the term 'fundamentalism' as historically and contextually specific to Protestant sects that
emerged in the USA in the early twentieth century. It is thus inapplicable
to phenomena as varied as long-standing revivalist currents within Islam
or the Hindu regressive ideology (*Hindutva*) that has plagued the Indian
political scene for more than a century.

With these various limitations and framings in mind, this volume is divided into three major parts. Part 1, Global 'sex' wars, seeks to map out some of the key political struggles that have emerged around sexuality, both locally and globally, over the course of the past two to three decades under conditions of intensifying globalization and, more recently, militarization. It is divided into three chapters. The first, 'Landscaping sexualities', looks at the explosion of discourses related to sexuality and the ways in which sexual politics has expanded and become more complex, almost in inverse relation to the disenchantment that currently prevails in politics at large in the contemporary world. It focuses on how movements of resistance to sexual oppression have gradually begun to evolve into more radical projects for social transformation at the local and regional levels, and are increasingly being pushed to engage at transnational levels as well. The second chapter, 'The real politics of "sex"', seeks to examine these political projects and the concerted resistance to them, organized by reactionary forces such as the Bush administration in the USA, in greater detail. While the repressive politics of US unilateralism has been one of the quintessential features of the early twenty-first century, it has hardly been unique and is, in fact, symptomatic of a far wider array of global sex wars focusing on issues ranging from lesbian, gay, transgender, and intersex rights, to trafficking and sexual slavery, sexual commerce and the rights (or lack of rights) of sex workers, and to the battlefields of abortion, sexuality education, and adolescent sexuality. Chapter 3, 'The sad "return of the religious"', builds on the previous two chapters, focusing on the return of religious fervour and the rise of religious extremism – linked, as it so often ironically is, to the quest for 'natural' certainties in the runaway world of contemporary globalization, where scientific and 'rational' certainties increasingly seem to be slipping away or out of reach.

In Part 2, Epistemological challenges and research agendas, we move from mapping the contemporary global politics of sexuality to examining the ways of knowing about sex – the sexual truths and certainties that have been constructed over time as we have sought to explore sexuality under the light of reason, as an object of scientific investigation and analysis. Part 2 is also divided into three chapters. Chapter 4, 'The modernization of "sex" and the birth of sexual science', focuses on the long-standing attempts to substitute religious doctrine and superstition with a 'scientific' understanding of sexuality – initially through sexology, psychiatry, psychoanalysis, and anthropology, and more recently through social science research and statistical investigation in fields such as social psychology, sociology, and demography. It also examines the gradual extension of the scientific gaze from a preoccupation with sexual deviance and diversity in Western societies, to a growing fixation with reproductive sexual practices and population control in societies across the globe. In Chapter 5, 'The social construction of sexual life', we explore the more recent critique of this scientific project by a more reflexive social analysis focusing on the historical and cultural construction of sexual experience. We examine the roots of this alternative approach in social history, anthropology, and sociology, as well as in the progressive political projects that began to emerge in the 1960s and expanded rapidly over the course of the next few decades. Here we focus on the ways in which a social and relational perspective has provided the foundation for the examination of sexuality in feminist research as well as gay and lesbian studies and transgender and queer theory. Building on this discussion, in Chapter 6, 'After AIDS', we look at the profound impact that the HIV epidemic has had in drawing research attention to issues related to sexuality, and to the ways in which both vulnerability and empowerment of different communities and individuals are shaped by a wide range of social inequalities in relation to class, gender, race, and ethnicity. We argue that focusing on the cultural and structural dimensions of sexuality is necessary in order to confront the continuing silences, invisibilities, and injustices resulting from the multiple forms of social exclusion, stigma, and discrimination that continue to contaminate the field of sexuality studies.

In Part 3, The promises and limits of sexual rights, we move from the terrain of epistemology to that of ethics and rethinking normative frameworks. We recognize the problematic status of rights-based discourse, and the historical baggage of racism and liberal individualism it carries. None the less, we argue that a focus on rights – as necessary but insufficient and as linked to a politics of social justice – offers, at the moment, the best available conceptual architecture for furthering the struggle to build a world in which sexual diversity and freedoms can be protected and expanded. In Chapter 7, 'On the indispensability and insufficiency of human rights', we explore a number of the most important critiques that have been developed in relation to human rights frameworks and the implications of such critiques for attempts to build a notion of sexual rights in particular. We look at both the limitations and the strengths of rights language, including its individualist and exclusionary legacies and, on the other hand, its rhetorical power and capacity to give those seeking social and erotic justice the possibility of some sort of redress or accountability on the part of governments and societies more broadly. In Chapter 8, 'Inventing and contesting sexual rights within the UN', we seek to push this argument further, picking up the discussion originally raised in Part 1 on the importance of the United Nations as a site for developing a new understanding and practice of human rights in relation to sexuality. We argue that what is most important about this development is not so much the discursive universe that has been constructed around sexual rights to date, but rather the process of construction – the ways it has brought together feminist, sexual and reproductive health, lesbian and gay, transgender, intersex, and human rights groups from every region of the world, to work closely together, across their many existing differences, in order to begin building a broader coalition around these issues.

In Chapter 9, 'Transnational debates: sexuality, power, and new subjectivities', we build on this discussion by examining several sites of ongoing contention within sexual rights thinking and advocacy. We focus on four key sites of debate: the separation of sexual health and rights from reproduction; sex work and sex trafficking; treatment access for HIV and AIDS; and the problematic principles of non-discrimination and equality. We suggest that these debates illustrate the complicated political interconnections and divisions currently producing the domain of sexual rights, and we try to examine the ways in which they call into question a number of unexamined assumptions that currently prevail in feminist and sex/gender identity politics. In Chapter 10, 'At the outer limits of human rights: voids in the liberal paradigm', we bring Part 3 to a close by going deeper into a number of key challenges to human rights that seem (at least to us) more intractable, where the liberal trappings of rights-based discourses create exclusions or conceptual blind spots that are so easy to resolve, including the very limitations of the category of the human. We argue that these dilemmas are all the more troubling in times of intense militarization and ethnic and imperial conflict, such as that which we currently inhabit.

Finally, in the Postscript to this book, 'Dreaming and dancing – beyond sexual rights', we try to bring these various strands of analysis together. Our goal here is not to provide some kind of grand synthesis – a task that is surely beyond the pretensions of this short volume – but rather to offer an assessment of the key challenges confronting us as we seek to advance a liberatory politics of sexuality. In particular, we emphasize the continued need for an understanding of sexuality as embedded in social, cultural, political, and economic structures, as well as an analysis of the politics of sexuality that recognizes the fundamental tension between local struggles and broader transnational arenas and debates. Without in any way resolving all the questions we have raised in the book, we offer at least some provisional conclusions about the ways in which struggles for erotic justice may be linked to, and integrated within, broader struggles for social justice.

Part 1

Global 'sex' wars

Chapter 1

Landscaping sexualities

The idea that sexuality, politics, and economics are connected is not new. In the early nineteenth century the writings and practices of Utopian socialists, such as Owen and Fourier, articulated economic justice and sexual liberation in their revolutionary principles and strategies. A few decades later Engels (1884) explored the subtle articulation between sex and economics in *The Origin of the Family, Private Property, and the State*, which socialist feminists like Emma Goldman and Alexandra Kollontai would later build on. At the same time the groundbreaking works of Darwin and Sigmund Freud laid the foundations for the development of a science of 'sex', establishing the notion of a sex drive and deeply influenced further theorizing and research. These developments also coincided with the 'invention' of homosexuality (see Chapter 4). A few decades later, in the late 1920s and early 1930s, Central European intellectuals and activists created the SexPol Association, interweaving Marxism and psychoanalysis to advance radical propositions about sexuality, economics, and power.[1] In the late 1940s, Simone de Beauvoir's critique of 'anatomy as destiny' (1953 [orig. 1949]) opened the path for conceptualizing 'man' and 'woman' not as separate biological entities but as contingent, cultural constructs. By the 1960s, the ideas emerging from SexPol reached the counterculture through the writings of Wilhelm Reich (1971, 1973b) and Herbert Marcuse (1966). Young feminists were now reading de Beauvoir and revisiting Marx, Engels, and Freud to more fully understand male control over women's sexuality, the political dimensions of the private sphere, and the meaning of bodies as potential foundations of political entitlements (Firestone 1970, Greer 1970, Millet 1979, Mitchell 1974, Rubin 1975).

This was the moment when an epistemological shift occurred that would deeply transform thinking about 'sex' (see Chapter 5). In the USA, as early as 1973, Gagnon and Simon (1973) started moving away from the previous conception of 'sex' towards a new approach that privileged the personal and cultural meanings that a sexual act has for the actor. During 1974 to 1975, feminists in the USA further developed the concept of 'gender' through a critique of prevailing naturalistic assumptions about male and female subjectivities, social roles, and sexual behaviour (Rosaldo and Lamphere 1974, Rubin 1975). Concurrently, sociologists such as Plummer (1975) and Gagnon and Simon (1973) argued that sexual life is embedded in social contexts and cannot be fully grasped unless other aspects of human interaction (e.g., class, labour, race, and family relations) are taken into account. A short while later, Michel Foucault (1978 [orig. 1976]) illuminated the placement of 'sex' as a pivot in the webs of power that pervade discourses, norms, and practices and that produce hierarchies, exclusions, and stigma in modern societies (see Chapter 5). From there, the discourses and conceptual frames that conceive 'sex' as an immutably natural drive would be systematically scrutinized and these novel theories would infuse new ideas into sexual politics.

Since then, as well, the world – in which sexuality and politics are constantly intersecting – has changed substantially. The political climate and geopolitical dynamics of the 1970s were determined by the overall logic of the Cold War, in which closed political regimes in the socialist world coexisted sometimes peacefully and sometimes not with a number of Western-supported (in particular, US-supported) dictatorships South, but also North, of the equator. Progressive political imagination was inspired by not only the socialist promises of equality but also by the ongoing impacts of the 1960s counterculture and its radical slogans, such as 'Make love not war'. In 1989, when the Cold War era ended, the process of change that came to be known as globalization accelerated across all continents. The scientific and technological revolution, which had been underway for some time, infused a new rhythm to capital accumulation, rapidly reshaping the material basis of society and the means of communication among individuals, social groups, and interacting cultures. As economies around the globe have become interdependent the relationship between economy, society, and the nation state has been transformed.

In geopolitical terms, the USA achieved unprecedented economic and military hegemony, which would become particularly problematic following the election of George W. Bush to the presidency in 2000 and even more salient after the attacks in New York and Washington on 11 September 2001. That infamous day made visible and influential worldwide the neo-conservative military, economic, and moral agenda that had been gaining strength in US domestic politics since the 1970s. Today the global scenario contrasts sharply with the optimistic predictions of the late 1980s that the end of the Cold War would see resources spent in warfare and for nuclear deterrence transferred to peaceful economic and human development and the deepening of democracy – the short-lived 'peace dividend' (UNDP 1990). While the tragedies and crimes of the 2003 Iraq war and subsequent occupation and the related militarization of geopolitics remain at the centre of the global stage, in the past decade new centres of economic power have emerged to contest US hegemony, revive nationalist agendas and popular sentiments, and produce new geopolitical skirmishes in the most diverse regions.[2]

When contemporary sexual politics sparked in the 1960s, political affairs were in large part contained within national boundaries, but this has changed dramatically. By 1979 Keynesian macroeconomic principles, which had emphasized the role of states in economic production and regulation, would be supplanted by the neo-liberal premises[3] of the so-called Washington Consensus, calling for drastic cuts in public spending, privatization, and trade liberalization. In subsequent decades, structural adjustment programmes (SAPs) derived from these policy guidelines fundamentally reshaped national economies. The detrimental effects of these policies affected almost all countries, including those in Western Europe as well as the USA, but were especially devastating in developing countries, particularly in Africa, and in the Eastern European economies in transition (Castells 1996, 1998, Harvey 2005, Rodrik 2000, Saad-Filho and Johnston 2005, Stiglitz 2002, Stiglitz et al. 2006; see also Chapters 6 and 10).[4]

At the same time, supra-state structures in the form of regional blocks and economic alliances became more robust or were created where they did not exist before – including the European Union, Mercosur (Mercado Común del Sur/Southern Common Market), Southern Africa Development Community (SADC), Asia Pacific Economic Community (APEC), Caribbean Community (CARICOM), and the African Union (AU). These new institutional and economic structures have been gradually reconfiguring state boundaries, not only in economic terms but also with regard to normative frames. Even more important, from the mid-1980s on, the so-called 'global governance complex' – the United Nations, the World Bank, and the International Monetary Fund (IMF) – became the focus of organized campaigns by civil society actors.

Since 1985, and with more intensity after 1990, the effects of the Washington Consensus were systematically criticized and civil society groups mounted demonstrations against the World Bank, IMF, and, later on, the World Trade Organization (WTO) and the Group of 7 (after 1994, the Group of 8)[5] wherever these institutions held their high-level meetings. Concurrently, the UN adopted a deliberate strategy to encourage the engagement of civil society in policy-making processes, in particular in a series of international conferences on its development agenda, known as the UN cycle of social conferences. These included the Children's Summit (New York, 1990), the Conference on Environment and Development (Rio de Janeiro, 1992), the World Conference on Human Rights (Vienna, 1993), the International Conference on Population and Development (Cairo, 1994), the World Summit on Social Development (Copenhagen, 1995), the Fourth World Conference on Women (Beijing, 1995), the

Second UN Conference on Human Settlements/Habitat II (Istanbul, 1996), the World Food Summit (Rome, 1997), the Millennium Summit (New York, 2000), the UN General Assembly Special Session on HIV/AIDS (New York, 2001), and the International Conference Against Racism, Racial Discrimination, Xenophobia, and Related Forms of Intolerance (Durban, 2001). Each of these global events mobilized a vast and diverse gamut of civil society actors, exposed them to global policy debates and dynamics, and brought to the attention of states situations of gender and sexuality-based inequality, discrimination, and violence. During the past ten to 15 years, therefore, the main policy debates and gains in the domain of sexuality – including those related to women's rights and HIV/AIDS – have played out in the intersections between national and global policy arenas.

Taking the 1970s as a point of reference, a key differential observed with respect to the dynamics of sexual politics is the increasing transnationalization of actors and issues, as well as greater connectivity across civil societies. Another striking distinction, however, is more sombre. In the 1960s and 1970s, sexual politics were deeply interwoven with Utopian socialist and radical ideas. In subsequent decades, a large number of Southern countries, a few European societies, and all of Eastern Europe and Central Asia experienced democratizing processes. In most Southern countries, these processes were characterized by great expectations of social justice and created openings for new political agendas, such as the struggle for gender equality, for women's human rights, and against other forms of sexuality-based discrimination.

Today, in sharp contrast, the loss of credibility in politics is widespread, and nationalist, communitarian, and religious forces have been reactivated practically everywhere, very often using the notion of culture as immutable to gain the hearts and minds of people (Castells 1997, Freedom House 2007, UNDP 2004). Across the world, discredited political processes and the revival of authoritarian politics have been related to growing inequalities, bad management, corruption, and the increasing inability of states to respond to urgent societal needs and aspirations.[6] The very term 'democracy' is now subject to ideological manipulation, with the most striking illustration being the use made of the term by US neo-conservatives to justify the invasions of Afghanistan, in 2001, and Iraq, in 2003. Concurrently, the effects of the 'war on terror' are infringing on civil liberties everywhere, including in long-established democracies, and restricting the activities of NGOs, particularly those engaged in the promotion and protection of human rights (AI 2007, HRW 2004c, IGLHRC and CWGL 2005).[7]

A variety of authors who have examined these trends emphasize the paradoxical features of our times (see, e.g., Appadurai 1996, Giddens 1990, 1992, 2000, Held *et al.* 1999, Touraine 1997, Touraine and Khos-

rohavar 1999). They call attention to the primacy of markets and techno-
science as the main forces behind the rapid changes the world is experiencing, underlining their negative impact on politics at large and, most
particularly, on the ability of states to retain their capacity to govern.
These authors also emphasize how such changes are negatively intersecting
with, and deepening inequalities within and across, countries as well as
class, race, ethnic, and caste divisions (Castells 1998, Guimarães 2005, Sen
1995, UNDP 2005). To a few observers, the most pervasive and perverse
trait of our times is the proliferation of situations of perennial emergency,
or 'states of exception', to which large sectors of the world population are
subjected in daily life (Agamben 2005; see also Chapter 10). A state of
exception implies the total abandonment of whole populations or individuals to pre-juridical conditions, expressions of societal fascism, 'terror-
ism', increased state policing, and other interventions by powerful
non-state as well as state actors. States appear to have lost their capacity to
provide for the well-being of their citizens, even as militarization is
increased, the security apparatus strengthened, and extra-constitutional
powers become pervasive.

While these analyses underline the key relevance of scientific and
technological development in capital accumulation, particularly in communications, information, and biotechnology, they also place strong emphasis
on the phenomenon of the 'return of the religious' in the form of dogmatism, fundamentalism, or extremism (Armstrong 2000, Castells 1997, de
Boni 1995, Derrida and Vattimo 1998, Sen 2005). Human history has
experienced many moments in which religious dogmatism drove social
conflicts and contaminated state rationales, but religious extremism can no
longer be portrayed as a phenomenon confined within certain communitarian, institutional, or national boundaries. Today dogmatic visions are
manifest in all dominant religious traditions and, practically everywhere,
politically organized religious extremists operate to influence legal norms
and policies, when they are not directly engaged in taking state power
through electoral politics. These forces are interconnected globally and
utilize the most up-to-date communication technologies to expand their
support base and exert pressure on state institutions (see, e.g., Almond *et
al.* 2003, Girard 2004, Jelen and Wilcox 2002, Mujica 2007). This trend,
which has been interpreted as a reaction to the growing uncertainties of
late capitalism (see Chapter 3), poses unpredicted political and conceptual
challenges with respect to the philosophical foundations and political
meanings of secularity. In addition, everywhere, religious revivalism
systematically targets emerging new 'sex' and gender orders as a strategy
to re-create 'tradition' and to allow space for dominant heteronormativity
and sexism to regain a sense of control (Imam 2000, Jung *et al.* 2001,
Saghal and Yuval-Davis 1992, Sen and Corrêa 2000, Sow *et al.* 2007).
Sexual and gender hierarchies – deeply rooted in ancient religious

doctrines and pre-modern cultures – reappear strongly in the discourse of dogmatic religious voices.

Further complicating the global mapping that situates 'sex' and sexuality in our time, the surge and expansion of HIV and AIDS, from the early 1980s, began to alter individual and public perceptions about sexual identities and practices. These complex intertwined dynamics created new forms of injustice and preventable death, and at the same time illuminated the webs of power underlying the interactions among 'sex', social hierarchies, and sociocultural change. This enhanced the contestation and redefinition of sexual identities and norms, the emergence of new family forms, and the destabilization of traditional notions of masculinity and of patriarchy itself.

The brave new worlds of 'sex'

One of the key features of life in the early twenty-first century is the appearance of a brave new world of sexual possibilities and choices. Riding on the waves of the information age (Castells 1996), and perhaps most visible in relation to the Internet, today's apparent proliferation of sexual options seems to extend far beyond what might have been imaginable only a few decades ago. As writers such as Giddens (1992), Plummer (2003), and Weeks (1995) have all highlighted, this explosion of intimate possibilities appears to be one of the defining characteristics of sexual life and experience under the conditions of late modern capitalism.

These striking transformations are at play everywhere in the world. At least at the level of discourse and media representations, images of these kinds of possibilities are available across the globe. As lived alternatives, however, they imply intricate dynamics in terms of personal relations but also in regard to state actions, religious domains, and contentious state–society interactions. As part of a global cultural imaginary, they are palpable in many arenas – the press and television, music, theatre, video, cinema, and the core domain of informational society, the Internet. Although these realms of media and popular culture are too vast and complex to be fully analysed here, they cannot be entirely left aside in any effort aimed at landscaping sexualities in the twenty-first century. We saw a foreshadowing of this moment in the atmosphere of the 1960s counter-culture, crystallized in the popular imagination as the era of 'sex, drugs, and rock-and-roll'. But the scope, scale, and rhythm of what is experienced today are unprecedented, as may be seen clearly in looking at film production. Sex and gender have been a leitmotiv of film production since the invention of cinema, and a number of films produced in the 1960s, 1970s, and 1980s delved deeply into explorations of heterosexual desire and eroticism.[8] Male homosexuality was portrayed in cinema from as early as the 1950s, and from the 1960s large audiences have been exposed to the gay and transgender themes and aesthetics of works by Pasolini, Fassbinder, and, more recently, Almodovar.[9] However, during the past decade, despite a growing regressive moral climate, an outburst of mainstream Hollywood and independent productions has raised the visibility of homosexuality and transgenderism in cinema.[10] At the same time, alternative 'LGBTQ' film festivals, as well as documentaries about sexuality in the most diverse cultures, are mushrooming worldwide.[11]

In the past 30 years, television and radio productions, in both industrialized and developing countries, have diffused new gender and 'sex' norms, which have been rapidly absorbed into the popular imagination and gradually translated into everyday practices with respect to issues such as family size, women's role, the use of contraception, and sexual liberation itself. The wildly popular soap operas produced in Brazil since the 1970s now constitute a major export item, seen in Europe, the USA, across Africa, and in parts of Asia including China (Faria and Potter 2002, Hamburger and Buarque de Holanda 2004). In the 1990s and 2000s music videos, the cable television network, Music Television, often using sexuality as a selling point, have traversed national and cultural borders capturing the imagination of young people in places as diverse as Mexico, Nepal, and Asia-Pacific, and sexual affairs are shown openly in most 'reality shows'. The US television series *Sex and the City*, watched by audiences worldwide, offers a fine ethnography of the transformations underway in the realm of heterosexuality and female sexuality in Westernized urban areas.[12] More recently, *The L Word*, portraying the daily lives of a group of Californian lesbians, started to soak up audiences previously addicted to *Sex and the City*. In addition, the series *Queer Eye for the Straight Guy*, which makes cultural jokes about the lack of taste and good manners on the part of heterosexual men, attracted huge audiences in the USA at the same time as neo-conservative morality took over the state.

In theatre production the most compelling illustration is perhaps *The Vagina Monologues*, which is often performed in combination with feminist activism such as the V-Day Campaign,[13] has appeared in countries as disparate as Serbia, Barbados, and China (Djordjevic 2006). The success and popular appeal of *The Vagina Monologues* has been enhanced rather than hindered by the controversy that often follows in its wake.[14] In the domain of popular music, since the 1960s rock stars have been reinventing genders and sexualities through lyrics, stage performances, and personal conduct, and in the world of fashion the transformation of gendered and sexual images is constantly at play on runways and in glossy magazines. The most compelling example is, perhaps, the 1980s unisex style that both reflected the deep transformation of gender roles and anticipated the instability and fluidity of queer politics that would follow.

Thus, a wide range of close intersections between sexual politics and cultural production has been evolving worldwide in recent decades. In many countries, lesbian, gay, and, increasingly, transgender initiatives have sparked social and sexual networks engaged with the arts and popular culture and, more often, the reinvention of lifestyles, as reflected in the long list of lesbian and gay-friendly cities, hotels, and beaches around the world, with San Francisco having long been the icon of this trend. In Brazil since the 1980s, HIV prevention work has been conducted in combination with transvestite and drag queen shows, other popular performances, and during Carnival. In Asia, *Prima Donna*, a performance piece mounted by a Malaysian sex workers' association to raise awareness about HIV/AIDS and human rights, is rapidly gaining fame across the region and beyond. In Thailand, the Empower Foundation uses traditional paper dolls known as Kumjing to call attention to the tragic marginalization of undocumented Burmese migrant sex workers. The exhibition, The Journey of Kumjing, is displayed at fairs and art exhibitions around the country and beyond its borders, and aims to persuade institutions and individuals to provide migrant sex workers with jobs and legal papers.[15] In Sweden, a group of young people recently created a theatre group to build awareness of sexual diversity and gender identity that, as surprising as it may seem, are issues not fully understood in that country and a cause of violence and discrimination.[16] For many years gay pride parades in a variety of countries have attracted millions of people with their mix of art, market economics, and politics.[17] At the global level, the Gay Games and Out Games are expanding the visibility of diverse sexual communities, and creating novel spaces to debate and claim human rights.[18]

Finally, since the early 1990s the Internet has become a critical space in which gender and sexuality norms are contested and re-created and sexual identities and cultures reinvented, politicized, and made more visible. Through it, gays, lesbians, and transgender and intersex persons have been able to overcome isolation and find solidarity networks in places where homosexuality and gender nonconformity are criminalized or strongly stigmatized. Second Life, the web game where players can recraft their bodies, sexual identities, and relations on the basis of individual desires and fantasies, is the epitome of these novel virtual realities of gender and 'sex'. The Internet is thus a key element in the accelerated transnationalization of sexual politics. Starting with e-mail in the early 1990s and moving into the new world of websites, portals, instant messaging, and Skype, the web provides the tools and spaces without which it would be impossible to sustain communication and action across local and global levels or to create new possibilities of dialogue between different cultural experiences.

But this novel and expanding frontier of sexual politics via the mass media, technology, and the culture industry is inevitably fraught with contradictions. These intense flows may suggest that social acceptance of alternative gender and sexualities is expanding almost everywhere. But this appearance contrasts sharply with public opinion polls showing that, in most countries, the majority of the population does not fully accept or support the rights claims of persons whose sexuality does not conform to dominant norms. Information, communication, and art forms project new ways of imagining and experiencing gender and 'sex' that openly conflict with norms and practices that still prevail in many local contexts – including places in the USA and Europe – and this provokes harsh conservative backlashes. Individuals and groups struggling for political recognition on the basis of local identities, meanings, and practices contest the Western imprint of cinema and cable TV images. Most importantly, the images and words proliferating through contemporary communication systems also carry with them extremist religious values, gender biases, homophobia, and incitement to violence. The most compelling illustration is the Internet itself, as a stage where the thorniest 'sex' issues of our time are enacted: exhibitionism, prostitution, trafficking, self-selling of bodies, pornography, paedophilia, and sadomasochism.

The novel and shifting spaces and interaction created by the Internet must be understood as one key dimension of public spheres in the twenty-first century, and if this is so it must be politically invested (Castells 1998). While the culture industry's thirst for profits is evidently eroding gender and 'sex' orders everywhere, the information and communication systems in which it is embedded constitute core devices of social regulation, market fetishization, state policing, and invasion of privacy. For those engaged in sexual politics it is vital to acknowledge as well how rapidly the informational revolution has been appropriated by 'religion', whether or not in its most extremist manifestations.[19] Bina Srinivasan's (2004) insights are illustrative of this paradox. She starts by developing a critical analysis of television messages and images for Valentine's Day, which in 2001 had flooded the city of Gujarat, India, where she was living:

> Valentine's Day is all about dynamo-driven advertisement, currency-laden romance. Love in the twenty-first century is about business, about creating illusions, raking in the profits, and laughing all the way to the bank.... Love is business. It is about money.
>
> (Srinivasan 2004)[20]

But when, three years later, in Colombo, Sri Lanka, she saw billboards calling for the boycott of Valentine's Day because it is against Buddhist culture, her focus shifted towards the challenge of sustaining a feminist position on sexuality and gender justice without falling into these convergent cracks.

Sexual politics: triggers and threads

The brave new worlds of 'sex' and gender, described above, are triggered by markets and embedded in consumerism and commodification. They contrast sharply with inequalities and threats to human security affecting exactly those whose human rights and basic needs most urgently need to be respected and fulfilled – millions of people who are today exposed to the images and expectations created by these complex flows cannot be entitled by the invisible hand of the market. Consequently, politics in its traditional sense – as resistance, protest, and engagement with the state and other powerful institutions – is more crucial today than it was 30 years ago.

Despite the climate of growing disenchantment with politics in general, sexual politics has expanded, diversifying and becoming more effective but also more complex. The paths leading to this expansion and maturation are characterized, among other things, by a variety of connections between theorizing and political action. In various contexts, North and South of the equator, the surge of feminist and lesbian, gay, and transgender groups was organically linked to sex research and theorizing, and in more than a few cases these connections would expand under the impact of HIV and AIDS. Even though the dissemination and absorption of new conceptual frames remains uneven across regions and communities, and conflicts continue to exist between academics and activists, these connections and dialogues should not be minimized. Last but not least, a number of contemporary 'sex thinkers' have been directly engaged with political activism.

In the course of the past three decades, contemporary sex theorizing has given the political actors of sexual politics a powerful tool with which to name and map the continuities, discontinuities, and instabilities through which bodies, sexualities, and genders are constituted in discourses, norms, and social practices (see Chapter 5). Concurrently, remarkable historical investigations into the regulation of sexuality in all human cultures have shown that sexuality was politicized long before modernity, in a wide range of circumstances.[21] European and US researchers devoted attention to the political and institutional processes through which sexuality became politically centred in the transition to modernity through the most varied angles. Researchers elsewhere have used the same lenses to investigate the reconfiguring of sex-gender systems (Rubin 1975) under the impact of economic modernization and rationalization in other cultural and political contexts, showing how everywhere the establishment of nation states strongly relied on the crystallization of resilient images and norms with regard to gender and sexuality.

Many studies have further illuminated the articulations and disjunctions between sex, gender, race, caste, and state transformation under colonial and postcolonial conditions. Contemporary anthropological research and theorizing pulled further at the threads originally woven by early twentieth-century pioneers such as Mead (1928, 1935, 1949) and Malinowski (1927, 1929), gathering a bulk of evidence about the variation of sexual meanings and practices across cultures, class, race, and sexual communities.[22] This extensive literature contributed to the destabilization of the dominant Western and non-Western systems of 'sex' classifications and hierarchies, and prompted a plethora of intense and productive cross-cultural dialogues around issues of sexuality and politics. A recently published interview with Judith Butler (2007) explores the multiple facets of the contemporary synergy between 'sex' and gender theorizing and transformative political praxis:

> *Gender Trouble* includes a critique of the idea that there are two ideal bodily forms, two ideal morphologies: the masculine and the feminine. I want to suggest that today the intersex movement is very engaged with criticizing that idea. Not all bodies are born in male or female. There is a continuum of bodies and it seems to me that trying to persuade medical and psychiatric establishments to deal with the intersex involves critique of the binary gender system. Similarly there continues to be extreme, sometimes very extreme, violence against transgender people. And it seems to me that *Gender Trouble* will always be important to try and open up our ideas of what gender is. So, I don't know if it's revolutionary, but maybe it still has something to say to those issues.
>
> (Butler 2007)

Last but not least the urgency of the HIV epidemic placed 'sex and gender norms under the looking glass, revealing that the transmission of a microscopic entity is, in fact, driven by social, cultural, political, and economic forces' (Garcia and Parker 2006, p. 16). A new wave of articulation between research and activism ensued, with strong arguments constructed in response to state and medical discourses that identified homosexuals and sex workers as the main carriers of a new and mortal disease. In this regard, the pandemic has helped to open or expand the space for these marginalized groups to denounce discrimination and claim rights in many contexts where the same assumptions that prevailed in the early 1980s are still alive. In addition, it has enhanced the emergence and development of solidarity networks that mobilized support for affected persons and groups across national boundaries, cultures, and lines of social stratification. As the third decade of the pandemic approached, the embodied realities of illness and the denial of access to services and treatment fully illuminated the intersections between sexuality, poverty, class, race, ethnicity, and other forms of discrimination and exclusion (see Chapters 6 and 8).

The complex and yet poorly understood synergy resulting from democratization, globalization, HIV/AIDS, and novel ways of 'thinking sex' allowed many other voices and bodies to emerge: sex workers, lesbian, gay and bisexual persons, young people, transgender and intersex people (who, as in the case of Indian *hijras* and Nepalese *métis*, often relied on their own traditions), and others marginalized on the basis of sexuality, gender, bodily difference, or some combination of these, such as single women, widows, and the disabled. Garcia and Parker (2006) situate the development of the 'sexual rights' movement in relation to the emergence and diversification of social movements in the past three decades and identify three distinct currents of interpretation.[23] They recall that while a large number of authors consider structural forces – economic crises and political opportunities – to be the main triggers of the surge of social movements, other analysts emphasize that in late modernity (or late capitalism) political contention does not emerge exclusively in the domains of interaction among civil societies, states, and economic powers. Political contestation may also, and often does, challenge the norms prevailing in sociocultural environments and redefine the society. These later authors emphasize the dynamics through which contention is framed, and the role of embodiment and emotions in political mobilization. Garcia and Parker (2006) consider (correctly) their frames to be more appropriate to investigate the motivations and directions of a movement that 'has been driven and thwarted by political opportunity structures (e.g. regime changes) as well as by the emotional desire for freedom and sexual autonomy' (p. 15). This political quest for freedom and autonomy must address the dissonance between the embodied practice of sexuality and the social categorizations used to define 'sex' and sexual conduct. Contemporary sexual politics may be portrayed as a web of social and cultural processes through which these categories are subject to contestation and reinterpretation by a large number of social actors. While these political initiatives claim respect for difference or specificity, they are also inspired by, and committed to, an ethics of the body – its integrity, health, pleasure, and freedom from violence – as defined not by 'experts' or medical or moral authorities but by those whose bodies and pleasures are most intimately affected (Petchesky 2003).

Another poignant feature of contemporary sexual politics is the gradual shift from the logic of resistance that dominated the first sexuality struggles of the 1970s towards a novel 'politics of project identities' (Castells 1997). For many years now feminists, lesbians, gays, HIV-positive persons, sex workers, and, more recently, transgender communities, have been openly engaged with legal reform, human rights work, and policy design, particularly in the domain of public health. The earliest examples of engagements with legal reform are found in the efforts made, since the 1950s, to eliminate laws criminalizing homosexual acts in those European countries that had not decriminalized them in the nineteenth century and in the USA, and in the early struggles for legal abortion (also in Europe and the USA) (see Chapter 2).[24] In the three decades that followed – despite the shifting and problematic trends observed in geopolitics and national politics – feminists and other sexual politics actors have expanded, deepened, and intensified their engagements with the state. Gains have been achieved in diverse countries in relation to new constitutional provisions that have advanced gender equality and, in the case of at least three Southern countries – Ecuador (1991), Fiji (1993), and South Africa (1994) – these reforms have included provisions that condemn discrimination on the basis of sexual orientation. Positive changes in constitutional anti-discrimination norms have also been adopted in a wide range of countries (Cameron 2002, ILGA 2007, Rios 2006).

From the late 1970s, these successful national initiatives sparked an increase in cross-border dialogues, and by the 1990s – fuelled by globalization, the UN international conferences, and the increasing use of the Internet – these connections expanded, matured, and became transnational. As a result an increasing number of sexual politics actors have started to engage in global policy arenas.[25] Whereas in the 1990s feminist networks were the more visible and active in these global spaces, ten years later many other voices would be heard in UN and related intergovernmental policy debates.[26] Jeffrey Weeks (2003) encapsulates this expanding and complex political dynamic in his recognition that we face new and unpredicted challenges in negotiating our way 'through the maze that apparently constitutes "sexuality", especially as we enter the world of "global sex"' (p. 2).

The maze goes global: the United Nations 'sex saga'

One main outcome of this global leap was the conceptual crafting and political legitimacy of new frames to address sexuality as a lawful domain of life to which human rights principles could and should be applied. Deriving directly from national struggles against discrimination and abuse, the use of citizenship rights language to address sexuality was boosted by globalization and new communication technologies, and connected to transformations under-way in the global human rights discourse. This inevitably transported these debates into the main international policy arenas, in particular, the series of UN conferences and evolving debates already mentioned above (Corrêa and Parker 2004, Girard 2007, Petchesky 2000, 2003).

The strategic relevance of the UN in this new cycle is not surprising given the history and mandate of the organization. The Commission on the Status of Women (CSW) was created in 1946, even before the UN itself was fully established. The principle of equality between the sexes enshrined in the 1948 Universal Declaration of Human Rights had its meaning and scope expanded in other United Nations instruments, such as the Convention for the Elimination of all Forms of Discrimination against

Women (1979), and in debates such as those initiated at the four world conferences on women (in Mexico City 1975, Copenhagen 1980, Nairobi 1985, and Beijing 1995). Between 1948 and the 1990s, women and 'sex' issues were also addressed by the health and population research and policy agendas implemented by WHO, UNFPA, UNICEF, and UNDP, even though the discourses deployed by these institutions remained strongly heteronormative, instrumental, and essentialist (Corrêa and Jolly 2006).

The full eruption of sexuality in the context of UN negotiations, policy, and normative documents had to wait, however, until the 1990s. While we will discuss these developments in greater detail in Chapter 8, within the context of the current discussion it is important to highlight that this breakthrough was triggered by a combination of trends and forces. One of them was clearly the HIV epidemic. Throughout the 1980s the UN and the World Bank barely addressed HIV, but by the early 1990s it had already been defined as a priority by the WHO. By the end of that decade a new UN agency, UNAIDS, had been established to address the pandemic as a main global development issue and the UN Security Council itself had taken up the matter of HIV as a 'threat to security'. At the same time, the UN 'sex saga' must be analysed against the background of other global trends that included optimistic assumptions on the part of the main international institutions that the post-Cold War period would be peaceful and more democratic. This optimism translated into a wide gamut of new policy initiatives such as the Human Development Report, launched by UNDP (UNDP 1990). But this period also included the widening of the UN cycle of social conferences, mentioned earlier, which provided a platform for gender and sexuality to gain policy status and public visibility. A number of these conferences were also subject to five-year and ten-year review processes (Cairo Plus Five, 1999; Copenhagen Plus Five, 2000; Beijing Plus Five, 2000; Cairo Plus Ten, 2004; Beijing Plus Ten, 2005) in which the controversies on gender and sexuality would intensify. However, the UN polemics around 'sex' would become particularly contentious following the election of George W. Bush in 2000, when the USA became a major obstacle to progress in this arena of policy debates.

In addition to debates evolving in the context of the major United Nations intergovernmental conferences, gender and sexuality related matters were, and still are, systematically addressed by other less visible permanent UN bodies such as the Commission on the Status of Women, the Commission on Population and Development, the annual WHO World Health Assembly, UNAIDS committees, human rights treaty bodies, and the General Assembly itself. The trends and complexities implied in these overlapping UN processes will be examined more extensively in Chapter 8. For now it is worth calling attention to the fact that although there have been a number of important advances in relation to acknowledging sexuality as a key dimension of human health and well-being (the ICPD Platform of Action), and in defining the human rights of women in relation to sexual matters (paragraph 96 of the Beijing Platform for Action), these groundbreaking definitions none the less remained, to a large extent, within a heterosexual conceptual frame (Corrêa and Parker 2004, Girard 2007, Petchesky 2003).

It is only even more recently that UN debates have begun to address issues related to sexual orientation. One of the earliest examples of this was the 1994 decision by the UN Committee on Human Rights in the *Toonen* v. *Australia* case, which led to the revision and abolition of sodomy laws in Tasmania. Since then infringements and abuses related to sexual identity and conduct have gained relevance in the debates and procedures of treaty bodies that monitor the implementation of human rights conventions on civil, political, social, and economic rights, on women and children, and on torture, and special rapporteurs on human rights have increasingly reported on perpetrations related to sexuality.

In 2003, a key moment occurred in the trajectory of sexuality debates at the level of UN treaty bodies when Brazil presented to the Human Rights Commission (HRC) a groundbreaking resolution on human rights and sexual orientation. Under heavy attack from the Organization of the Islamic Conference (OIC), the vote on the resolution was postponed to the 2004 session of the Commission. This delay allowed for a quick and intense mobilizing of lesbian and gay rights organizations in support of the resolution (APDC 2004), but even so, in 2004, under an OIC threat to boycott an Arab–Latin American trade summit scheduled for later the same year, Brazil retreated from retabling the text (Girard 2007, Pazello 2005). Despite this setback, sexual rights advocates have expanded and deepened their efforts, initially, in the Commission itself, and, after 2005, in the Human Rights Council, created to replace the HRC, with the same policy status as the Economic and Social Council (ECOSOC) and the Security Council.

This persistence is paying off. In December 2006, during the third session of the council, Norway, supported by 54 other countries, tabled a statement on human rights violations based on sexual orientation and gender identity.[27] And, in March 2007, the Yogyakarta Principles for the Application of International Human Rights Law in relation to Sexual Orientation and Gender Identity was launched at the fourth session of the Council and was positively received by many member states (see Chapter 7).[28]

The 'eternal return' to nature

The panoramic overview outlined above tells how, in the course of the past 30 years, sexuality theory, research, and political activism have been sustained, renewed, and diversified across national and cultural boundaries. Despite imbalances across regions, political instabilities, and the growing influence of religious dogma, 'sex' and gender norms were extensively reconfigured in most countries and, importantly, positive legal reforms have occurred in a variety of settings. Even so, essentialist conceptions of sexuality remain pervasive. Today, as in the past, scientific discourses and hard evidence are constantly deployed in academic studies and media outlets to 'prove' the natural imprint of human sexual behaviour and its intrinsic connection to reproduction. Indeed, these arguments have only become more sophisticated with the late twentieth-century breakthroughs in genetics and molecular biology, as illustrated by Dawkins' theory of the 'selfish gene' (1976) and Wilson's treatise *Sociobiology* (1975) (see also Chapter 4). Both authors 'explain' all human behaviour, and most particularly sexual behaviour, as a vehicle to ensure that successful genes survive and are represented in the next generation. Since their thesis was made public in the mid-1970s, Dawkins and Wilson have gained much public visibility and popular credibility, and such views are pervasive in mainstream institutions. Two recent and compelling studies of the World Bank have captured the depth of sex essentialist and heteronormative imprints in the dominant discourse of the institution (see Bedford forthcoming, Camargo and Mattos 2007). As described by Camargo and Mattos, there is a strong tendency in World Bank documents to medicalize sexuality, particularly its HIV/AIDS programmes and policies. This is part of the overall technocratic approach to health taken by the Bank, but, because of the silencing of sexuality in the Bank's public discourse, what is reinforced is an essentialist biological conception of sexuality that delegitimizes any claims based on rights (Camargo and Mattos 2007, p. 372).

For decades, sex theorists as well as those working in the biological field have contested 'scientific' arguments that push sexuality and gender back towards nature (see, e.g., Elredge 2004, Fausto-Sterling 2000, Gagnon and Parker 1995, Hubbard 1990, Weeks 2003).[29] But such critiques rarely receive significant media or other coverage – and even when they do they encounter much resistance because sex essentialism is so deeply ingrained in mentalities, discourses, and practices. Thus, just as biomedical views of sexuality are hegemonic in societies at large, versions of the same leitmotiv often appear among those who are themselves engaged in sexual politics. Large sectors of the feminist movement remain attached to a limited conception of gender as a binary descriptor of relations between men and women, in which gender is interpreted as a cultural layer superimposed over biological differences.

In recent years, too, various segments of the gay community have incorporated the notion of a 'gay gene' into their political discourse. Not infrequently, in public controversies about homosexuality, sexual rights advocates resort to 'scientific evidence' demonstrating the existence of same-sex relations among animals as their main argument to call for equality under the law. Sex essentialist theories are extremely appealing and pervasive because, as Weeks (2003) has analysed so insightfully, 'they provide clarity where social scientists may see complexities, while others recognize only contingency' (p. 47). Moreover, the intelligibility of biological explanations for sex and gender converges with a long-standing cognitive *habitus*, which, as suggested by Bourdieu (1998, 2002), is not easily destabilized by Cartesian political pedagogies.

The entrenched and resurgent appeal of sex essentialism has been and remains a main obstacle in the path of those who aim to expand the boundaries of political thinking and action in relation to sexuality, health, and human rights. It is particularly problematic in a historical conjunction when religious dogmatism is intensively engaged in the deployment of moral and philosophical arguments to revitalize natural conceptions of gender and sexuality. In the most diverse settings, simplified prescriptions – often extracted from 'sacred books' – are disseminated to attack women's personal, sexual, and reproductive autonomy and the integrity of persons of nonconforming sexualities.[30] These trends, observed at the grassroots level, are linked with systematic efforts at higher doctrinal levels to establish and revive naturalistic conceptions of gender and sexuality.

Feminists involved in the process leading to the Beijing Conference on Women in 1995 remember that in the final preparatory meeting the term 'gender' was bracketed during the negotiations under the pressure of the Holy See and a few Islamic countries. Meanwhile, pamphlets were distributed to official delegates by the Coalition for Women and the Family, a right-wing NGO, charging that 'there is a "gender feminism", often homosexual, which strongly promotes the idea that gender is something fluid, changing, not related naturally to being a man or being a woman. According to such feminist-homosexual ideology, there are at least five genders!'[31] (quoted in Girard 2007, p. 334). It soon became clear that this manoeuvre was grounded in a close study of feminist and queer studies texts and theories of gender, not only as culturally constructed, but also as containing the potential for multiple expressions. In particular, the Vatican had seized upon a paper by Anne Fausto-Sterling (1993) entitled 'The five sexes' and inferred from its premise a doctrine collapsing gender with sexuality and homosexuality.

The scope and depth of this doctrinal attack on 'gender' would become fully evident almost ten years later when, in August 2004, the Vatican Congregation for the Doctrine of Faith issued its 'Letter to the Bishops of the Catholic Church on the Collaboration of Men and Women in the Church and in the World' (Vatican 2004). The introduction analyses the evolution of feminist thinking without once mentioning the term 'feminism', and asserts that this thinking has experienced a substantive shift from a confrontational position between women and men to a new approach:

In order to avoid the domination of one sex or the other, their differences tend to be denied, viewed as mere effects of historical and cultural conditioning. In this perspective, physical difference, termed sex, is minimized, while the purely cultural element, termed gender, is emphasized to the maximum and held to be primary. The obscuring of the difference or duality of the sexes has enormous consequences on a variety of levels. This theory of the human person, intended to promote prospects for equality of women through liberation from biological determinism, has in reality inspired ideologies which, for example, call into question the family, in its natural two-parent structure of mother and father, and make homosexuality and heterosexuality virtually equivalent, in a new model of polymorphous sexuality.

(Vatican 2004, p. 1)

The intellectual sophistication reflected in this doctrinaire piece of writing is not, however, exclusive to Vatican thinkers. Similar endeavours are underway in the context of other religious traditions, as portrayed in the writings of the Egyptian Islamic female scholar Ezzat (2002), who insists that since the 1940s feminists, through their influence on the UN, created a 'new Leviathan', which is now being imposed on women who want to retain their difference and family values:

The non-discriminatory, sex-neutral category that includes provisions, which reject a conceptualization of women as a separate group and rather reflect on men and women as entitled to equal treatment. The idea here is that biological differences should not be a basis for the social and political allocation of benefits and burdens within a society. ... With the 'coming out' of the lesbian and gay movements and the powerful theorization on lesbian epistemology, many women became intimidated, nay, confused. Within the same line of thinking, in the last (secular) analysis, one should not define the family according to some fixed, biased, pre-modern measures! The classical family structure, according to gay and lesbian discourse, is to be renegotiated; a new form and understanding of 'a family' must be given. Against that, if one expresses a different perspective from that of the gay movement, the mildest accusation would be homophobia, the strongest would be fundamentalism.

(Ezzat 2002, p. 1)

Powerful adversaries of gender equality and sexual pluralism are therefore devoting much intellectual energy to contesting contemporary sex and gender theories, and their arguments are now pervasive in national and international policy arenas. While in 1995 the right-wing contestation of the term 'gender' did not reach the final Beijing negotiation, five years later, in 2000, during the negotiations leading to the creation of the International Criminal Court, the Rome Statute of the ICC (which is correctly considered to be one of the most important contemporary human rights instruments) adopted the following definition of gender: 'For the purpose of this Statute, it is understood that the term "gender" refers to the two sexes, male and female, within the context of society. The term "gender" does not indicate any meaning different from the above' (Article 7, quoted in Miller 2006, p. 6).[32]

It is ironic, therefore, that these same theories are not always taken seriously by progressive voices working in the physical and social sciences. One striking illustration is highlighted by Richard Dawkins himself. Considering his more recent writings – in particular his book *The God Delusion*, which has become a bestseller worldwide – that contest religious extremisms and the very idea of God, in the complex politics of our times, Dawkins could be a potential ally of sexual politics activists who systematically resist and criticize the growing influence of religious dogmatism in state policies. However, Dawkins remains strongly attached to the premises of biological essentialism and never enters into dialogue with authors who emphasize the socially and culturally constructed 'nature' of sex and gender.[33] It is also rather incongruous that, as we have seen, a wide range of activists directly involved in crucial sexuality and gender struggles still do not fully understand the theoretical frames contesting sex essentialism. The recognition of this paradox is, in fact, one important motivation for this book, as we are convinced that one of the main challenges to those committed to sexual rights is to expand the reach of contemporary thinking on sexuality towards the front lines, where the skirmishes and battles of late modern sexual politics are evolving on a daily basis.

Chapter 2

The real politics of 'sex'

In his series of studies on the history of sexuality, Michel Foucault suggested that to more precisely investigate the relationship between sex and politics the focus should be on the extremes of power, on what might be described as its outer limits, and on the ways in which the workings of power flow through every social system (Foucault 1978, 2003). This conceptual turn was crucial in diverting researchers and activists from those sites considered to be the main (if not the only) sources of power – the state, capital, and religious authorities – in order to examine other places where sexuality and politics constantly intersect in more subtle ways. But this should not be interpreted to mean that state instruments to punish sexual conduct have disappeared.

Since 1791, when the French Revolution abolished the crime of sodomy, a long and winding road leading towards the decriminalization of same-sex relations was inaugurated. However, this trajectory was slow and uneven across countries. Significantly, the reforms introduced immediately following the French Revolution did not occur exclusively in Europe. Data collected by Ottosson (2007) shows that by the late nineteenth century 12 countries had already abolished the crime of sodomy: seven European countries, five recently independent Latin American nations, and Turkey and Japan. By 1950, seven other countries had reformed punitive legislation, four of them in Europe and two in Latin America.[1] The next spate of reforms, from the 1950s through the 1970s, became linked in the political imagination with the sexual revolution then underway. In Western Europe, laws criminalizing homosexual practices were almost completely abolished during the period, including entrenched Anglo-Saxon laws that had not been shaken by the revolutionary spirit of 1789. The second wave began in quite unexpected places – Greece, Thailand, and Jordan – and expanded into the socialist world, where such practices were decriminalized in Bulgaria, Croatia, Czechoslovakia, Hungary, Montenegro, and Slovenia before reaching Canada, Germany, the United Kingdom, and Norway.[2]

This trend continued into the 1980s – starting with Colombia and Portugal – and since then sodomy laws or similar codes have been abolished in another 29 countries. The rhythm of these reforms intensified after the mid-1990s, reflecting the effects of political transition in the socialist world but also of democratizing processes in Latin American countries and in South Africa. The list of countries that have decriminalized same-sex relations in the 1980s and 1990s also includes New Zealand, Ireland, China, Russia, the Bahamas, and Cape Verde.[3]

Today, although many countries have left behind codes penalizing same-sex relations, criminal laws are still in place in 86 countries. In 47 of these countries, existing laws apply exclusively to sexual relations between men, while in the others they apply to both male and female same-sex relations.[4] In most of Africa and the English-speaking Caribbean and some countries in Asia and the Pacific, these laws are a legacy of the British Empire and remained largely untouched after independence, even in countries where the critique of Western imprints has been strongest. Ramasubban's analysis of the current struggle in India against section 377 of the penal code that criminalizes sodomy illuminates this striking paradox:

> Section 377 remained unchallenged in independent India until the advent of HIV/AIDS towards the close of the twentieth century, nearly 50 years after the British left the country. It remains on the statute books nearly 40 years after the anti-sodomy law was abolished in Britain itself. The paradox is that an archaic and outmoded law of colonial origin embedded in nineteenth century Victorian norms of morality, and what some sexual-rights activists describe as culturally alien Judaeo-Christian values, is being defended by the independent, modern Indian state, not to mention large sections of civil society that perceive such sexual practices as violating Indian culture.
>
> (Ramasubban 2007, p. 91)

However, similar legislation is also in place in African countries colonized by France, Germany, and Portugal. And, in the Islamic world, same-sex relations – usually codified under the broad juridical term *zina*, which covers a wide range of conduct considered to be unnatural – are also subject to criminal punishment in the majority of countries and, in seven of them, punishable by death.[5] In addition, in many countries where same-sex relations are not typified as a crime, persecution and prosecution still occur based on codes that criminalize 'debauchery', 'prostitution', or 'public immorality', or such relations are still prohibited among public officials, particularly the military.[6] We would also point out here that the absence of laws criminalizing same-sex relations does not guarantee the rights of sexual and gender nonconforming persons.

In the first decade of the twenty-first century, even a superficial glance at the main hubs of power – states, the global governance complex,

transnational capital flows, and military geopolitical strategies – is sufficient to grasp the extent of the interlocking of politics and 'sex'. We begin
by charting this novel phenomenon in the USA since, despite the shifting
geopolitical scenario briefly examined in Chapter 1, it still occupies a
central position in the so-called concert of nations.

'Sex' in the 'New American century'[7]

George W. Bush inaugurated his first administration in January 2001 by
reinstating the Mexico City Policy, also known as the Global Gag Rule,
which prohibits overseas recipients of funds from the United States Agency
for International Development (USAID) to research, provide, or advocate
for abortion.[8] In February 2003, the Bush administration announced the
President's Emergency Plan for AIDS Relief (PEPFAR). Concurrently the
National Security Directive against Trafficking in Persons was made public
and an interagency task force established to manage the trafficking policy.
A few months later the Congress approved the PEPFAR guideline in the
HIV/AIDS Global Act of 2003[9] and, in December 2003, the Trafficking
Victims Protection Reauthorization Act (TVPRA) passed into legislation.

By May 2007, PEPFAR had directed some US$15 billion in US foreign
assistance towards the prevention and treatment of AIDS in the most
severely afflicted regions (Stout 2007); it has done so by insinuating the
heteronormative, conjugal, and procreative model of sexuality so dear to
the hearts of the US Christian Right into the criteria for receiving funding.
In both the legislation and regulations authorizing PEPFAR as well as in its
practical implementation, this has meant: (1) a policy promoting the
'A-B-C' (abstain, be faithful, use a condom) approach to HIV prevention,
but with a clear emphasis on 'A' and a subtle if not direct discouragement
of 'C' (the legislation requires that at least one-third of all funds be
devoted to abstinence programmes); (2) priority in the distribution of
funds to 'faith-based' (usually Christian) organizations over secular or
public health-based ones, whether or not those groups have any experience
in AIDS treatment and prevention; and, (3) stigmatization and disqualifica-
tion of advocacy groups that are composed of, or reach out to, sex
workers, even though these groups have been among the most effective in
developing prevention strategies that work and have virtually halted the
spread of HIV among sex workers in many communities. The December
2003 regulation on international trafficking – the TVPRA – also includes
the so-called Prostitution Loyalty Oath, which inhibits foreign organizations that support sex workers' rights from receiving funds.[10]

Similar guidelines, including the A-B-C guidelines, were adopted into
domestic policies to the detriment of more comprehensive sexuality education programmes. The Bush administration has also increased financial
allocations for the promotion of marriage under policy guidelines defined

by the 1996 Welfare Reform Bill (di Mauro and Joffe 2007, Girard 2004), and research institutions were pressured to use flawed, allegedly scientific, research to discredit the efficacy of condoms in preventing HIV and other sexually transmitted infections (STIs). In May 2003, conservative members of Congress tabled a constitutional amendment to ban same-sex marriage.[11] In the months that followed, two judicial decisions occurred that incensed the religious Right: the Supreme Court overturned sodomy laws in the state of Texas and the Massachusetts Supreme Judicial Court decided that gay couples had the right to marry under the state constitution. President Bush openly declared his opposition to the Supreme Court decision and announced his support for the constitutional amendment, a position that would be made explicit in his 2004 State of the Union address (Girard 2004).[12] Regressive domestic developments have also occurred in relation to abortion, including a ban on the late-term abortion procedure that the religious Right has successfully labelled 'partial-birth abortion'.[13] The ban was approved by the Congress in October 2003 and confirmed by the Supreme Court in early 2007 in *Gonzalez* v. *Carhart* (CRR 2003).[14] By 2004, USAID operations had already become very stringent with respect to the implementation of the A-B-C and prostitution clauses in both the PEPFAR and TVPRA regulations. The Department of Justice argued that the same restrictions could be applied to US-based organizations even though the US Constitution prohibits interference with the free speech of US physicians and civil society organizations (CHANGE 2005b; see also Chapter 10).[15]

This is not the first time in US history that state and society find themselves engaged in sex wars. At least since the nineteenth century recurrent ideological and moral battles around sexuality sparked anxieties and social strife.[16] One notorious example was the Comstock Act of 1873, which made it illegal to send any obscene, lewd, and/or lascivious material through the mail, including contraceptive devices and information (Beisel 1997, di Mauro and Joffe 2007, Gordon 1976). In the McCarthy era of the 1950s, supposed homosexuals were witch-hunted as communist infiltrators seeking to erode national morality (Miller 1995; see also Chapter 18). Immediately after the 1973 Supreme Court ruling, *Roe* v. *Wade*, which legalized abortion, religious conservative forces started to organize against it. A decade later these forces would be strong enough to influence policies adopted by the Reagan administration, which included the restriction on international abortion funding that would be revived in 2001 (Petchesky 1990).[17] In fact, policy measures of the Bush administration in relation to abstinence-only programmes and the promotion of marriage build upon and deepen the provisions enshrined in the text of the 1996 Welfare Reform Bill, approved by a Republican Congressional majority but also sanctioned, without much debate, by the Clinton administration (Girard 2004). Even when placed against this historical backdrop, the intensity of the sex obsession that impregnates current US policies is exceptional.

Although a complex gamut of trends and forces underlies the surge and evolution of contemporary US neo-conservatism, including the contradictory effects of globalization on US society and hegemony,[18] one key contributing factor to the 2000 and 2004 electoral triumphs of the neo-conservatives was the political strength accumulated since the 1970s by the religious Right. The many positions on sexual politics obsessively deployed by the Bush administration are clearly intended as payback to the religious Right for its consistent electoral support. However, they must also be seen as core components of the neo-conservative geopolitical strategy in that they are deliberately used to project, domestically and internationally, an image of the USA as a nation blessed by the Judaeo-Christian god. As Jacques Derrida (1998) foresaw, the global 'war on terror' is intentionally scripted as a new form of religious war that pits Christian crusaders against Islamic jihadists. And a key signifier of Christian righteousness (deeply contaminated now, of course, by the events of Abu Ghraib – see Chapter 10) is its claim to sexual morality.[19] Last but not least, Bush's obsession with sexual matters has also served to divert society's attention from other critical areas, such as the lies and failures of the Iraq war, increasing social inequalities, the erosion and escalating costs of health care, and the impacts of global warming.

Since 2001, a number of authors have critically scrutinized the military, economic, and geopolitical effects of US neo-conservative policy agendas (see, e.g., Halper and Clarke 2004, Johnson 2004, Risen 2006). However, they have not sufficiently scrutinized the neo-conservative discursive and financial complicity in sexuality issues. In contrast, advocates involved in sexual politics immediately understood the geopolitical scope and potentially detrimental effects of Bush's 'many positions on sex' both within and outside the country. Since early 2001, groups and networks engaged in global policy debates have closely monitored and resisted the positioning and strategies of US delegations in related negotiations, such as the 2001 UN General Assembly Special Session on AIDS and the 2002 Asia Conference on Population and Development (Freitas 2001, Girard 2007, Sen 2005). In addition, as early as 2004, the negative impacts of PEPFAR and TPVRA began to be felt in the most diverse settings, and a year later public conflicts involving USAID and recipients of US HIV/AIDS prevention funds broke out in Brazil and India (see also Chapters 3 and 9).

The victory of the Democratic Party in the 2006 Congressional elections seemed to signal the beginning of a new cycle in US politics. Despite disappointing retreats by the Democratic majority on many fronts (for example, treatment of 9/11 detainees, warrant-less wiretaps, conservative presidential appointments, funding for the Iraq war), and although positions on sexuality and abortion vary widely among Democrats, important initiatives have taken place at the Congressional level. Systematic pressure is being brought to bear on the PEPFAR conditionalities[20] and, as this book was being finalized in September 2007, the US Senate passed an amendment to the State and Foreign Operations appropriations bill, to repeal the Global Gag Rule, by a vote of 53–41 (CHANGE 2007). Nevertheless, the complete transformation of policies currently being implemented will require many other legislative and normative reforms and, most principally, the containment of regressive forces in the society itself.

It is also crucial to keep in mind that the global impacts of Bush's prescriptions on sex have been widespread and deep. Although it would be an over-simplification to say that the myriad sex wars underway globally are merely an effect of US policies, the moralistic geopolitical climate of the past seven years has, practically everywhere, inspired conservative states and social forces to push for their political and religious agendas. In addition, in a large number of cases the Bush administration's guidelines and prescriptions have been incorporated into national policy frames. Even if these policy frames become modified in the future under a different leadership in Washington, the full reorientation of programmes adopted under the influence of USAID will, as we know, take much longer.

Here, there, and everywhere...

The worldwide proliferation of sex wars in recent years cannot be attributed exclusively to Bush's regressive policies. The so-called 'Queen Boat' episode that occurred in Egypt in May 2001, when the Bush administration had barely begun its obsessive investment in sexual matters, illustrates the point (Bahgat 2001, HRW 2004c). In Egypt, as in many countries, the law allows same-sex relations between consenting adults, but in practice homosexual and transgender persons are persecuted and prosecuted on the basis of laws that criminalize promiscuity, prostitution, and immorality (Ottosson 2007). The episode in question started when a police squad raided a nightclub on a cruise vessel docked in Cairo and detained more than 30 men. As described by Long (2004), the media portrayed these men as members of a 'devil-worshippers' organization' devoted to the practice of 'perverted activities' and 'pornography' and reported that the police found the 'satanists' naked and holding a marriage ceremony for two male youths. The treatment they received from the police and justice system infringed a wide range of human rights principles:

> Fifty-two men were tried before an Emergency State Security Court, one boy before a juvenile court. All were charged with the 'habitual practice of debauchery,' and nearly half convicted. Most of the men had been tortured in detention. The lives of all were ripped apart.... Despite charges that the 'cult' was caught at the Queen Boat, only 30

of the 53 who ultimately went to trial were arrested there. Most of the rest were picked up on the street, through informers, in the days before.

(HRW 2004b, p. 1)

In the wake of the episode police informers multiplied, the police invaded private homes, hundreds of people were imprisoned and tortured, and the emerging gay community has practically disintegrated (Long 2004). This brutality is explained by the many paradoxes of society traversed by rapid changes that are, as elsewhere, deeply transforming sex and gender orders (Bahgat and Afifi 2007). Egypt's 30-year state of emergency gives the police extensive arbitrary powers, and the state deliberately targets gender and sexuality issues to distract attention and satisfy those sectors of society influenced by Islamic revivalists. However, as analysed by Human Rights Watch, the episode also involved an obscure dynamic of personal persecutions and family vendettas.[21]

In contrast, in Uganda, the interconnections between internal dynamics and the US influence are blatant. Since the 1980s, the country has experienced a constant decline in HIV infection rates and has been considered a 'success story' in spite of evidence that stringent fiscal constraints adopted under IMF rules have increased internal inequalities, limited social investments, and created greater dependency on foreign funds to sustain the response to the epidemic (Action Aid 2004, Okidi and Mugambe 2002). Girard (2004) recalls that prior to 2003, analysts who assessed Uganda's HIV and AIDS policies emphasized its multiple approaches to prevention, which included condom promotion (Epstein 2007, Pankhurst 2002, Richey 2005). Girard quotes David Serwadda, director of the Uganda Institute for Public Health, who said: 'We must not forget that abstinence only is not always possible for people at risk, particularly women' (2004, p. 10). However, following the approval of the Global AIDS Act in 2003, the US government systematically manipulated data on Uganda in order to use it as scientific evidence on the efficacy of abstinence-only strategies and, later on, to restrict the provision of condoms through USAID. In 2005, various sources denounced the shortage of condoms in the country and suggested that this could account for the disturbing increase in HIV infections among married women (CHANGE 2005a).

Although the negative US influence on country policies is flagrant, it is not the only factor favouring regressive discourses and interpretations of Uganda's HIV policies. In the mid-1980s President Yoweri Museveni became known worldwide for his policy commitment to HIV and AIDS, an attitude that contrasted positively with the denial then prevailing among other African heads of state. But the history behind Museveni's commitment casts a different light on his motivations. Richey (2005) reports that in 1986, when Museveni came to power, 60 top military cadres were sent to Cuba for military training. A few months later, at a conference in Zimbabwe, Cuba's president, Fidel Castro, informed Museveni that 18 officers in the group had tested positive for HIV. The author analyses how this encounter, which motivated the priority given to the epidemic, partially explains Uganda's 'military approach to AIDS as a threat against which people must mobilize and fight' (Richey 2005, p. 100).[22] However, it should be noted that this top-down model converges with the ways in which Ugandan politics evolved in the following years. Museveni, in power for more than 20 years, has always been socially conservative and he constantly manipulates moral and religious issues in order to retain power (Jacobson 2006).[23] In addition to adopting, without critique, Bush's policy guidelines for HIV and AIDS, Museveni frequently deploys homophobic rhetoric, and the Ugandan police systematically prey on persons whose sexuality does not conform to dominant norms. Amnesty International (AI 2003) reported the dramatic effects of discriminatory speeches combined with police persecution on the lives of LGBTQ people in Uganda:

> In March (2002) President Museveni said in a speech to the Commonwealth Heads of Government Meeting in Australia that the relative success of the fight against AIDS in Uganda was because the country has no homosexuals. In August the Minister of Ethics and Integrity ordered police to arrest and prosecute homosexuals. Security agents continued harassing members of the LGBT community throughout 2002, and several were arrested because of their sexual orientation.
>
> (AI 2003, p. 1)

Not surprisingly, in 2005 new legislation was adopted defining marriage as a union between a woman and a man and, a year later, the newspaper *Red Pepper* publicly accused 13 women of being lesbians (AI 2006). It should be noted that this virulence is not restricted to homosexual behaviour. For instance, in 2004 a performance of *The Vagina Monologues*, planned as part of the V-Day Campaign (see Chapter 1, n. 13), was suspended by a governmental ordinance.[24] The International Gay and Lesbian Human Rights Commission, working in collaboration with the local organization Sexual Minorities Uganda, has compiled a report of other systematic abuses and violations, which was presented to the African Charter on Human Rights Commission in May 2006 (IHRC and SMU 2006).[25]

As happens elsewhere, as sexual rights gained visibility in Uganda, homophobia escalated. In August 2007, in response to a news conference held by Sexual Minorities Uganda to call upon the government to let them live in peace, evangelical and born-again Christian leaders created the Interfaith Rainbow Coalition Against Homosexuality. This group then organized a public demonstration to deliver a document to the Minister of Ethics and Integrity requesting stronger government action against what the coalition described as 'a well-orchestrated effort by homosexuals to intimidate the government' (Roubus 2007).

Nigeria provides another example of the growing politicization of sexuality issues in the sub-Saharan region. Since independence in the 1960s the country has experienced a series of conflicts and a sequence of dictatorships, the last of which ended in 1998 to 1999. In the turmoil following this latest transition to democracy, one manifestation of the persistent tensions between regional political forces and the central government was the re-establishment of Sharia laws in northern states where the Muslim population is in the majority. Between 2001 and 2002, when a Sharia tribunal accused two women, Saffyia Tungar-Tuddu and Amina Lawal, of adultery (*zina*) and condemned them to death by stoning, the cases received global visibility (Imam 2005; see also Chapter 3).[26] In 2003, when a major dispute erupted within the global Anglican Church about the nomination of a gay bishop in the US state of New Hampshire, branches in the global South threatened to sever ties with the Anglican Communion Office in London. The Nigerian archbishop, Peter Akinola, played a vocal role in this potentially schismatic move.[27]

From 2003, as PEPFAR guidelines became more stringent, HIV prevention programmes at the country level have been shifting towards abstinence-only approaches. This move has set back pioneering efforts to implement sound sexuality education policies, which had been underway since the mid-1990s when Nigerian feminists and other civil society actors started pushing for the implementation of the ICPD and Beijing agendas (Esiet forthcoming; see also Chapter 1), and local religious communities connected to US-based evangelical churches often support abstinence-only programmes. In January 2006, the impact of transnational conservative streams became clear when the minister of justice presented a bill to Parliament proposing a ban on same-sex marriage. The bill is entitled the 'Act to Make Provisions for the Prohibition of Relationship Between Persons of the Same Sex, Celebration of Marriage by Them, and for Other Matters Connected Therewith' and is clearly inspired by the constitutional amendment proposed in the US Congress in 2003 (see above and Girard 2004). However, it goes further, calling for a five-year prison term for any person who 'goes through the ceremony of marriage with a person of the same sex', 'performs, witnesses, aids, or abets the ceremony of same-sex marriage', or 'is involved in the registration of gay clubs, societies, and organizations'; and it prohibits any public display of a 'same-sex amorous relationship' (Global Rights 2006, HRW 2006a, 2006b, 2007a, IGLHRC 2007a, 2007b). Human Rights Watch considered the draft act to be a flagrant infringement of international human rights law:

> [It] ... violates Nigeria's commitments under international human rights law. These commitments include the International Covenant on

Civil and Political Rights (ICCPR), to which Nigeria acceded without reservations in 1993, and which protects the rights to freedom of expression (article 19), freedom of assembly (article 21), and freedom of association (article 22). The ICCPR affirms the equality of all people before the law and the right to freedom from discrimination in articles 2 and 26.

(HRW 2006b, p. 1)

During 2006 the bill proceeded slowly through Parliament. Then, in February 2007, as general elections scheduled for April approached, a Senate public hearing was called to discuss it, and conservative sectors made a strong push for a vote to be taken before the end of the legislative session. As the bill gained greater visibility in the global media, Nigeria's conservative sectors became more vocal and aggressive, and Nigerian human rights and LGBTQ groups had to fight hard to gain access to the parliamentary proceedings.[28] An effective mobilization effort was launched, linking local and global activists, key actors in the human rights field, and religious leaders (IGLHRC 2007a, 2007b, HRW 2007d, UN 2007). Despite the formidable obstacles and risky political pitfalls these groups faced, the bill was not tabled before the end of the legislature, and tensions eased temporarily. Then in August 2007, 18 men were arrested in the city of Bauchi, in northern Nigeria, and charged with sodomy and attendance at a same-sex marriage. Some were released on bail, and the charges were reduced to indecent dressing and vagrancy. Among those expressing their concern with the arrests and subsequent imprisonment, Reverend Rowland Jide Macaulay, a progressive Nigerian pastor, condemned the arrests as a clear violation of human rights. However, when the accused men attended the first court hearing, local religious and communitarian groups protested against the change in the charges and release of the accused men, bringing traffic to a halt as they hurled insults and stones at the court building. Conservative sectors and the media used the episode to call for the immediate approval of the Same-sex Marriage Prohibition Act (Masike 2007).

In South Asia, India has also been the stage of major public controversies about sexuality in which state actors are directly engaged. Between 1999 and 2003, policy makers and communitarian Hindu purity groups, backed by the then ruling Bharatiya Janata Party (BJP) and its Hindu revivalist, or *hindutva*, constituents, have, as in Uganda, intensified virulent speech and actions in relation to gender and sexuality (Butalia and Sarkar 1995, Chakravarti 2000, Narrain 2004, Sow *et al.* 2007; see also Chapter 3). It is important to situate this trend within the deep social, cultural, and economic transformations occurring in India as well as the rapid expansion of HIV and AIDS. These combined and complex forces have enhanced the surge and expansion of a lively and diverse movement for sexual rights, as well as increasing the backlash against them. In the late 1990s, public debates on sexuality gained strength through the voices of a diverse range of new actors: feminists, gays, lesbians, *khotis*, and *hijras*.[29] Against this contradictory and shifting background, groups advocating for the rights of alternative sexualities joined efforts around a public interest litigation campaign to challenge the legality of the anti-sodomy law in section 377 of the India Penal Code.[30]

Another vibrant expression of sexual politics in India is the plethora of sex worker associations and NGOs providing services related to prostitution, particularly HIV prevention and treatment (Kotiswaran 2001, *The Times of India* 2005).[31] In the Indian context, though large numbers of women and girls are engaged in sex work, *hijras* depend heavily on commercial or transactional sex, and the 'trade' also involves *khotis* and men (CREA *et al.* 2005, Nanda 1994, Seshu 2005). Since the 1980s, feminist and sex worker organizations have debated the reform of India's prostitution law.[32] Three incompatible views contend in these debates, echoing divisions – including among feminists – over sex work in other contexts and at a global level: one that equates prostitution with slavery and calls for the abolition of all commercial sex; an opposing view that defends legalization and sex workers' rights (labour, health, education); and a third position which recognizes that sex workers should not be criminalized but calls for the punishment of clients, as exemplified by the 1998 Swedish law (Collet 2006, Ditmore 2007, Kempadoo 1998; see also Chapter 9).[33] The current global conservative climate in relation to sexuality issues and, most particularly, sex work, has given visibility and strength to the abolitionists (Kempadoo 2005).

In India until very recently, no relevant state actor had publicly expressed a position on the subject. However, after the Congress Party regained power in 2004 – a shift that would enlarge the policy space for the litigation against section 377 – in October of 2005, a public announcement stated that key sections of government were about to propose legislation criminalizing clients of sex workers (*The Times of India* 2005).[34] This policy proposal, though supported by internal social forces, reflected the growing strength worldwide of both the abolitionist position on prostitution and the Swedish legal model.

In the months preceding the proposal, the Prostitution Loyalty Oath imposed by USAID (see above) and the activities of US-based NGOs engaged in rescuing children from brothels prompted major public clashes. In May 2005, in Sangli, where the successful Sangram programme supporting female sex workers is based, Restore International, one of these 'rescue' NGOs mobilized a police raid in the red light district. Thirty-eight women and girls and 18 brothel keepers were taken to the police station. The raid was followed by a vicious online campaign accusing Sangram of trafficking minors, and press articles reported that USAID had stopped funding the organization because it had thwarted the 'rescue' efforts (Sangram 2005).[35]

Not surprisingly the new policy approach to prostitution, which aims to criminalize clients, was met with protests by sex worker organizations and, since 2005, the proposal has lost visibility. This may be due to the fact that national policy debates on HIV and AIDS gained new contours and became more clearly articulated with the efforts aimed at repealing section 377.[36] During the 2006 UNGASS five-year review in New York, the India delegation aligned fully with those countries that resisted the USA, the Vatican, and other conservative forces in the debates around sexual and reproductive health and rights and HIV and AIDS policies. Then, in July, immediately before the International Conference on AIDS held in Toronto, the head of India's National AIDS Control Organization (NACO) called publicly for the elimination of section 377, arguing that the law makes vulnerable groups clandestine and thereby compromises prevention and treatment measures. At that stage the repudiation of section 377 had gained high-profile supporters, such as film actors and other celebrities and well-known intellectuals such as the Nobel Prize-winning economist, Amartya Sen.

Experiences in China and Vietnam provide a quite distinctive illustration of the interplay between sexuality, politics, and morality in which religion is entirely absent. In both countries, although the logic of compulsory secularity established under communism prevails and criminal laws condemning same-sex relations have been abolished, nonconforming sexual identities and conducts are still perceived as socially deviant. The environment for sex work is similar, if not worse, since communist regimes strongly condemned such activity as a remnant of capitalist values and made it illegal and a constant focus of state control and violence. What is distinctive in both cases is that, though religious forces are entirely absent from the political scene, conservative sexual morality is not. Rather, it is embedded in the state itself.

In China, despite decriminalization, same-sex relations are still deeply stigmatized, and state violence against sexual and gender nonconforming behaviour and expressions is widespread. For instance, in December 2005 the police raided the first Chinese lesbian and gay film festival, and this open state violence was broadcast live on national television. At the same time, under the impact of the rapid economic transformations experienced since the 1980s, sex work is today a fast-growing 'industry' that is very often controlled by the local authorities of the Communist Party. This mix of corruption and communist morality that characterizes commercial sex activities quite often leads to public actions to shame and stigmatize prostitutes in order to isolate them from institutional actors involved in the trade. In 2006, a group of 100 sex workers and their male patrons were paraded in Shenzhen (Guangzhou Province) in an incident that replicated the practice of public humiliation extensively applied during the Cultural Revolution (1966–1976) but outlawed in the early 1980s (HRW 2005). HIV and AIDS activism is also subject to stringent state regulation, and restrictions are often placed on individuals and organizations who work with populations stigmatized because of their sexuality or because they criticize the state response to the epidemic.[37]

In the case of Vietnam, a study by Le Minh and Nguyen (2007) examined how *Doi Moi*, the economic reform policy of the 1990s, initially opened novel spaces for policy proposals on reproductive health, gender equality, and civil society participation to gain legitimacy in social and official circles. But this brief moment of détente vanished in the 2000s, when increased HIV rates and anxieties, spurred by economic liberalization and renewed neo-Malthusian concerns, restricted political and policy spaces. This in turn re-created a crisis climate in which the state perceived HIV and AIDS and fertility as potential threats to economic growth and national security. In this new phase, family planning guidelines once again became more stringent, HIV was strictly defined as a social risk issue, and the openings for civil society participation were restricted.

Even when the factors determining the many restrictions on sexual and reproductive rights in Vietnam are predominantly specific to the country's political and policy environment, transnational influences are still present. The policy shift described above coincided with the influx of international funds for HIV and AIDS from PEPFAR and the Global Fund, which implied the reduction of domestic financial investments to respond to the epidemic. In addition, though religious doctrine does not play any role in Vietnam's internal policy definitions, the 'moral' rationales of US policy converge with the government's own moralistic conception of HIV as the outcome of 'social evils', namely prostitution, drug abuse, and homosexuality.

When the focus shifts to Eastern Europe, the landscape of sexual politics appears deeply intertwined with the many paradoxes affecting the region in the post-communist era, including a clear return to religious values and the influence of religious actors in public policy formation. In the 1950s, abortion had been legalized in the Soviet Union and the Eastern European countries under its influence, but a turn towards restrictive policies has marked the period since 1989, in particular Poland.[38] As noted earlier, laws penalizing same-sex relations had also been abolished in various countries of the region long before these reforms were completed in Europe or the USA – in Poland in 1934 and in six other countries before 1980 (see n. 2). As most countries in the region have acceded to the European Union, they have been required to comply with its human rights standards. However, these formal legislative gains and the potentially beneficial effects of EU accession contrast sharply with aspects of the prevailing political and policy climate.

In Poland in 2004, when a bill to legalize civil unions for same-sex partners was partially approved, the sponsoring senator was heavily attacked
from within and outside Parliament. In 2005, when an extreme right-wing
coalition, led by the Law and Justice Party, won the parliamentary majority, the climate worsened. The twin brothers, who became president and
prime minister, have declared on various occasions how proud they are of
being allied with Bush in the 'war on terror'. Consistent with this perspective the prime minister publicly declared, immediately after his nomination,
that if a person tried to 'infect' others with his/her homosexuality the state
should intervene in 'this violation of freedom' (Reuters 2005). Then, in
early 2007, the deputy minister of education announced that the government was preparing a bill to 'punish' anyone who 'promotes homosexuality' in schools and education establishments. Teachers, principals, and
students who violate the law could face dismissal, fines, or imprisonment
(HRW 2007b).

The loss of legal abortion and the escalating climate of state-sponsored
homophobia was consistent with the prevailing political climate in Poland,
as illustrated by the October 2006 law requiring all senior civil servants,
university professors, lawyers, headmasters, and journalists born before
1972 to fill out a form with the question: 'Did you secretly and knowingly
collaborate with the former communist security services?' This information is given to their immediate superiors and processed by the Institute of
National Memory, responsible for issuing a certificate of political purity.
As Ramonet (2007) remarks in an article published in Le Monde Diploma-
tique: 'This mad law, which is causing uproar in the European Union,
makes the McCarthyites of the United States in the 1950s look like ama-
teurs at the practice of anti-communism' (2007, p. 1).[39]

But Poland is not an exception. In 2005, the Latvian Parliament
approved legislation defining marriage as a union between a woman and a
man in order to block same-sex marriage or civil union bills from being
tabled (Araloff 2006). It also refused to pass legislation on non-
discrimination on the basis of sexual orientation, which all European
Union member states are required to adopt. From 2004, a sequence of
conflicts was sparked in Poland, Latvia, Moldavia, and Russia when local
authorities issued ordinances prohibiting gay and lesbian pride parades
while at the same time skinheads and other right-wing groups brutally
attacked gays, lesbians, and transgender persons. In practically all these
cases, LGBTQ groups contested the prohibitions before national or European higher courts, but these litigations will not automatically eliminate
repressive state measures and societal violence.[40]

In 2006, the conflicts surrounding the Moscow gay pride parade, which
gained significant global visibility, illustrate the deep connections between
state actors and religious forces in a country where compulsory secularity
has been the rule for almost 80 years. The mayor's decision to prohibit the

parade had the open support of the Patriarch of the Orthodox Church and the long-distance approval of the Vatican (Long 2006). Despite systematic protests and legal contestations after the 2006 conflict, in 2007 major clashes erupted once again in Russia as well as in the other countries of the region (HRW 2007c, HRW and ILGA 2007).

The bird's-eye view offered in the previous pages shows that the interplay between sexual morality, secular laws, and the growth of politically oriented religious forces is not just rapidly shifting – it is also exceedingly complex. Everything suggests that, as we will examine in Chapter 3, calling for a return to stricter secular rules will not be sufficient to provide a solid base for the full development of and respect for sexual rights. The experience of Turkey, as illuminated by Ilkkaracan (2007), provides a sharp illustration of these complexities. Her study examines the harsh debates evolving between 2002 and 2004 during the Campaign for the Reform of the Turkish Penal Code from a Gender Perspective. The campaign was launched by feminist organizations, seizing the opportunity of Turkey's accession to the European Union to mobilize against restrictions contained in the criminal law with respect to honour, virginity, sexuality of youth, and sexual orientation. These debates evolved while the Islamist AKP Party governed Turkey, but this does not fully explain the political tensions triggered by the campaign. As important as the immediate political environment was the penal code adopted in 1926, when, under Kemal Ataturk, Turkey was modernized on the basis of strong secular principles, and the application of Sharia law was abolished. As Ilkkaracan makes clear, the reformed law retained strong elements of traditional sexual morality, in a secular guise, and its legacy created inevitable obstacles for the penal code reform:[41]

> Despite the apparently opposing views of modernists and Islamists on women's role in society, in fact, they competed zealously to construct a patriarchal ideal of female sexuality and to maintain and reconstruct mechanisms to control women's sexuality and bodies. The modernists attempted to confront the social anxieties triggered by women's participation in the public sphere through the construction of the modern Turkish woman, emancipated and active in the founding of the new republic as mother, teacher, and political activist, yet also modest and chaste.
>
> (Ilkkaracan 2007, pp. 250–251)

Another relevant trait of the Turkish debate is that, as in other cases, it cannot be fully apprehended without taking into account the influence of transnational trends. One determining factor in the debates was that progressive alignment with European Union criminal laws is a criterion for accession, EU officials adopted public positions with regard to the Turkish

Penal Code Reform. Conversely, feminist groups decided to launch the campaign precisely because the EU requirements, while requesting changes with respect to the abolition of the death penalty, pre-trial detention provisions, and the expansion of the scope of freedom of expression, did not directly address gender equality or articles concerning sexuality. Most importantly, immediately before the new draft of the code was approved by Parliament, the conservative government announced it would table a new bill to criminalize adultery. EU officials reacted immediately and publicly and, in order to prevent the process of accession from being derailed, the government retreated from tabling the proposal. Ilkkaracan (2007) observes that the EU intervention, although converging with the Turkish feminist agenda, mobilized internal conservative reactions.[42]

Abortion trenches[43]

A dominant worldwide trend towards greater access to pregnancy termination has prevailed since the 1995 Fourth World Conference on Women in Beijing, when countries adopted a recommendation that they should revise punitive legislation.[44] According to an updated policy briefing on abortion reforms by the Centre for Reproductive Rights (CRR 2007), 17 countries have eliminated legal barriers, and in six countries reforms went further to allow abortion without restriction within the first 12 to 14 weeks of pregnancy: Albania (1996), Cambodia (1997), Nepal (2002), Portugal (2007), South Africa (1996), and Switzerland (2002). In addition, there have been state-level reforms in Australia and in the Federal District of Mexico (April 2007),[45] while struggles aimed at legalizing abortion or to make abortion accessible in circumstances permitted by law are ongoing in a large number of countries.[46]

The Centre for Reproductive Rights (CRR 2007) has reported major legal reversals in three countries – El Salvador, Nicaragua, and Poland – and also examines other cases where less dramatic restrictions on access to abortion have occurred. However, it is significant that, in the past 12 years, the number of countries in which further restrictions to abortion have been approved is minimal when compared to the expanded access to abortion experienced elsewhere. Moreover, the majority of progressive abortion reforms were approved after 2000 at the same time as anti-abortion arguments and funding restrictions were being amplified. In light of that fact, the contexts where major setbacks have occurred may be portrayed as critical trenches from which anti-abortion forces expect to regain terrain. The trajectory of the abortion debate in Nicaragua and Poland, in particular, illuminates how contemporary trends can, and should, be traced back to the geopolitics of the 1980s. Bernstein and Politi (1996) analysed how, in the final period of the Cold War, Pope John Paul II and the US president, Ronald Reagan, devised geopolitical strategies to defeat communism that combined the destabilization of Nicaragua's Sandinista regime, the silencing of progressive Catholic voices in that country, and support for the Polish transition through a Church alliance with the Solidarity Movement.[47]

In Nicaragua, a first effect of these manoeuvrings as they involved sexual politics was the reform of the penal code during the Chamorro administration. This legal change, adopted in 1992, included a provision to criminalize same-sex relations among both males and females and meant that Nicaragua became the only country in Latin America where same-sex relations are still criminalized (see nn. 1 and 2). Throughout the 1990s there developed a series of battles related to abortion that would intensify under the impact of the Cairo and Beijing conferences.[48] In 2003, Rosita, a nine-year-old Nicaraguan girl who was living with her Catholic parents in Costa Rica, was raped and became pregnant. The family travelled back to Nicaragua and requested judicial authorization for an abortion. The parents were not only threatened with excommunication by Catholic bishops, but an international petition campaign was also launched calling on people to back the bishops. Some 28,000 people signed the petition but, after a series of diverse judicial skirmishes, the abortion was performed.

Then, in May 2006, a large public demonstration was organized in Managua calling for same-sex relations to be decriminalized and this suggested that the political in relation to sexual and reproductive rights was improving. However, in October, immediately before the presidential elections, a march organized by the Catholic Church called upon the Congress to abolish a therapeutic abortion clause that had been enshrined in the penal code since the nineteenth century. This move was rather unusual, since a full reform of the penal code was already being debated in Parliament. However, it had the open support of Daniel Ortega, the Sandinista leader (and ex-president), who was running for the presidency.[49] In an interview by Gago (2006), Monica Baltodano, the former Sandinista commander and the only woman who was part of the high command that ousted the dictator Anastasio Somoza, gave a negative analysis of the episode:

> Ortega got just 30 per cent of votes using obscure manoeuvring and will experience difficulties in governing. Consequently he has become still more conservative than he is so as to appease the bankers, the Church and the United States. The elimination of the abortion clause is a brutal backlash promoted by a political force that has shown more commitment to reactionary positions than a right-wing party that may have won the elections.
>
> (Gago 2006, p. 1)

The abolition of the abortion clause prompted an intense local and international mobilization. A case was presented to the Constitutional Court requesting the provision be re-established, but as of August 2007 no decision had yet been handed down, and there were already strong signs that the judges were sharply divided.[50] Two months later the full penal code reform was completed and while the sodomy law has been abolished, the 2006 elimination of the therapeutic abortion clause was retained.[51]

In the case of Poland, Nowicka (2007) recalls that the first attack on abortion rights occurred in 1988, even before the 'fall of the walls' – the end of the Cold War and the breakup of the Soviet Union. This early push would be followed by 11 further attempts between 1989 and 1991. Then, in 1993, a new law was passed that eliminated access to abortion on 'social grounds', restricting the access to legal abortions to those women who could pay for the procedure, and leaving poorer women limited to the choice of unsafe procedures.[52] In 1993, just 200 procedures were performed in public hospitals. Nowicka identifies the conditions then prevailing in the political environment as one main factor behind this backlash: 'Many members of the anti-communist opposition became actively involved in the anti-abortion campaign, which was strongly supported by the Roman Catholic Church hierarchy and had the personal backing of Pope John Paul II' (Nowicka 2007, p. 170). However, in 1996, Parliament approved another bill that reinstated the 'social ground' provision, but then President Lech Walesa vetoed it. Although a case was presented to the Constitutional Court to undo this veto, in 1997 the judges confirmed the President's position. A new wave of activism occurred in 2003, when a left-wing coalition gained the majority in Parliament. During the electoral campaign the coalition had promised to re-table a liberalizing provision, but after the victory its leaders retreated, claiming that the legislative reforms required for Poland to gain access to the European Union must take priority.

Nowicka (2007) identifies multiple obstacles faced by abortion rights activists in Poland. She reminds us that abortion was legalized under communism without a struggle: abortion was never a right for which women themselves fought. Since gender equality was guaranteed by the communist regime, a climate was created in which, apparently, there was no need for a women's movement. Polish culture considers the family and the community to be more important than the individual, and celebrates women as self-sacrificing 'mothers of the nation'. Since the late 1980s, the adversaries of abortion have systematically used the argument that abortion is one of the evil remnants of communism. The period during which the Law and Justice Party governed Poland has created even greater barriers to making abortion accessible once again in Poland. It has also led Polish officials to systematically raise extremely conservative positions with respect to other critical areas of the human rights agenda, such as health and the death penalty.[53]

Even so, civil society organizations have systematically raised their voices against the threats and reversals pushed by conservative forces both within the country and in key international arenas. One successful effort is the case of Alicja Tysiac, who was refused access to abortion under the existing Polish law. Tysiac's case was presented to the European Court of Human Rights, which, in March 2007, handed down a decision recognizing that her rights had been infringed by the Polish state under the privacy clause contained in the European Convention on Human Rights. Although the Polish government appealed against the decision its arguments were rejected and, in October 2007, the Court upheld its previous decision and ordered the Polish government to compensate Ms Tysiac for the failure to protect her rights. Moreover, during the 2007 electoral campaign the newly created Women's Party gained global visibility with its billboard portraying seven naked women behind the slogan, 'The party of women. Poland is woman'. Significantly, the party's leader, Manuela Gretkowska, declared that she had decided to create the party when the government announced that it would further restrain access to abortion.[54]

Chapter 3

The sad 'return of the religious'[1]

Discourses and actions deployed by dogmatic religious voices and groups are a major influence in determining the contours of sexual politics in the early 2000s. The need to better understand the origins, resources, scope, and direction of the religious turn in contemporary politics is important. As we argued in the Introduction, terminology such as the 'growth of fundamentalism', the most widely used descriptor of the phenomenon, is both problematic and ahistorical, and its widespread usage requires deconstruction. It is also important to situate religious extremism, which many authors in the USA particularly define in terms of 'the religious right', in relation to, and separate from, religiosity and spirituality at large, and to examine more closely how these forces intersect with political, cultural, and economic influences. Finally, since many voices are trying to reactivate secularity and *laicité*[2] as a response to the policy inroads of religious conservatism, our discussion must also revisit the trajectory of secularization as well as its potentialities and limits.

'Fundamentalism': a misnomer?

The origins and evolution of the term 'fundamentalism' are intrinsic to the sequential waves of evangelical revivals in the USA beginning in the early days of independence (Armstrong 2000, Imam 2000). The leaders of the so-called 'Second Awakening' of the late eighteenth and early nineteenth centuries called for a return to the Bible to contest the growing influence of deism that promoted 'atheism and materialism'. Drawing their adherents mainly from the poorer and less educated sectors, these early reformers believed Enlightenment values revered 'Nature and Reason instead of Jesus Christ' (Armstrong 2000, p. 107).[3] In the second half of the nineteenth century, another wave of Protestant revivalism gained followers among the middle and upper classes. Some of its factions expressed liberal views on individual rights, equality, and women's status and engaged in the anti-slavery struggles, but others became increasingly attached to the truth of the scriptures and were vocal and virulent, particularly following the publication of Darwin's (1859) *The Origin of Species*. Their reaction was directed less towards Darwin's theories than towards the writings of British Anglican thinkers gathered around the journal *Essay and Review* who welcomed Darwin's work and explored new approaches to biblical reading – the so-called 'superior critique', which would rapidly influence liberal religious circles in the USA. In their view, the miracles reported in the scriptures should be interpreted as literary allegories and the same rational rigour applied to the critique of other texts extended to the Bible (Armstrong 2000, p. 116).

The destruction resulting from the American Civil War (1861–1865) was frequently interpreted by dogmatic preachers such as John Darby as a biblical sign of the approaching final war between God and Satan. Consequently, between the 1870s and early 1890s a series of religious conflicts ensued that led to accusations of heresy and expulsions within Protestant denominations.[4] These coincided with sex-related moral panics leading to the approval of the Comstock Act (1873), which criminalized the mailing of 'obscene, lewd, and/or lascivious' materials, including contraceptive devices and information. The law was named after the anti-obscenity crusader Anthony Comstock, founder of the New York Society for the Suppression of Vice, and was used to prosecute a number of feminist pioneers and progressive religious thinkers, among them the birth control pioneer Margaret Sanger.[5]

By the early 1900s, conservative religious groups in the USA were advancing their Manichean vision by establishing Bible colleges and schools across the country, developing dogmas to guide Christian communities, and publishing pamphlets to persuade the general public that salvation required a return to the original truth of the scriptures. By 1910 the very notion of Bible fundamentalism – meaning the return to the foundational sacred text – was well established. Less than a decade later these groups would depict the First World War and the 1917 Russian Revolution as signs of the apocalypse announced by late nineteenth-century preachers and would interpret the creation of the League of Nations as a symptom of the pagan Roman Empire being revived (Armstrong 2000).[6] By the late 1920s Bible fundamentalism had expanded its ranks and achieved influence over public policies – for instance, a number of states banned the teaching of evolutionary theory in public schools and introduced, instead, the teaching of creationism, creating a controversy that still festers today. These restrictive laws triggered the 1925 Dayton case in Tennessee, when the teacher John Scopes was prosecuted for teaching evolutionary theory.[7]

Armstrong (2000) points out that North American religious upheavals of the late nineteenth and early twentieth centuries differed from those of the past in that they were neither territorially bound nor confined to groups outside mainstream religion and politics. These new groups broke through their original boundaries, challenged the secular establishment, and organized to influence or even seize state power. As observed by the international network, Women Living Under Muslim Law (WLUML 1997), this systematic striving for political power remains a feature of contemporary manifestations of religious dogmatism, albeit with sharp distinctions.[8] Most notably, while in the US the movements of the nineteenth and early twentieth centuries sprang exclusively from evangelical circles, the 1979 reactivation was a political initiative crafted by a small group of Republican operatives with extremely conservative positions, not only on 'moral matters' but also on national security and defence and state intervention in the economy. Their strategy to gain power included the mobilization of Christian conservative sectors, and Jerry Falwell, the evangelical pastor and co-founder of the Moral Majority, was an ideal ally to achieve this objective.[9] The Moral Majority's self-defined mission was to counter the liberalism and secularism of US society in the 1960s and 1970s. It recruited supporters among Pentecostals and dissident members of traditionally liberal Protestant denominations as well as conservative Catholics, including members of the Church hierarchy.

When today's North American Christian Right is compared to other manifestations of religious dogmatism, the distinctions are even more pronounced. Catholicism may also be portrayed as a 'religion of the book' and therefore the scriptures may be used to mobilize conservative public positions on a wide range of issues, including gender and sexuality. For instance, the condemnation of sodomy found in Leviticus, through the writings of the Jewish theologian Philo (AD 30–40), penetrated early Church doctrines before reaching Roman legal frames to become 'the model for laws decreeing capital punishment for homosexuality in Europe and in as much of the world that came under Europe's sway down to the end of the eighteenth century' (Crompton 2003, p. 34).

Dogmatic Catholic views on sexuality and gender often converge, therefore, with those propagated by other Christian voices. However, the centralized institutional nature of Catholicism, its deeply grounded tradition of incorporating and Christianizing other philosophical and religious streams, its ability to adjust to temporal changes, and, most principally, to persecute, prosecute, and eliminate dissent, create a distinctive environment in the emergence and evolution of dogmatic doctrinaire currents. These revivals of tradition are best characterized as slow, virulent, and painful internal Church struggles. The most recent started in 1980, when conservative sectors demolished the new doctrinal edifice created by Pope John XXIII after the 1962 Vatican II Council, through intricate political manoeuvres and the prosecution and exclusion of dissident voices.[10] As always when reactionary shifts occur, the so-called guardians of the doctrine installed in the Vatican stronghold are responsible for interpretation. Catholic dogmatic revivals are never a simplistic 'return' to the literal reading of the Old or New Testaments, but a new stage in the theological reinvention of tradition. For example, contemporary Vatican doctrines on homosexuality are more complex than the definitions found in Leviticus in that they interweave Old Testament references with more sophisticated religious and philosophical arguments that directly or indirectly respond to contemporary feminist, lesbian, gay, and transgender positions. Thus, we must always understand waves of religious extremism in dialectical relation to the social movements that provoke them.

Differences may also be observed in how the Catholic Church asserts political power. Dogmatic Catholic forces often operate outside the structures of power from which they have been excluded. In Mexico, for example, the ruling Partido de Acción Nacional (PAN) originated in the 1920s' Catholic rebellions – the so-called *Cristeros* – against the anti-clerical measures adopted by the leaders of the 1910 Revolution (Ortiz-Ortega 2005), and the Polish Catholic conservative revival of the past 20 years is a reaction to the period of communist compulsory secularity (see Chapter 2). But elsewhere, what stands out is the remarkable ability of the Catholic Church to operate strategically from both within and outside state systems, a political expertise acquired in the course of almost two millennia during which the powers of the Church and the state were conflated in Western politics. Until recently, this fusion remained palpable in a few European countries (e.g., Ireland, Portugal, and Spain) and across Latin America, even though rules of separation between state and Church were widely established by the late nineteenth century. In most Latin American countries, the Church hierarchy has direct access to the highest policy-making levels, and representatives of dogmatic Catholic currents are easily installed in, or elected to, high-level policy-making positions. When greater force is needed to influence policy definitions, the extraordinary mobilizing machinery of Catholic institutions can be activated to organize popular petitions and demonstrations.[11]

As noted above, feminist activists and researchers, devoted to analysing and resisting the arguments and actions of the Muslim Right, were the first to raise concerns about the indiscriminate use of the term 'fundamentalism'. They recognized that Islamic and Christian fundamentalists shared certain commonalities: the striving for political power; the calls for a return to the fundamentals of faith and tradition corrupted by modern excess; and the open attacks on any assertion of female or sexual autonomy. However, because the term originated in the West, Muslim feminists are reluctant to apply it to the Islamic world. They also contest the mainstream media's deliberate and systematic conflation of 'Islam' and 'fundamentalism', which constitutes a main source of stigmatization of Muslims, women and men, who do not share or support extremist views (Sow *et al.* 2007).

Muslim feminists maintain that 'Islam' (a religion) and 'Muslim' (a culture) must be distinguished to deconstruct this Western essentialist vision and illuminate variations in rules and practices, like the much debated custom of veiling (Imam 2000), or the tremendous differences among diverse Islamic sects and Muslim histories and geographies (Armstrong 2000). Although the religious and ethical principles of Islam are enshrined in a sacred text that cannot be contested, 14 centuries of Islamic history have meant deep transformation and, because of that, the *ulemas* (Muslim theologians) can resort to other sources to interpret the law according to the conditions of the time. In practice, Islamic rules have been reconstructed and adapted to the multiple conditions in which Muslim communities live: 'Once the five pillars – creed (*shahada*), prayer, fast, alms, and pilgrimage to Mecca – of Islam are fulfilled, a number of rituals and practices may change, according to culture' (Sow *et al.* 2007, p. 1). Imam (2005) concurs, listing the multiple sources of interpretation: the Qu'ran; the *sunnha* (traditions of the prophet) recounted in the *hadith*; the *ijma*, a consensus about what the law is, which is attained through *qiyas* (analogy); and *ijtihad* (interpretive reasoning). She also reminds us that among Sunni – who constitute 80 per cent of all Muslims – there are four schools of jurisprudence that disagree about many issues, including questions relating to gender and sexuality. Finally, she refers to the ever-evolving disputes regarding the authenticity of sources, the reliability of procedures, and, most principally, 'whose consensus is to be accepted: should it be the *ulema*'s ruling? Or, should it be the communities' consensus, which women are also part of?' (p. 76). Her conclusion is that:

> the stereotype of a single, unified, divinely revealed 'Islamic law' is false, whether in terms of historical and empirical accuracy or as jurisprudential principle. However this principle has been useful to Muslim conservatives and the religious right as well as to Islamophobes in the West.
>
> (Imam 2005, p. 76)

The widespread assumption equating Muslim political culture with theocracy must be critically revisited as well. Western ideas of secularity spread across the Islamic world from the early nineteenth century, often, as in the case of Egypt, through force of arms, but also through measures adopted by Muslim rulers and political leaders (Armstrong 2000, Ilkkaracan 2007). Although these secularizing waves provoked sharp religious reactions, they also inspired educational reforms such as the creation of schools for girls and the establishment of secular political parties (Delaney 1995, Ghosh 2002, Ilkkaracan 2007).[12] Secularization expanded further in the twentieth century, initially through the indirect rule established by European colonizers and later, in the final phase of decolonization (1950–1970), general principles of secularity were adopted in a range of Islamic countries including Algeria, Egypt, Indonesia, Iran, Iraq, Jordan, Libya, Pakistan, Senegal, Syria, and Tunisia. In fact, the contemporary surge of Islamic religious and political forces is largely a response to the secularization promoted by authoritarian and corrupt regimes, which was almost immediately contested by religious forces, in particular Shia groupings, most famously in Iran (Armstrong 2000, Bahgat and Afifi 2007, Sow *et al.* 2007).

Secularization has been partial and contradictory in the Islamic world because the legal weight of Sharia remained largely uncontested, especially with respect to personal codes, family law, and norms regarding sexuality. Most Muslim countries did not modify significantly the colonizers' model, leaving arbitration of a wide range of matters to pre-existing Islamic courts. Even in Senegal – which, in the 1970s, became the first Muslim country to initiate a secular reform of the family code – the new family law retained polygamy and gender inequality in inheritance. Such patchwork juridical frames facilitate the religious Right in pushing for the reintroduction of Sharia norms. In settings where Islamic law coexists and conflicts with secular constitutional principles, the discrepancies between the two 'systems' create complex juridical conflicts (Imam 2005, Nussbaum 1999). Given that repressive laws on gender and 'sex' are embedded in existing legal systems, the Islamic Right – differently from the Christian Right – does not exclusively target the state. As described by Sow *et al.*, these forces are strongly engaged in ongoing surveillance of people and the enforcement of modest dress and comportment:

> It is thus the obligation for women to wear the veil or longer skirts in public spaces, the obligation for individuals to fast or not to eat in public at the time of Ramadan, to pray in an ostentatious manner in public. Refusal to keep to these codes of conduct can be the source of conflict, indeed of violence. One remembers the lynching, indeed assassination, by Islamic groups in Algeria, of women who refused to wear the veil, who are single, live alone or seem to be 'too free' [and] of journalists and intellectuals judged to be too liberal.
>
> (Sow *et al.* 2007, p. 6)

The inception and evolution of Hindu extremism is even more persuasive in terms of revealing the caveats of 'fundamentalism'. Unlike Christianity and Islam, Hinduism is a polytheistic religion with no single authoritative text; alongside the Vedas, the many sacred texts are constantly reinterpreted by diverse streams of thought, mysticism, and asceticism. The notion of prophets or prophecies, so central to Christian fundamentalism, is also alien to Hindu tradition. As emphasized in Sow *et al.* (2007, p. 8),

> Hinduism is a very dynamic and fluid religion open to a personal interpretation by the individual practicing Hindu within the para-

meters of core values like tolerance, love and compassion, and a strong ethic of what is right and what is wrong broadly termed as '*dharma*'.

In this context it is important to recall that Indian history and culture comprise a complex mosaic of ethnicities, languages, cultures, and faiths that conflict, but have also coexisted peacefully, at different historical junctures. Hinduism is also a religious or spiritual justification for the caste system, which rigidly stratifies its followers by birth, allows no space for social mobility, and is structured according to strict rules of endogamy.

Hindu revivalism began in the late nineteenth century alongside the struggle for India's independence. While the Congress Party, created in 1885, was civic oriented and gradually built a broad political base, including Muslims, Sikhs, Christians, Jains, and varied castes, the ideology of Hindu nationalism was crafted by members of the Brahmin and other high castes to conserve Hindu values and the hierarchical social order, and to develop the latent power of the Hindu community around modern ideas of industrialization, state restructuring, and corporatism. This combination of tendencies, as mentioned in Chapter 2, became known as *Hindutva* or 'Hindu-ness' (Swamy 2003). By the mid-1920s voluntary male organizations known as Rashtriya Swayamsevak Sangh (RSS), combining family language (*sangh parivar*) and a militia (*shakha* or cell), were created. Their leaders, though inspired by Fascist ideologies, did not construe the notion of Hindu purity on race-based rationales alone, but developed a sophisticated narrative that fused race and culture and drew on religious symbols (Taminnen 1996).[13] In the analysis developed by Sabrang and the South Asia Citizens Web, this formula 'avoids race while introducing a notion of purity through the back door':

> By defining belonging through a territorially contained notion of culture, it becomes possible to denote some minorities as within the ambit of 'the Hindu' and others as outside it. A large number of minorities – Sikhs, Buddhists, and Jains, for instance – are objects of integration. So, also, Dalits and *Adivasis* (tribal communities that do not share Hindu traditions) though historically oppressed by upper-caste Hindus are, in this definition, not excluded from the nation. The idea here is to redefine these minorities as 'Hindu' – where a certain specific upper-caste Hinduism (Sanatan Dharma) is the hegemonic pure form and all others are at varying distance from this purity. In contrast, Muslims, Christians, Parsis, and Jews, are clearly defined as outside the fold of the Nation, not because they have not been part of India for centuries but because their cultural signifiers are seen as lying external to the territorial nation.
>
> (Sabrang and the South Asian Citizens Web 2003, pp. 26–27)

Hindu revivalism became more conspicuous in the political reconfiguration of modern independent India after an ex-member of the RSS assassinated Mahatma Gandhi in 1948. As a result, RSS and other Hindu unity organizations were outlawed and remained in the shadows until the mid-1980s, when they regained strength as a Hindu nationalist response to regional autonomist movements in the northeast, Punjab, Tamil, and Kashmir. Note, too, the murders of Indira Gandhi (in 1984) and her son and successor Rajiv (in 1991) in episodes related to regional upheavals, and that caste-related tensions erupted in various places in the same period (Chakravati 2000). Today *Hindutva* is more diversified, encompassing the traditional RSS network as well as Vishwa Hindu Parishad (VHP), Bajrang Dal (BD), Shiv Sena and other similar organizations that include women's wings, and the Barathya Janata Party (BJP), which formed a coalition government with 23 other political parties between 1998 and 2004. Organizations outside India that are funded by Hindu expatriates must also be included because, as we show later in this chapter, they played a key role in the 2002 Gujarat genocide, the most recent and tragic communalist strife registered in India.

Hindutva's main discursive strategy to generate 'unity' reinvents Hindu history to circumvent cultural and religious plurality and the tensions deriving from the rigid caste system.[14] Although religion may be portrayed as a secondary element in the *Hindutva* ideological frame, it is ubiquitous in the discourse and actions deployed by member organizations; gods, goddesses, temples, and other 'religious' or spiritual expressions are instrumental means to achieve political ends. For instance, in the past few decades persistent communal strife has occurred in Ayodhya (Uttar Pradesh) concerning the remnants of a temple dedicated to the hero god Rāma over which, it is said, Barbur, the first Mughal emperor, built a mosque. In 1988, the BJP launched a popular movement to demand that the temple be reconstructed, and although it retreated from the initiative soon after, the Mosque was destroyed by a mob in 1992.[15]

In recent years, *Hindutva* leaders have introduced Hindu divinity images and prayers in public schools. Most importantly, the majority of *Hindutva* discourse uses the spiritual notion of *dharma* to maintain rigid caste hierarchies and gender and 'sex' boundaries, reviving the socially grounded idea that if one does not respect caste duties he/she is acting against the natural order. The notion of purity is another key pivot sustaining the caste system through the rigid rules of caste endogamy, spatial segregation, and stigmatizing corporeal rules, like those assigning to Dalits the most abject activities, such as scavenging. These rules determine, among other things, the distribution of basic economic resources, such as water, schools, and clinics. Thus various authors who have analysed Hindu revivalism conclude that it cannot be qualified as either religious dogmatism or fundamentalism but should be portrayed as a fascist-inspired 're-creation of the religious' (Sow *et al.* 2007).

The trajectories described above compel us to maintain a critical distance from simplified arguments seeking to conflate 'fundamentalism' and 'Otherness', and not to lose sight of the West itself as a territory also plagued by past and present manifestations of religious extremism. They also constitute a strong warning against indiscriminate and inaccurate uses of the term 'fundamentalism' – even as we identify commonalities among regressive 'returns of the religious' with their thirst for political power and obsession with 'sex' and gender. Armstrong (2000) reminds us of the other trait shared by religious extremists past and present: they have thrived on the basis of 'the corruption' of doctrines, institutions, and practices they hold dear, whether through aligning themselves with science and technology, absorbing Western secular ideas, or making alliances with secularists to struggle against the colonizers. While re-creating golden ages and reviving old imageries, traditions, and legal prescriptions, religious and cultural revivalist forces in the twenty-first century make use of the same political language and political instruments utilized by the corrupt leaders and institutions they publicly scorn, including electoral politics and effective and extensive use of communication technologies. In Derrida's (1998, p. 24) words:

> Like others before, the new 'wars of religion' are unleashed over the human earth (which is not the world) and struggle even today to control the sky *with finger and eye*: digital systems and virtually immediate panoptical visualization; 'air space', telecommunications satellites, information highways, concentration of capitalistic-mediatic power – in three words, *digital culture, jet*, and *TV* without which there could be no religious manifestation today, for example, no voyage or discourse of the Pope, no organized emanation of Jewish, Christian or Muslim cults, whether 'fundamentalist' or not.

'Sex' and 'religion' on the front lines

Having presented this overarching frame, we now examine three sites where sexuality is caught in the spirals of the sad 'return of the religious': the Vatican discursive deployments on 'sex', the reintroduction of Sharia law in Nigeria, and the Gujarat genocide of 2002 – three distinctive landscapes that illuminate the intricate ways in which culture, politics, and economics traverse current 'sex wars'.

Vatican 'prosopopeia'

Vatican doctrine on sexuality strongly influences the current politics of sex and, as noted by Derrida (1998), is now 'cyberspacialized'.[16] The subordinate placement of women and the suspicion of sexuality are deeply rooted in Christianity, appearing in the New Testament's split between flesh and spirit, and becoming more pronounced in the consolidation of Christian definitions with both Jewish conceptions and Platonic ideas (Jantzen 1995, 2000). The resulting sexual morality confined sex within the boundaries of marriage and reproduction, grounded Catholic ideology on femininity and motherhood, and, simultaneously, implied the radical condemnation of non-conjugal, non-procreative expressions of desire and eroticism. Augustine, whose writings are a key source of Christian theological teaching, even argued that if Adam and Eve had not sinned, procreation would take place without desire or bodily exchanges.[17]

Since these early times, Catholicism has perennially revived suspicion of the flesh, and on numerous occasions made 'sex' a primary target – for example, during the Inquisition, particularly in Spain, Portugal, and Latin America (Crompton 2003).[18] Over the past three decades, as sexual politics matured, Catholic theological positions have become more dogmatic with respect to women's role, contraception, abortion, condoms, family, youth, and homosexuality. More recently, under the combined impact of HIV and AIDS, LGBTQ rights claims, and internal paedophilia scandals, the Vatican has intensified its doctrinal propaganda regarding homosexuality, as illustrated by a series of sequential papers published between 2000 and 2004. After Cardinal Ratzinger was installed as Pope Benedict XVI in 2005, two other substantial documents, directly or indirectly related to homosexuality, were published – 'Instruction Concerning the Criteria for the Discernment of Vocations with regard to Persons with Homosexual Tendencies in view of their Admission to the Seminary and to Holy Orders' (Vatican 2005a) and an encyclical letter, 'Deus Caritas Est' (the first edict of Benedict XVI) (Vatican 2005b). In May 2006, the Pope condemned same-sex marriage using arguments based on these documents (Vatican 2006). One main theme is that heterosexuality is natural, blessed, and transcendental in contrast with homosexuality, as defined by the 'Catechism of the Catholic Church':

> Basing itself on Sacred Scripture, which presents homosexual acts as acts of grave depravity, tradition has always declared that 'homosexual acts are intrinsically disordered'. They are contrary to the natural law. They close the sexual act to the gift of life. They do not proceed from a genuine affective and sexual complementarity. Under no circumstances can they be approved.
>
> (Vatican 2004, ch. 2, para. 2357)

The same approach is adopted in the 'Instruction' (Vatican 2005a), which prohibits those who practise homosexuality, present homosexual tendencies, or support 'gay culture' from admission to seminaries and holy orders. However, these negative positions coexist with language calling for respect and non-discrimination for these same persons, in a bid to recapture the Christian morality of love for the 'Other'. More crucially, the Vatican doctrine, as deployed today, recognizes same-sex desire as a possibility in the human experience even as it radically condemns same-sex acts. Carrara points out the paradox of this moral formulation:

> Homosexuality is not condemned by Catholicism provided it remains as desire, provided it is not put into practice. This is a strange position if one takes into account the very tradition of Catholicism, which does not restrict sins to acts, but also includes certain thoughts and desires. Desire defines homosexuality, but in the Church's view if you do not practice it, although you continue desiring, you are not sinning, because desire is not a sin because it belongs to the realm of nature.
>
> (quoted in Castilhos 2007, p. 1)

In 'Deus Caritas Est', the term 'homosexuality' is never used, but the subject lurks beneath the sophistication and seduction of the argumentation. The encyclical letter revisits the scriptures, Plato, Aristotle, Aquinas, and even Nietzsche to address the multiple and elusive Western conceptions of love (*Eros*), friendship (*Philia*), and charity (*Caritas*), and develops a complex reasoning on the meanings of justice. The text first distances itself from a world where the name of God is associated with vengeance, then briefly examines post-Enlightenment contestations of the Church position, before shifting to a convoluted exercise aimed at responding to the question: 'Did Christianity really destroy *Eros*?' In response, the text reaffirms that the love between men and women in marriage, and leading to procreation, is natural and fulfils divine purposes, while other manifestations of *Eros* are associated with hubris, self-denigration, objectification, and 'prostitution'. Not surprisingly one of its main conclusions is that *Eros* needs to be disciplined and purified if it is to provide more than fleeting pleasure.[19]

The paradoxes of 'Deus Caritas Est' are not as evident as those identified in other Vatican papers deploying 'sex' doctrines, but they are present none the less. Would the Vatican engage in such an impressive intellectual exercise if the Church doctrine on love, particularly erotic love, were fully safeguarded against deep social transformations in the realm of sexuality today and ample evidence of sexual diversity in the past?[20] In May 2006, when the Pope railed against 'confusing marriage with other types of unions based on a love that is weak' (Bloomberg 2006, p. 1), the true impetus behind the Vatican's renewed deployment of discourses on meanings of love became transparent. The Italian philosopher Gianni Vattimo responded to this declaration in a statement that further illuminates the paradoxes of 'Deus Caritas Est':

The homosexual question that the Pope himself insists on locating at the core of his preaching has a more essential meaning. Not by chance it implies the discussion of all the sexist and sex-phobic politics that have dominated the Church, especially in modernity. Originally sexism and sex-phobia are not Christian traces but have been entrenched in Christianity as the gift of Constantine.

(Vattimo 2006, p. 1)

Vattimo recalls that the image of 'human reproduction imitating heaven on earth' appearing both in the encyclical letter and the declaration cannot be traced back to the Christian tradition but comes directly from Aristotle. He argues that if the Vatican had instead searched and valued its own 'traditions', as found in the experiences of the first Christians, the results would be radically different. These early communities were egalitarian and mainly formed by women, children, slaves, and foreigners, depicted as inferiors by Greek and Roman thinkers. Had the Pope pulled that lost thread he might have been driven to appreciate families that are not 'natural', and to contest the 'natural' hierarchical placement of persons in social hierarchies. He also suggests that illuminating the contradictions of the doctrine is necessary but not sufficient; it is also important to locate the discourses of the Pope and the Church in relation to their stated positions in world affairs.

The Pope's own words and actions often contradict the goodwill manifested in recent theological discourses about love. At the University of Regensberg, Benedict XVI quoted a fourteenth-century Christian emperor who said that Muhammad had brought the world only 'evil and inhuman' things, thereby raising fury across the Islamic world (September 2006); while visiting Brazil in 2007 he affirmed that Christianity had not alienated indigenous people in the Americas, which triggered strong reactions across the region (May 2006); and he was photographed with a Polish priest widely known for his view that Auschwitz was not an extermination site but a labour camp (August 2007) (BBC World 2006, Gaspari 2007).

A less well-known gaffe, directly related to sexuality, occurred during the Vatican's Holy Friday celebrations in 2007, when violence against women was depicted as a renewal of Christ's suffering. While this was aimed at demonstrating the Church's concern with gender-based violence, the meditations on the subject, prepared by Monsignor Gianfranco Ravasi, refer to female genital mutilation in old Christian ethnocentric terms: 'all those women who have been abused and raped, ostracized, and submitted to shameful tribal practices' (Vatican 2006, p. 1). Finally, in April 2007, when abortion was legalized in the Federal District of Mexico, the Church threatened parliamentarians with excommunication. Similarly, before and during the Pope's visit to Brazil, Church authorities equated women who seek abortions with terrorists. These strikingly ethnocentric and quasi-inquisitorial pronouncements openly contradict the religious doctrine of enlarged reason and love for the 'Other'.

Northern Nigeria: Sharia front lines

Mernissi (2000) reminds us that, unlike Christianity, Islam views sexual instinct as a gift of God's wisdom, which is not good or bad per se; if unregulated it may lead to destructive acts, but if 'used according to God's will, the desire of the flesh enhances life on earth and in heaven' (p. 20). While Islamic conceptions of 'sex' coincides with Christian doctrine in naturalizing sexual drives, directing them towards marriage and repro-duction,[21] and condemning masturbation and homosexuality, Islam does not deny women's sexuality but rather portrays it as more powerful and dangerous than men's (Accad 2000, Ilkkaracan 2000, Imam 2000, Ilkkaracan and Seral 2000, Mernissi 2000). Moreover, as Imam (2000) emphasizes, practices relating to women's sexuality vary widely across the Islamic world. While honour crimes are pervasive in the Mediterranean region, including Christian Greece, Arabia, and South Asia, they are vir-tually unknown in sub-Saharan Africa and South-East Asia. Female genital mutilation, or clitoris amputation, is practically the norm in coun-tries such as Egypt, Sudan, the Gambia, Mali, Eritrea, and Somalia, but is not practised in other Muslim countries. In contrast, the practice is quite extensive in some non-Muslim cultures, including Christian Ethiopia and a range of communities in Nigeria, Sierra Leone, and Kenya. Ilkkaracan's (2000) research on female sexual norms in Turkey has also revealed that such practices as bride price, honour killings, polygyny, forced or arranged marriages, marital rapes, abortion, and extramarital relations vary widely depending on cultural and religious traditions prevailing at local levels.

Against this backdrop of diversity in religious norms and practices regarding sexuality, we now examine the reinstatement of Sharia law in 12 northern Nigerian states in the late 1990s and early 2000s, when five women were prosecuted for the 'crime' of *Zina* (the broad category used to address all 'unnatural' sex acts; in these cases, adultery) and condemned to death by stoning. All cases were the focus of strong opposition by Nigerian women's rights and human rights organizations.[22] Those of Safiya Tungar-Tudu and Amina Lawal, who were both accused of adul-tery, achieved global visibility because international human rights net-works, in particular Amnesty International, mobilized Internet campaigns and media exposure.[23] Imam's analysis (2005) links the reintroduction of Sharia in northern Nigeria to similar developments in Iran, Libya, Pak-istan, and Sudan. She traces the trend to its roots in British colonial prac-tices that systematically manipulated ethnic and religious identity politics to control the territories. Colonial administrators left behind a political modality that local leaders seized upon to mobilize state resources for specific communities, to the exclusion of others.

Imam (2005) also examines how contemporary religious extremism in northern states of Nigeria, as elsewhere, is a by-product of World Bank structural adjustment programmes. By demanding debt repayment and shrinking social budgets, these programmes left state machineries incapable of responding to basic social needs. Sharia was not reintroduced because of pressure from Islamic activists; it was the initiative of discredited and corrupt politicians (governors) who, seeking greater popularity without the necessary financial resources, decided to exploit an issue with great emotional and political appeal. As Imam observes, the use of Sharia for political objectives worked because 'traditional' prescriptions often resonate with poor people, who experience religion as a protection against distress. Moreover, given the prevailing insecurity, many sectors expected the adoption and enforcement of Islamic criminal laws to end corruption and speed up judicial processes in which individuals were often held in endless pre-trial detention. Here we might usefully apply Rubin's (1984) insight that in times of social crisis and uncertainty 'sex' becomes an easy target.

The local 'populist' strategies and resurgent Islamist identity politics Imam describes occurred in a context of growing Islamophobia worldwide and the 1999 electoral victory of Olusegun Obasanjo, a born-again Christian, which the mainstream media depicted as a sign of a religious war between Muslims and Christians. In the same period, Nigerian Protestants and evangelicals were becoming more vocal in promoting conservative positions on sexuality. However, as Imam emphasizes, even as religious conservatism gained strength nationally, and amid widespread support for Sharia in northern states, many Muslims aligned themselves with the protests as members and supporters of women's and human rights organizations working on Sharia cases.

Another key dimension of northern Nigeria's political and policy environment concerns the intricacy of the juridical system. The national constitution is secular. It stipulates that all death penalty cases are eligible for review by the Supreme Court, and that appeals from state-level Sharia courts must be heard by a panel of at least three federal judges versed in Islamic law. But these provisions refer strictly to civil procedures, and it is not clear if they cover criminal laws recently created by state legislatures. Imam points out that in the *Zina* cases women's rights activists and their allies opted to defend the accused under new Sharia criminal codes, in Sharia courts, instead of at the higher juridical levels. This choice was partly to protect the accused and delay the executions, but also to avoid alienating the majority of the Islamic community, who support Islamic criminal laws. This strategic decision also created an opportunity for women's rights advocates to expose the biases and deficiencies of Islamic courts with respect to women's rights. By promoting alternative views on Islamic law, the advocates aimed to erode the monopoly claimed by the religious Right and other conservative voices.

> To respect the beliefs, tenets, and practices of both local cultures and international human rights agreements requires a double 'claim and critique' strategy. This consists of claiming ownership of both local cultures and international human rights discourses (including the right to participate in the defining content of each), while privileging neither local nor international as automatically superior, and thus being able to criticize both.[24]
>
> (Imam 2005, p. 66)

Gujarat: 'othering', 'sex', and the desecration of bodies

The 2002 Gujarat genocide was triggered by the burning of a train coach, which was immediately and publicly interpreted by the BJP governor as an attack by Islamic terrorists funded by Pakistan (U.S. Congress 2002). A wide range of observers described the Hindu retaliation that ensued as a meticulously planned pogrom against members of the Muslim community:

> Between February 28 and March 2, thousands of attackers descended on Muslim neighbourhoods clad in saffron scarves and khaki shorts, the signature uniform of Hindu nationalist groups, and armed with swords, sophisticated explosives, and gas cylinders. They were guided by voter lists and printouts of addresses of Muslim-owned properties – information obtained from the local municipality.... The groups most directly involved in the violence against Muslims include the Vishwa Hindu Parishad (World Hindu Council, VHP), the Bajrang Dal, the Rashtriya Swayamsevak Sangh and the Bharatiya Janata Party (BJP) that heads the Gujarat State Government.
>
> (HRW 2002, p. 1)

Communal strife had been escalating in Gujarat since 1998 when the BJP gained political control of the state. The following year the Human Rights Watch annual report highlighted violence perpetrated against Christians and tribal groups, and noted a deliberate strategy by *Hindutva* groups to take control of the state machinery and communities (HRW 1999). Most analysts agree that the Gujarat genocide was unusual in its novel configuration of actors and its orchestrated brutality. Over three days, some 2000 Muslims were killed and another 150,000 evicted from their homes and thrown into refugee camps (Citizen's Initiative 2002, IIJG 2003, NHRC 2002, Sow *et al.* 2007). Indian and international women's rights and human rights organizations responded quickly, going to Gujarat, identifying the individuals responsible, providing support to victims, and pushing for action by national and international human rights bodies. As a result, the US Congress's Commission on International Freedom of Religion held a hearing in June 2002 (U.S. Congress 2002). Civil society groups and independent experts identified links, including the transfer of resources, between *Hindutva* groups in Gujarat and the expatriate Hindu community in the USA and elsewhere (Sabrang and South Asia Citizens Web 2003).

Any portrayal of the Gujarat genocide as a faraway communal strife spurred by backward uneducated community groups is not merely a simplification but a blatant distortion of the international implications of the atrocity.[25] Mukherjee lists other significant aspects of the episode:

> What makes Gujarat unique ... is the open and active collusion of the state and its institutions and its machinery, including the police. The BJP and its allies were in power in the state during that time. A second unique feature was the mobilization by Sangh Parivar civil society organizations of women, the Adivasis, and the Dalits, who provided support for the horrific violence perpetrated on the Muslims. Thirdly, from being an urban phenomenon, riots spread to villages in the rural areas. Fourthly, violence was perpetrated in the most cold, calculated, and systematic way on the Muslims with the aid of technology like cell-phones and computer printouts.... The marauding mobs wreaking violence were not *lumpens* or hired criminals. They were ordinary men and women from everyday life – men who could torture, rape, rip pregnant women apart, dismember foetuses and then burn them while women openly acquiesced and found nothing wrong in these macabre acts of perverse sexual violence.
>
> (in Sow *et al.* 2007, p. 14)

To understand the gender and sexuality dimensions that erupted in Gujarat requires a closer examination of *Hindutva* discourses, which have persistently promoted the image of the Muslim 'Other'. From its inception, *Hindutva* ideology has defined Muslims not as infidels or aliens, but as invaders (Swamy 2003); 'virile' Muslim men who raped and molested Hindu women. After independence and particularly in the context of the post-1980s *Hindutva*, the invader image was contradictorily interwoven with the systematic depreciation of Muslims as backward, illiterate, procreating an excessive number of children, depleting resources, and failing to produce enough for the society. Sarkar interprets this discursive fluctuation as the 'infinite elastic revenge':

> Therefore, Muslims of the past must pay for what the Muslims of the present are doing, just as Muslims of the present are paying for past

sins. If past, present, and future have to unify, then the production of an appropriate historical memory is crucial for the generation of a new political culture.

(Sarkar 2002, p. 158)

The *Hindutva* corollary of the sexualized Muslim invader is the weak and 'effeminate' Hindu man who was unable to resist and protect the nation (and women's bodies). This construct automatically casts as weak, abject, and impure the various expressions of non-heteronormative sexuality that have always existed in Indian culture, as expressed by the tradition of the *hijras*, whose origin is directly related to Ardhanarishvara, hermaphrodite manifestation of Lord Shiva.[26] The re-creation of Hindu masculinity in terms of the 'celibate hero who will rescue the emasculated nation' has been, therefore, one centrepiece of *Hindutva* ideology. It is manifested in the military model of the *shakha* and the warrior-style dress of its militiamen but also through the words and deeds of BJP politicians and in television productions, with portrayals of God Ram and Chandragupta, the Mauryian King, in the image of the Hindu hero.

Chakravarti's (2000) analysis of these productions notes the complex and contradictory handling of gender and sexuality by Hindu extremism. Although male heroes and male bonding overshadow women, female characters are also agents of resistance and liberation against the 'invaders'. Chakravati draws an analogy between this paradoxical construction and the real politics of *Hindutva*: though saffron is a sign of celibacy, saffron leaders used a sexually charged rhetoric to incite their militiamen. She concludes that *Hindutva* ideological reconstructions 'can draw from the cultural repertoire of the past ... but have very contemporary political functions' (p. 266). Gupta's (2005) analysis of Uttar Pradesh in the early twentieth century reminds us that the deliberate sexualization of Muslims by the Hindu Right is not restricted to men but is extended to women, who are depicted as both irresistible and uncontrollable. Narrain (2004), on the other hand, examines how the Hindu Right uses another centrepiece, 'the pure Hindu nation', to cast 'queer' sexuality as 'either impure (*hijras* and *kothis*) or alien (gays and lesbians), or both' (p. 159).

These perspectives are crucial for expanding the boundaries of the postgenocide critical narratives. Despite the brutal violations perpetrated against women's bodies, the gender dimensions of the carnage did not receive immediate or prominent attention in governmental assessments, or even in the reports of the mainstream human rights network. To bridge this gap, a group of Indian feminists invited a team of international women's rights activists to visit Gujarat and collect testimonies from survivors and relief workers, both women and men (IIJG 2003). While some observers interpreted the killing of children and the savage attacks on women's reproductive and sexual organs as reflecting the anxiety of Hindu

men about Muslim fertility rates (Sow *et al.* 2007), the IIJG's interpretation reflected the use of women's bodies as battlegrounds in the struggle to
define India as a Hindu state. However, as Petchesky notes, the IIJG
report, even when it calls attention to ideological *Hindutva* constructions
of masculinity,

> does not investigate acts of sexual violence against Muslim men, gays,
> and lesbians, or *hijras* themselves, or the ways in which it indirectly
> alludes to such acts: the public shaming of Muslim men forced to watch
> as their mothers, wives, and daughters are raped; and apparently the
> genital mutilation and rape of Muslim men by Hindu men (IIJG 2003,
> pp. 39–40). The battle of communities, of religions, becomes in part an
> onslaught, not only against the enemy's women and their wombs, but
> also against the circumcised by the uncircumcised penis.
>
> (Petchesky 2005, p. 11)

Petchesky raises another key aspect: although the actors and factors in the
Gujarat genocide are highly context specific, the sexualization of ethnic,
armed, and 'religious'-laden conflicts is not exceptional. This phenomenon
may be identified in historical events and current realities: the sexual violation and emasculation of slaves in ancient and modern times; the burning
of male and female 'sodomites' during the Inquisition; the sexual tortures
performed under dictatorships and in prisons around the world today; the
body violations and desecrations reported in all major ethnic and civil conflicts in the late twentieth and early twenty-first centuries, as in Angola, the
Balkans, Burundi, Cambodia, Darfur, Liberia, and Sierra Leone; and, the
horrors of the Abu Ghraib prison in Iraq in 2004 (see Chapter 10).

Religion and secularity: the battle over morality

One of the most astute thinkers of the twentieth century, Hannah Arendt,
is a source of inspiration for those concerned with the thorny problems of
justice, plurality, and identity in the complex political conditions of late
modernity. In this analytical context, it is interesting to recapture a lecture
given by Arendt to the American Association of Catholic philosophers in
1973. As reconstructed by Cohen:

> Arendt said that for the first time we live in a world in which the
> stability of moral authority is missing ... especially Church authority.
> For centuries the authority of the Church had kept the oscillations of
> will in suspension and refraining from actions through threats of
> damnation, but now, she said, almost nobody – certainly not the
> masses – still believes in this authority.
>
> (in Levinas 2003, p. 25)

At that time, a wide spectrum of Western observers – liberal, Marxist, radical, and even some progressive religious streams – would agree with her prognosis. This 'spirit of the time' reflected the gradual but steady secularization, since the eighteenth century, of societies rooted in the most diverse political and religious cultures. It also signalled transformations underway in religious institutions and doctrines, in particular the shifts in Catholicism since the Second Vatican Council.[27] This certainty, of inexorable secularization, echoed eighteenth-century philosophers' imagery of reason overcoming superstition and Hegel's God descending to Earth in the form of reason, politics, and the state. Or, yet more radically, Marx's widely repeated definition of religion as the opium that feeds alienation, Nietzsche's affirmation that God was dead, and Freud's interpretations of religious attachment as a psychic phenomenon.

By the late 1970s, these certainties would be deeply shaken. In 1978, as mentioned above, John Paul II was elected Pope and started dismantling the progressive doctrines and new institutional architecture previously announced by Pope John XXIII. In 1979, the Iranian Revolution and the victory of Ayatollah Khomeini illuminated the breadth, strength, and depth of Islamic revivalism, which had been at work for much longer in many 'secularized' countries but, until then, went unseen by most Western political analysts. A few years later, John Paul II and the CIA's William Casey were demolishing communism in Poland and liberation theology in Latin America (Bernstein and Polliti 1996), while in India the resurgence of *Hindutva* had begun. Concurrently, in some countries experiencing democratization, such as Brazil and the Philippines, the Catholic Church was lobbying for the right to life at conception to be included in the new constitutions under debate (Corrêa 2006).

In 1989, when the Cold War ended, a fire-storm of reactions to 80 years of 'compulsory state religion' was ignited almost everywhere in the former Soviet Union and Eastern Europe (Gadamer 1998, p. 201). Once again the distortions of top-down secularization became the object of critique.[28] Over the past 30 years, perceptions of and discourses on the connections between religion and politics have changed drastically. In the words of Vattimo,

> Perhaps not by its essential nature, but *de facto*, given the conditions of existence in modernity (the Christian West, secularized modernity, a *fin de siècle* state of anxiety over the impending threat of new and apocalyptic dangers), religion comes to be experienced as a return.
>
> (Vattimo 1998, p. 79)

Vattimo and many other observers see this 'return of the religious', particularly among popular sectors, as motivated by the insecurity that was already palpable during the Cold War but would intensify after 1989, as welfare policies eroded, awareness of environmental risks expanded, the power of science and technology as well as commoditization became glaring, and localized tensions and armed conflicts mushroomed. Susan Sontag (quoted in Armstrong 2000) observed that the contemporary return of the religious must be examined in light of the complex processes of change under way, as ordinary people start searching for simple and safe ways of interpreting the meaning and direction of human existence.

The current state of world affairs has also motivated many thinkers to ask new questions: Are the connections between manifestations of religious extremism traceable to what has been experienced in many settings throughout modernity? What are the common features and discrepancies between past and present experiences? Can we really describe what is witnessed today as a 'return of the religious'? Should it not be more precisely interpreted as a 'return of religion repressed'? Or are we being challenged to go beyond the 'philosophies of suspicion' that for a long time viewed religion as a residue, a leftover (Trías 1998)? Conceptually, this implies that 'religion' and 'spirituality' need to be extricated from the 'return of the religious' in the form of dogmatism and extremism. This requires a more systematic engagement with authors who are wrestling with the subject, but also the recapturing of past and contemporary political and sociological literature devoted to the analysis of religion and its connections to politics and social and cultural structures. Particularly relevant are the works of those who have examined belief systems, such as Weber (1993) and Durkheim (2001). For those engaged with sexual politics it is also crucial to revisit the remarkable research of anthropologists who have delved into the complexities of religious language and meaning, since they open up new possibilities for analysing sexual norms and the construction of sexual prerogatives and rights (see, e.g., Asad 2003, Geertz 1973, 1983). Also critical are the contributions of authors who have examined the role of religious values and institutions in the development of social movements and networks engaged in the work of 'solidarity', 'relief', and social service intrinsic to modernity (Bourdieu 1993).

Another approach is to contest religious doctrine from within the religious community. Feminist theologians and the Catholics for a Free Choice network have been doing so for decades, and the WLUML network develops its political analysis and action from a perspective located both outside and within Islamic religious traditions, as exemplified in its strategy of questioning the distortions of Sharia in Nigeria while avoiding attacks on religion. In recent years various streams from within Protestantism, Judaism, Buddhism, and Hinduism have started discourses across religious boundaries, as illustrated by the online Religious Consultation on Population, Reproductive Health, and Ethics, or the Conference on Women and Religions in a Globalized World, in Thailand, in 2004.[29]

As the influence of religious dogmatism and extremism on laws and policies has expanded in various quarters of the world, there have been mounting calls to restore the principles of secularity and *laïcité*. In Latin America such initiatives have blossomed and gained visibility in recent years; for example, various regional campaigns (such as the 28th of September Campaign for the Decriminalization of Abortion, Campaign Against all Forms of Fundamentalism, and Campaign for an Inter-American Convention on Sexual Rights and Reproductive Rights) have produced an array of popular materials; in Mexico GIRE (the Information Group on Reproductive Choice) sponsored a series of conversations on civil rights in Mexico; and a regional network of researchers has been established to investigate *laïcité* and freedom.[30] Freedman reflects, in general terms, the main conceptual and political motivation behind these initiatives, even when positions and analyses may vary:

> The persistence of juridical norms and institutional practices [such as the subsidizing of abstinence-only programmes by the US government] make us believe that the defence of *laïcité* is not an anachronistic objective, is not something belonging to the past. We call attention to the fact that it is necessary to struggle for a state grounded in principles of *laïcité* in order to eliminate the religious overarching vision that still prevails in the exercise of political power and in the implementation of public policies. This will permit that abusive infringements are avoided, which have as their consequence the restrictions on determined individual rights, as well as the consolidation of certain cultural values and patterns within civil society itself, which are guided by particular religions and impose relations of subordination and domination.
>
> (Freedman 2005, p. 43)

Given all we know about the regulation and disciplining of 'sex' by secular institutions and the deeply embedded place of the religious in political thinking, it is necessary to ask whether a restoration of secularity and *laïcité* would automatically resolve the dilemmas and tensions. An array of critical writing about religion and secularity in the post-Cold War and post-9/11 world underlines how the idea of a 'secular space' or 'public (civic) sphere', untainted by religion or any form of faith, is as much of an illusion as the imagined religious Utopia untainted by politics – whether the Rapture, the Second Coming, the *umma*, or the Zionist dream.

Jakobsen and Pellegrini (2003) challenge 'the current commonsense view ... that morality is based on religion and is primarily about regulation' – especially regulation of sex. Instead, they propose that 'morality in the public sphere' ought to be 'plural and open to debate' rather than settled; a conversation among diverse religious traditions and those without religious faith, rather than the monopoly of any one tradition

(p. 11). But to admit this is to admit that the idea of a strict separation between the 'secular' and the 'religious', or between 'public' and 'private' spheres, was always a discursive construct that hid a much messier and long-standing intercourse between the two. Jakobsen and Pellegrini (2003) also revisit the ambiguities and stigmatization inherent in the concept of 'tolerance', and trace that concept to the long history of normalizing Protestant Christianity in Western Europe following the French Wars of Religion (1562–1598). The principle of *cuius regio eius religio* – that each monarch would declare his own religion – was, from its origins, bound up with presumptions about superiority and inferiority, and the codification of social hierarchies.[31] For example, the 1689 Act of Toleration in England – a protective covenant for Protestants – left Catholics, Jews, Muslims, and atheists outside the bounds of protection from persecution. Indeed, the very notion of 'tolerance' – whether of religious or sexual nonconformity – implies objectification, or minoritization, of the 'Other'; 'being allowed to live in peace' falls far short of enabling conditions for full, democratic citizenship and 'free exercise of differences'. Jakobsen and Pellegrini also show how the US version of secularism, from its roots through the ascendancy of the Christian right in recent decades, has entailed a contradiction between the First Amendment clause on religious freedom and a dominant political culture that bases 'religious toleration ... on the assumption that America is, at heart, a Christian nation' (2003, p. 109).

Other recent scholarship traces the mythic dichotomy between Church and state, or the myth of an exclusive secularity to the particular genealogy of Western nation states and the very self-construction of Europe and 'the West'. Asad (2003, 2005) connects secularization, and particularly the French concept of *laïcité*, with the European state's claim to be the bearer of peace, order, and tolerance as it imposed political rule, both internally and through colonialism's 'civilizing mission' (2005, p. 2; 2003, p. 100). Derrida (1998) identifies the idea of 'religion' being a 'singular' something, 'a separate institution', as altogether 'Graeco-Christian, Graeco-Roman' – i.e., Western. This concept, argues Derrida, with its linguistic roots in Latin and Greek, actually conflates an 'irreducible duality', or the 'two veins ... of the religious' – 'the experience of belief' and 'the experience of ... *sacredness* or of *holiness*' (pp. 36–37).[32] The purpose of his argument is to show how the binary 'Reason *and* Religion' or 'Science *and* Religion' inherited from the Enlightenment and perpetuated by modernity from Voltaire through Marx, Nietzsche, Freud, and Heidegger actually obscures the necessary and intrinsic component of faith, *doxa*, or 'witnessing' inherent in any system of knowledge or reason. 'Tele-techno-scientific critique and reason' can only exist on the basis of 'an irreducible "faith", that of a "social bond" or a "sworn faith"'; 'a performative of promising ... without which no address to the other would be possible'. But this means that 'the imperturbable and interminable development of critical and techno-scientific reason, far from opposing religion, bears, supports, and supposes ... *that religion and reason have the same source*' (pp. 28, 44, our emphasis).

Derrida's argument has a political purpose in its critique of what he calls 'globalatinization', 'the Christian prevalence that has imposed itself globally within the said Latinity' of 'religion' (Derrida 1998, p. 38). The Graeco-Romanized notion of 'the religious' as a separate, delimited sphere – its other and equally Christian side is 'the secular' – conceals the religiosity of global capitalism and the ways in which its 'cyberspatialized' technologies and 'expropriative and delocalizing' effects constitute 'war by other means'. Thus, according to Derrida, today's 'wars of religion', and all the excesses of religious fundamentalisms, must be understood as reactions to 'globalatinization' – whether it takes the form of neocolonial policies 'in the name of peace' (e.g., loans and structural adjustments), 'unequal access ... to the same world market', or military interventions (pp. 24, 43, 63, 65).[33] To speak of a 'resurgence' of religion or to associate religious fundamentalism exclusively with radical Islam is to ignore the enlightenment roots of Christianity's universalizing project as well as the 'mystical', even 'messianic', foundations of all authority, including the presumably modern and democratic.

Derrida (1998) deploys the metaphor of the desert as an abstract space that opens up 'an invincible desire for justice' and the possibility 'of a universalizable culture of singularities' (p. 18). Like the mountain Mohammed climbed and Moses came down, or the leap out of the void made by all the social contract theorists, the desert that promises infinite justice and 'universal rationality' is born of faith. But the desert is also a real, twenty-first-century place, and one of unimaginable destruction. Writing even before the *declared* 'war on terror' and the invasion of Iraq, Derrida moves abruptly from metaphor to a Žižek-style 'desert of the real' (2002): 'the Middle-Eastern desert, ... this borderline place [where] a new war of religions is redeploying as never before' (pp. 18–19). Now, with the neocrusade called the 'war on terror', globalatinization is no longer 'religion that does not speak its name' (p. 53). War and politics march openly as faith by other means.[34]

These reflections and insights suggest that while religion has always claimed a special knowledge and jurisdiction when it comes to sexual morality, the modern state has consistently appropriated and redefined 'religion' as a domain of public morality. This is true despite, or because of, the various contradictions among secular views – think of the UK or Israel with their democratic rhetoric alongside an official national religion; the USA with its constitutional doctrine of separation and anti-establishment together with its silent privileging of Protestant Christianity; France with its strict *laïcité* since 1905, in contrast to Germany, which allocates public funds to support religious schools, instructional training,

and hospitals (Ewing 2002); India's formal secularism alongside its main-
tenance of religious courts; and so on.[35]

Asad (2003, 2005) illuminates the extent of this confusion as 'the *interdependence* of religious and secular elements', and the many ways in
which 'the secularist ideological order separating public politics from
private belief' breaks down (2003, pp. 62–65, 155). In an analysis of
laïcité and the dispute over veiling or headscarves in public schools in
contemporary France, he deconstructs this concept, not on the basis of
'minority rights' or 'free exercise of religion', but rather by showing how
secularism operates as an instrument of state power. That is, the state
determines what constitutes 'religion', or 'religious' symbolism or practice,
by virtue of its unique power to define 'what properly belongs to the
public sphere'. Thus, although 'the French secular state today ... disclaims
any religious allegiance and governs a largely irreligious society', banning
the veil does in fact make a kind of religious law through 'an exercise in
sovereign power ... to dominate the entirety of public space' (Asad 2005,
pp. 2–3, 6).

Asad's main concern is with the mystifications inherent in the concept
of the secular, insofar as it presumes a unified public sphere with its own
cohesive culture in which all citizens are 'equal' and all 'minorities' are
subsumed. As Marx showed in *On the Jewish Question* (1843), this universalizing conceit of liberal modernity conceals a host of inequalities and
exclusions, including, in France, a long colonial and postcolonial history of
Islamophobia (Asad 2003, pp. 177–178; 2005, pp. 6–7). Of course, the
recent conflict over veiling in France is a story not only of racism and
ethnic containment but also of gender and sexual power. Asad's analysis
shows that underlying this controversy is the contest between the French
state and the French Islamic communities – both dominated by men and
heedless of the desires of young Muslim women – over who shall protect
the bodies and sexual virtue of women and girls in public space (2005, p.
4).[36] It is an important argument, since the usual claim on behalf of liberal
and feminist values is that any sort of covering, whether *hijab* or *burqa*, 'is
a symbol of fanaticism and the submission of women', thus associating a
ban on headscarves or veils with modernity and ending women's oppression. As Ewing (2002) points out, in the name of these liberal values, girls
have been forced to violate their beliefs, and some women in France,
Turkey, and Germany have lost their jobs as public schoolteachers (pp.
69–72).

Likewise, Jakobsen and Pellegrini (2003) question whether the USA has
ever been a 'secular' society or whether the 'separation' doctrine has ever
been more than a rhetorical façade. They document the ways in which
'conservative Christianity' and sometimes 'Christian theological pronouncements' and prohibitions infuse US sexual policies: 'the secular
state's regulation of the sexual life of its citizens is actually religion by

other means' (pp. 3–4, 13, 19).[37] The evidence is most compelling in rulings by the US Supreme Court, and most spectacularly in its decision upholding Georgia's sodomy statute in *Bowers* v. *Hardwick* (United States Supreme Court 1986). Justice 'Burger's invocation of "Judaeo-Christian moral and ethical standards"' in that notorious (and now obsolete) majority opinion, flew in the face of the obligation 'to uphold the principle of church–state separation'. Rather, the 'recasting of specific religious laws as generically moral ones' amounted to '[dispensing] religion in the place of justice'. But Jakobsen and Pellegrini point to a more insidious effect of the hyphen in 'Judaeo-Christian'. By collapsing 'Jewish difference into Christian tradition', while failing to cite any Jewish theological or scholarly sources and ignoring the vast disagreements about homosexuality within both Judaism and Christianity, it uses the hyphenation to construct an artificial 'religious pluralism' (pp. 31–32).

In *Lawrence* v. *Texas* (United States Supreme Court 2003, p. 10), Justice Kennedy's opinion for the 6–3 majority overturned the ruling in *Hardwick*, explicitly repudiating Burger's construction of a long-standing 'Judaeo-Christian moral and ethical' tradition condemning homosexuality between 'consenting adults acting in private'. Citing the scholarship of historians showing the lack of any consistent opposition to, or even concept of, homosexual persons in 'the history of Western civilization', as well as the strong pattern of non-enforcement of sodomy statutes in US law, the *Lawrence* majority opinion would seem to reinforce the doctrine of separation between religion and law and between private and public domains. Grounding its ruling firmly on the principles of liberty, privacy, and protection from governmental intrusion into personal (family, sexual, contraceptive, marital, procreative, affective) decisions and relationships 'by unmarried as well as married persons', it quotes its own prior decision upholding the right to abortion in *Planned Parenthood of Southeastern Pennsylvania* v. *Casey* (1992): 'Our obligation is to define the liberty of all, not to mandate our own moral code.'

In fact, the *Lawrence* decision demonstrates the negative as well as the progressive aspects of privacy and liberal tolerance. Justice Kennedy wants to dignify homosexuals as individuals with rights to an identity and to intimate relationships, but not homosexual sex. 'To say that the issue in *Bowers* was simply the right to engage in certain sexual conduct,' he writes, 'demeans the claim the individual put forward, just as it would demean a married couple were it to be said marriage is simply about the right to have sexual intercourse' (United States Supreme Court 2003, p. 6).[38] The liberal doctrine of privacy and tolerance, which is central to secularity, serves here to desexualize sexuality and efface individuals in relationships.

The problem is not that 'the secular' or 'public' space has been taken over by religiosity, since everything discussed above suggests that the wall between them was always an imaginary and rhetorical one. As Jakobsen and Pellegrini (2003) put it, 'the problem is not religion' but authoritarian or totalitarian religion; the absence of 'the freedom not to be religious and the freedom to be religious differently' (p. 12), and the equation, in both conservative religion and conservative politics, of 'morality' with sexual normativity. Historically, and in many diverse cultural and geographical contexts, sexual oppression, racist or colonial domination, and religious persecution have gone hand in hand – whether in the form of confinement of women; hate crimes against gays, lesbians, and transgender people; sexual violence against Muslims or other religious or ethnic minorities; or the sexual codifications and brutalities committed by Christian European conquistadors. At the same time, we have to remember that religious beliefs and practices – whether Hindu, Muslim, Jewish, Christian, or some other form – include as many diverse perspectives (liberalism, conservatism, feminism, patriarchalism) as do political movements.

Many current feminist scholars, echoing Derrida, emphasize that 'religions are inherently multi-vocal' and 'always have been', in a way that makes the very concept of 'religion' much too static and 'institutional' to convey what religious people experience through their faith. Castelli (2005) warns against the tendency to reify, ossify, or decontextualize religion as something separate from social life. When we do so, we ignore the critical fissures and debates taking place within religious movements and affiliations, especially over gender and sexuality, as well as the fact that progressive movements for peace, civil and human rights, and sexual freedom have always gained strength from religiously identified groups and activists. Or, as Lila Abu-Lughod (2005) suggests, we evade the troublesome tension between supporting religious freedom and attacking religious law. From this 'multi-vocal' perspective, Eck (2000) points out the absurdity of homogenizing 'the Islamic world', much less branding all Muslims as terrorists. Imam (2000) and Ilkkaracan (2000), in cataloguing the tremendous diversity in Muslim practices and interpretations of the Qu'ran across geographical regions, underline the need to look at contextual specificities, especially in regard to women's sexuality and dress and gay, lesbian, and transgender identities. These scholars remind us that, for religious believers, faith constitutes not an isolated compartment but a 'way of life'. The manner and interpretation are always matters of negotiation and struggle – of power relations.

In fact, in the great majority of cases, the continual breaching of the supposed 'wall' between public and private, secular and religious, is chiefly about regulating sexuality and gender. Foucault (1980) describes the nineteenth-century shift in attitudes towards hermaphrodites and the ultimate decree that 'henceforth, everybody was to have one and only one sex' (p. viii). Interestingly, this edict of non-toleration of poly-sexual identity required the complicity of medical (secular) and religious authorities, hitherto fierce rivals over 'morals' jurisdiction (Foucault 1980, pp. viii–xii). This codification of 'one true sex' through the partnership of science and religion merely prefigured a long history of public pronouncements on normative bodies and sexual behaviour in which medical and moral, and secular and religious discourses become thoroughly muddled. In the following section, we look at competing secular discourses on sexuality in the twentieth and twenty-first centuries, taking into account Derrida's warning against an overly dichotomized view of 'Science and Religion' since both are steeped in faith.

Part 2

Epistemological challenges and research agendas

Chapter 4

The modernization of 'sex' and the birth of sexual science

What Derrida (1998) described as the 'return of the religious', and its impact in shaping sexual politics in the twenty-first century, is hardly an altogether novel development. On the contrary, as Foucault and others have pointed out, the social articulation of sexuality since at least the Middle Ages had been organized primarily by religion: 'The Middle Ages had organized around the theme of the flesh and the practice of penance a discourse that was markedly unitary' (Foucault 1978, p. 33). What in fact has been most striking about the articulation of sex and sexuality in recent centuries is the extent to which a relatively unified and profoundly hegemonic religious discourse has been broken apart by a range of new discursive formations:

> In the course of recent centuries this relative uniformity was broken apart, scattered, and multiplied in an explosion of distinct discursivities, which took form in demography, biology, medicine, psychiatry, psychology, ethics, pedagogy, and political criticism. More precisely, the secure bond that held together the moral theology of concupiscence and the obligation of confession ... was, if not broken, at least loosened and diversified.
>
> (Foucault 1978, p. 33)

By the mid- to late nineteenth century, these emerging discursive practices had begun to offer an alternative scientific vision of sexuality and its consequences based less on accepted moral precepts than on empirical investigation and observation (Bozon and Leridon 1996).

In Part 1 of this volume, we emphasized the key political debates related to sexuality, health, and human rights that have emerged globally in recent years. We pointed out the ways these debates have been shaped by a broader range of social, cultural, and economic factors impinging upon diverse global arenas in which both discursive interventions and political actions take place. As we made clear, the politics of sexuality in the global era can only be fully understood in relation to this contemporary context, but there are also historical genealogies that must be examined and accounted for if we are to build a more just sexual order and more emancipatory sexual politics. Although the broader context of recent debates (e.g., rapid globalization, unilateral US hegemony) may be quite unique, some key aspects, such as the tensions between religious and secular visions and the challenge to the legitimacy of how we know what we know about sexuality, are deeply rooted in developments evolving over the past 300 years in relation to the ways sexuality has been conceptualized and questioned.

In Part 2, we want to highlight three moments or movements, in relation to what Gayle Rubin (1984) once called 'thinking sex', that are especially important for understanding the terms of reference for many contemporary debates: (1) the emergence, during the late nineteenth and early twentieth centuries, of sexology as part of a search for a 'scientific' understanding of sexuality and sexual behaviour; (2) the growth, after the mid-twentieth century, of what has been described as a 'social constructionist' (or 'deconstructionist') challenge to scientific certainty about the nature of sexual life; and (3) the massive expansion of research and discourse on sexuality that took place following the emergence of HIV and AIDS globally in the 1980s and 1990s. Together, these three interrelated developments laid the groundwork for the differing understandings of sexuality that underlie many of the most contentious debates around contemporary sexual politics. They have thus conditioned the possibilities not only for changes in discourse but also for moving from research and epistemology to practice, intervention, and action.

Sexuality and science

It is impossible to do justice to the historical development of research and analysis on sexuality and sexual behaviour in the space available here. What we will emphasize is the extent to which many of the contemporary debates between religious and secular visions of sexual life and sexual values are rooted in a long tradition, dating back to the mid-nineteenth century, of the study of sexuality throughout Europe (Gagnon and Parker 1995). In the closing decades of the nineteenth century and the early decades of the twentieth century, the emerging field of 'sexology' was a revolutionary attempt on the part of a small number of Western researchers and activists to bring sexuality under the domain of what was then understood as 'science'. This intellectual movement was managed principally by members of the new secular scientific professions that were taking shape and gaining force.

This is not to say that the discursive practices of this emerging sexual science were completely free or independent of the normative strictures of earlier times. On the contrary, it was precisely during this period that the majority of what would come to be known as 'the perversions' was articulated in the writings of the key founding fathers of sexology, Karl Heinrich Ulrichs, Richard von Krafft-Ebing, Magnus Hirschfeld, Havelock Ellis, Sigmund Freud, and their various successors (see Bozon and Leridon 1996, Weeks 1985, 1986). As Weeks has noted,

> the aspiration to fully scientific status gave the embryonic sexology a prestige – and more important a new object of concern and intervention in the instinct and its vicissitudes – that has carried its influence, definitions, classifications, and norms into the twentieth century.
>
> (Weeks 1985, p. 66)

Weeks suggested that there were two decisive moments in the emerging scientific discourses around sexuality and the sexual instinct. The first was the work of Charles Darwin and the impact of Darwinism in the mid- to late nineteenth century. With the publication of *The Origin of Species* (Darwin 1859), and then even more clearly with the publication of *The Descent of Man, and Selection in Relation to Sex* (Darwin 1871), the claim that sexual selection (the struggle for partners) acted independently of natural selection (the struggle for existence) suggested that the most important indicator of biological success could be found in reproduction. This, in turn, helped to bring about new scientific interest in 'sexual aetiologies' – in the origins of individual behaviour – and in the dynamics of sexual selection (Weeks 1985, p. 67). The biology of sex – of the sexual impulse and the differentiation between the sexes – thus became a focus for scientific attention and sexuality came to be located in nature as opposed to morality.

The grounding of sexuality in nature, in relation to the evolution of the species, was a central step in articulating an understanding of sex and the sexual instinct as biologically rooted – and of reproduction as the essential goal of sexual behaviour. If biology was destiny, however, it was only the point of departure for a normative framework that was capable of rivalling religious strictures in its role of organizing and controlling sexual conduct. As Weeks has argued, the publication of Krafft-Ebing's *Psychopathia Sexualis* (Krafft-Ebing 1939 [orig. 1886]), while perhaps not as broadly influential as Darwin's controversial texts on evolution, was every bit as powerful in articulating a scientific vision of sexual normality and deviance: 'it was the eruption into print of the speaking pervert, the individual marked, or marred, by his (or her) sexual impulses' (Weeks 1985, p. 67).

The case studies published by Krafft-Ebing grew from the 45 case histories and 110 pages originally published in 1886 to 238 cases and 437 pages by the twelfth edition in 1903, and became a model for the scientific work on sexual behaviour that followed over the next century (Weeks

1985). Together with the natural, biological grounding of the sexual urge or instinct, then, this detailed cataloguing of sexual pathology took shape as the nineteenth century's lasting legacy to the transformation of sexual experience and knowledge. The creation of new sexual discourses and practices by doctors, social workers, and researchers, who viewed themselves as reformers and progressives committed to the cause of modernization based on scientific principles, brought new legitimacy for the investigation of human sexuality as a central scientific undertaking (see Weeks 1985, 1986).

By the beginning of the twentieth century, at a time typically associated with the rise of modernity in Western Europe, a whole new collection of 'liberal' or 'liberated' ideas took hold of the new middle classes all over the European continent. New views about sexuality were articulated, especially in opposition to the perceived repressive doctrines of the Victorian period, and sexuality begun to take shape as an exemplary form of social resistance among avant-garde social and political groups (see Gagnon and Parker 1995, Robinson 1976). Within this context, the scientific study of sexuality began to take shape as a kind of emancipatory political process: a search for empirical evidence that might not only explain, but also simultaneously depathologize, sexual diversity. This process was consistently grounded in what may be described as an underlying 'essence' that can be identified and interrogated scientifically. As Robinson (1976), Weeks (1985, 1986, 1991), and others have pointed out, for much of the sexological tradition, this essence was typically rooted 'in nature'. As put by Connell and Dowsett, it has been based on 'the assumption that a given pattern of sexuality is native to the human constitution' (Connell and Dowsett 1999, p. 179).

Over the course of the late nineteenth and early twentieth centuries, the development of this 'naturalist' perspective moved in two important directions. On the one hand, in the work of thinkers such as Sigmund Freud and his followers Havelock Ellis, and other psychiatrists and psychologists, the clinic and the clinical case study became the point of departure for documentation of the widest possible range of sexual practices and proclivities, and for a complicated, and often contradictory, debate about their status as normal or abnormal aspects of our underlying human nature. On the other hand, in the work of scientists and social scientists such as Bronislaw Malinowski, Margaret Mead, and their contemporaries, as well as researchers such as Alfred Kinsey and his colleagues, observational and ethnographic studies and, increasingly, population-based survey research, formed the basis for empirical data collection and documentation of the wide range and diversity of human sexual experience across cultures and populations (see Gagnon and Parker 1995, Robinson 1976, Weeks 1985).

Freud's work, of course, has been particularly influential, with a reach that extends far beyond sexuality and sex research in shaping contemporary Western thought. It is also highly complex, with various nuanced developments over time. Freud's major impact on sexuality research, however, like Ellis', is found in his conceptual innovations, methodological approach, and, in particular, his focus on clinical cases and case reports as the *materia prima* for scientific investigation and analysis:

> The type of scientificity was redefined, but the basic claim could only be reinforced, when sexology moved out of a forensic into a clinical context. The Western *scientia sexualis* ... reached its first climax when Freud's key volumes appeared in 1900 and 1905, and Ellis's in 1897. Freud developed a flexible but profound therapeutic and research technique; he produced also a detailed developmental model of human sexuality, bringing childhood sexuality into focus. His most influential arguments demonstrated the protean character of sexual motivation and the significance of sexuality for human psychology generally.
>
> (Connell and Dowsett 1999, p. 181)

Perhaps Freud's key innovation was his argument 'for broadening the meaning of sexuality' (Weeks 1985, p. 71), which required a rethinking of Krafft-Ebing's 'perversions'. Freud argued that the so-called perversions could be understood as acts that either extend sexual practices beyond the conventionally appropriate regions of the body (typically, the genitals) or else linger on practices (such as foreplay) that are considered appropriate if they lead in the end to genital sexuality. In his 'Three essays on the theory of sexuality' (1905), Freud affirmed that what had been described by earlier writers as perverse manifestations of sexual desire characterizing a sick minority should, in fact, be incorporated into the acceptable range of human sexuality as common or typical of normal sexual expression:

> No healthy person, it appears, can fail to make some addition that might be called perverse to the normal sexual aim; and the universality of this finding is in itself enough to show how inappropriate it is to use the word perversion as a term of reproach.
>
> (Freud 1905, p. 160)

It was this understanding, particularly when translated into the concept of universal 'polymorphous perversity', together with the 'bisexuality' of infancy, that made Freud's psychoanalytic framework so groundbreaking and potentially revolutionary as a way of conceptualizing human sexual potential. Yet he also outlined a developmental process – from oral, to anal, to genital sexuality – which seemed to assume a 'normality' (or at least a 'normalization') that undercut the radical starting point of his own theory of desire. In his famous letter to the mother of a young homosexual man, for example, while he sought to assure her that homosexuality should not be considered a vice or an illness, he none the less concluded that: 'We consider it to be a variation of the sexual function produced by a certain arrest of the sexual development' (Freud, in Jones 1961, p. 277).[1]

In introducing a notion of development (which might somehow be arrested), together with the conceptualization of developmental phases, psychoanalytic theory demonstrated a degree of internal contradiction, when compared with its more radical potential, that would continue to pose serious problems over an extended period. As Weeks has suggested:

> For Freud the growth of each individual from infancy to mature adult sexuality repeated the (hypothetical) development of the race as a whole from primitive sexual promiscuity and perversity to monogamous heterosexuality. This was not the product simply of evolution but of cultural imperatives. It was the tragic destiny of humankind to necessarily forgo the infinite range of the desires in order to ensure survival in a world of scarcity. Each individual, like the race itself, had to attain the 'tyranny of genital organization' in order to survive, while appropriate object choice became less an act of volition and more of a cultural demand. In the end, therefore, a heterosexual and reproductive imperative is reinserted into Freud's account. Once a goal directed version of sexuality is introduced, however surreptitiously, then the whole laboriously constructed edifice of sexual variety begins to totter.
>
> (Weeks 1986, p. 73)

In spite of its radical potential, then, Freudian psychoanalysis – like other foundational discourses that contributed to the development of sexology as a scientific project – constructed what was still a unitary model of sexuality. It offered a normative vision of sexual desire and sexual behaviour that was fundamentally heterosexual, procreative, and essentially male. Female sexuality was effectively secondary, responsive to male desire and practice. While the open-ended possibilities of polymorphous perversity were clearly different from the more restrictive systems of earlier writers such as Krafft-Ebing, and the complexity of the conceptual architecture created in psychoanalytic theory was more sophisticated than much of the sexological tradition that would continue to develop over the course of the twentieth century, neither Freud nor the majority of his followers would fully escape the marginalization (and, more often than not, the pathologization) of abnormal or non-normative sexual expression.

At roughly the same time that Freud and his followers were creating psychoanalysis, Havelock Ellis was developing the foundation for what he would describe as the psychology of sex. Together with Freud, and in many ways more clearly, Ellis has been associated with what Robinson has described as 'the modernization of sex' (Robinson 1976). Indeed, Ellis, even more than Freud, is a paradigmatic figure defining what Robinson suggests is the ethos of this tradition – filling a role in relation to modern sexology similar to that of Weber in relation to modern sociology or Einstein in relation to modern physics (Robinson 1976). In six volumes of his *Studies in the Psychology of Sex*, originally published from 1897 to 1910 (Ellis 1936; see also Ellis 1932), Ellis articulated and defined nearly all of the major scientific and moral categories that would become the focus of subsequent theorization. The lasting impact of his thinking, and its role in articulating the fundamental philosophical basis for much of what would become the 'naturalist' tradition in sex research, was already apparent in the opening pages of *Sexual Inversion*, Volume I of *Studies in the Psychology of Sex*.

The first chapter of *Sexual Inversion* showed the extent to which Ellis incorporated two of the key characteristics that Robinson has identified as being central to the 'modernist' tradition in sexuality research. One argument, based on animal behaviour, was later used most effectively by Kinsey; another, focusing on cultural relativism, was soon adopted by researchers such as Malinowski, Mead, and a host of other anthropologists. Ellis noted that homosexual behaviour had been observed in diverse animal species – in particular among birds – and it had existed in nearly all known human societies. He also suggested that homosexuality was treated with indifference by the majority of non-Western peoples, thus calling into question the notion that homosexuality was somehow unnatural (Robinson 1976; see also Weeks 1985, 1986).

This emphasis on the inborn nature of sexual inversion, and of the other forms of sexual behaviour he would examine over the course of his career, contrasted with earlier interpretations of the acquired nature of such practices. This set Ellis in direct opposition to the earlier generation of writers, most clearly to Krafft-Ebing but also to Freud, who had localized the acquisition of sexual proclivities and the construction of sexual identities in psychic mechanisms such as the Oedipal complex. Throughout his work, Ellis sought to legitimize socially stigmatized or prohibited sexual practices by demonstrating their relationship with what might be seen as 'normal sexuality' and by viewing such practices as part of the wide range of sexual possibilities open to human beings. Indeed, he preferred to avoid the concept of sexual 'normality' altogether, substituting for it the idea of a 'continuum' of sexual behaviours – a strategy that allowed him to categorize the so-called 'perversions' as nothing more than an exaggeration of more statistically frequent behaviours (Robinson 1976).

Ellis followed this basic strategy in later studies on 'auto-eroticism', the 'sexual impulse', 'tumescence' and 'de-tumescence', 'sadism' and 'masochism', and so on. While his work lacked the theoretical elaboration of psychoanalysis, Ellis' understanding of such diverse expressions in human sexuality as fundamental in the immense natural variation characteristic of the species provided perhaps an even more vital contribution to the development of a sexual science. His work aimed to document empirically the full range of human sexual behaviour and to use this empirical documentation as the point of departure for creating an atmosphere of tolerance, one of the lasting marks of sexology as a science.

Anthropology, ethnography, and cross-cultural research

While Freudian psychoanalysis and Ellis' psychology of sex were the most important bodies of work in the late nineteenth and early twentieth centuries bearing directly on the conceptualization and investigation of sexual experience, the cross-cultural research of a number of early anthropologists offered another important source of information on sexuality. These early analyses were caught between their capacity to document sexual diversity and their search for underlying, universal, scientific truths. As Connell and Dowsett have noted, a very similar ambiguity also exists in early anthropological works on sexuality, which along with psychoanalysis became perhaps the most significant body of evidence regarding sexual diversity:

> Ethnographers brought back to the European and American intelligentsia accounts of sexual customs so varied but so comprehensible that it was impossible to regard them simply as exotica, as primitivism, or as simple variants on the European pattern. As the Newtonian universe shrank the Earth from being the focus of creation to being merely one of a number of bodies following gravitational laws, so ethnography shrank Western culture from the status of norm, or historic pinnacle, to being one among a large number of comparable cultures which simply had different ways of handling questions of sex.
>
> (Connell and Dowsett 1999, p. 184)

While the early anthropological investigation of sexual customs in search of broader cross-cultural patterns was widespread (see, e.g., Goldenweiser 1929; see also the discussion in Vance 1999), Malinowski's work was perhaps the most systematic and influential in the search for an underlying uniformity that might explain the variability of cross-cultural patterns documented in the ethnographic literature. In classic studies such as *Sex and Repression in Savage Society* (1927) and *The Sexual Life of Savages* (1929), drawing on his extended fieldwork with the Trobriand Islanders in Melanesia, Malinowski's writings situated sexual practices in a broader social and cultural context. Yet, as his work evolved, it incorporated sexual desires and behaviours into an understanding of kinship systems as a cultural response to the social need for reproduction (Malinowski 1944, pp. 75–103). It also reduced the diversity of sexual customs, as documented in the ethnographic record, to the various ways in which cultures solved the common problem of a naturally given need (see Connell and Dowsett 1999). Much like Freud or Ellis, then, Malinowski's work sought to uncover laws of society that would be comparable to the laws of nature delineated by the natural sciences. He saw culture as a mechanism for the satisfaction of human nature – for meeting 'basic instinctual needs' (Weeks 1986, p. 22).

Just as the work of psychoanalysis and sexology was wedded to the search for scientific understanding and universal laws, then, the early anthropological documentation of sexual diversity across cultures was particularly important in contextualizing Western cultural patterns, morality, and normativity more broadly. By recognizing the fundamental diversity of sexual practices and arrangements cross-culturally, it also offered a potentially useful and fundamentally sympathetic reading of sexual difference and diversity in Western societies. Perhaps the most popular example of this process – of cross-cultural research findings being used to hold up a mirror for Western practices – was Margaret Mead's examination of 'coming of age' in Samoa (Mead 1928). This was followed by a series of other studies (see, e.g., Mead 1935, 1949) focusing on cross-cultural differences in the organization of gender and sexuality, particularly in the Pacific Islands and Melanesian societies. Mead's work was especially influential in the USA because it demonstrated that American values related particularly to the regulation of adolescent sexuality were by no means universal or necessary (see Weeks 1985). Much of this same mode of analysis was later applied to explain differences in the ways diverse societies organized gender relations and the division between the sexes, but with considerable ambiguity and contradiction in the formulation of both underlying human nature and cross-cultural variability.

The anthropological work of Malinowski, Mead, and others (see, e.g., Bateson 1947, Honigman 1954, Murdock 1949) was thus central to highlighting the widespread cultural diversity of sexual customs across cultures. While these accounts were for the most part highly specific, grounded in detailed ethnographic accounts of local customs among particular peoples in highly determined places, they provided the necessary data for broader attempts at scientific generalization. Beginning in the 1930s, for example, researchers based at Yale University in the USA had begun to bring together individual ethnographic accounts (of not only sexuality but also the full range of anthropological topics) in what came to be known as the Human Relations Area Files. This archive was classified by subject matter and geographic area and based on thousands of books, articles, and related documents written by observers ranging from travellers and missionaries to anthropologists and ethnographers. These data made possible cross-cultural comparative analysis such as the work of Clellan Ford and Frank Beach in their study *Patterns of Sexual Behavior* (Ford and Beach 1951). In reviewing the ethnographic record, Ford and Beach found significant variations in sexual customs and practices across cultures. They concluded that no single society could be seen as representative of the human species; different societies held widely different views on the sexual impulses of children or the appropriateness of masturbation, on the acceptability of same-sex relations or the existence of sexual relations between humans and other animals, and so on.

None the less, most analysts saw such variability as a superficial variation in culture and customs that could be reduced to some kind of underlying natural or even biological similarity. It was understood less as a question of fundamental difference than as an overlay of local customs shaping an underlying natural essence – what Vance has described as a 'cultural influence model': 'In this model, sexuality is seen as the basic material – a kind of universal Play-Doh – on which culture works, a naturalized category which remains closed to investigation and analysis' (Vance 1999, p. 44). This model emphasized the importance of cultural norms and of learning culturally defined patterns as central to what may be described as the cultural regulation of sexuality, suggesting significant cross-cultural variation as a central part of the anthropological record of human societies. It thus rejects a simplistic essentialism, emphasizing behavioural variations and cultural differences:

> Culture is viewed as encouraging or discouraging the expression of generic sexual acts, attitudes, and relationships. Oral–genital contact, for example, might be a part of normal heterosexual expression in one group but taboo in another; male homosexuality might be severely punished in one tribe yet tolerated in another. Anthropological work from this period was characterized by a persistent emphasis on variability.
>
> (Vance 1999, p. 44)

At the same time, it also seemed to interpret away such variability in the search for underlying patterns or universals that are ultimately almost always assumed to be biologically determined – an underlying 'sex drive' or 'impulse'. Although this drive or impulse may be shaped by culture, it is none the less a force of nature that is awakened through the natural maturation process of puberty that often escapes social control or regulation and manifests itself differently in men and women (Vance 1999, p. 44).

In the end, as Vance, Weeks, and others have suggested, this anthropological articulation of variability was also submerged within the search for scientific explanation. It offered a useful counter to the hegemony of Western cultural patterns and accepted normative prescriptions. However, it provided little in the way of a foundation for a more radical sexual politics capable of calling into question inequality or oppression in sexual relations or in articulating a vision of sexual self-determination and freedom.

Surveying sexual behaviour

Around the time of the First World War, the growing interest in making sexuality an object of science had begun to translate into important new initiatives that would continue to shape the field in the mid-twentieth century. Indeed, the War itself was a watershed in the study of sexuality, shaping some of the most important research in the field. Even Malinowski's groundbreaking ethnographic work among the Trobriand Islanders might never have been carried out if he had not been marooned in Melanesia with the outset of the War and unable to travel for an extended period. Less serendipitously, in part as a result of social disruptions caused by the War in Europe, the centre of gravity for sexuality research and analysis shifted increasingly to the USA, and a set of new institutional contexts began to emerge that would have a major influence on the development of sex research for a number of decades (see di Mauro 1995).

The earliest surveys of sexual behaviour in the USA started in the 1890s (Ericksen and Steffen 1999). Early sex surveys were mainly conducted by social scientists and physicians, and were in large part justified by the perceived need for data on sexual behaviour in order to provide scientific grounding for a preventive health agenda. Such an agenda was intended as the basis for more effective sexuality education, aimed ultimately at controlling 'inappropriate' sexual behaviours and the spread of venereal disease (di Mauro 1995; see also Brandt 1987, Ericksen and Steffen 1999). In 1913, in large part due to concerns about the possible health impacts of prostitution and at the urging of John D. Rockefeller, the American Social Hygiene Association was created. In conjunction with this, a research arm known as the Bureau of Social Hygiene Association was financed by Rockefeller to support studies on prostitution in the USA and Europe (see Bullough 1985, 1994). The Bureau of Social Hygiene received more than $5.8 million over the next 30 years, primarily from the Rockefeller family's various charities, to support the 'study, amelioration, and prevention of those social conditions, crimes, and diseases which adversely affect the well-being of society, with special reference to prostitution and the evils associated therewith' (Aberle and Corner 1953, p. 4; see also Bullough 1985, 1994).

In 1916, the US National Academy of Science created the National Research Council to address crises in scientific research and research infrastructures brought about by the disruptions of the First World War. Intended as a conduit for research funding, the Council worked with staff

members from the Bureau of Social Hygiene after the war to set up a programme for funding research in sexuality that the Rockefeller group was
interested in supporting (Bullough 1985). In October 1921, participants at
a conference organized by the Medical Division of the National Research
Council, with funding provided once again by the Rockefellers, voted to
make support for sex research a Council priority:

> The impulses and activities associated with sex behaviour and repro-
> duction are fundamentally important for the welfare of the individual,
> the family, the community, and the race. Nevertheless, the reports of
> personal experience are lacking and the relatively raw data of observa-
> tion have not been collected in serviceable form. Under the circum-
> stances where we should have knowledge and intelligence, we are
> ignorant.... The committee is convinced, however, that with the use of
> methods employed in physiology, psychology, anthropology, and
> related sciences, problems of sex behaviour can be subjected to scient-
> ific examination. In order to eliminate any suggestion that such
> inquiry is undertaken for purposes of propaganda, it should be spon-
> sored by a body of investigators whose disinterested devotion to
> science is well recognized. For these various reasons, the committee
> recommends that the National Research Council be advised to organ-
> ize and to foster an investigation into the problems of sex.
>
> (Zinn 1924, pp. 94–95)

In November 1921, the Committee for Research in Problems of Sex was
established within the Division of Medical Sciences of the National
Research Council and quickly became the major source of funding for
research on sexual behaviour. Between 1922 and 1947, the Committee
received approximately $1.5 million to support the fields of endocrinology
and biology for the 'scientific study of sexuality as a biological phenomenon distinct from the limited study of human social problems of a sexual
nature' (di Mauro 1995, p. 5). More than $1 million in funding was also
provided to five US universities for sex research projects approved by the
Committee (Bullough 1985, di Mauro 1995).[2] After 1948, following a
reorganization of the National Research Council, the Rockefeller Foundation continued to provide support for the Council's sex research activities,
while its other research activities were funded by the US government. From
1948 to 1954, when it ceased to fund sex research (see below), the Rockefeller Foundation added another $600,000 for sexuality-related research
(Aberle and Corner 1953, Bullough 1985, p. 118).

Research supported by the Committee during the 1930s and 1940s
ranged from studies of hormones and the biology of sex to studies of sexuality and personality, but by far the most important and visible work it
backed was the survey research of Alfred Kinsey and his colleagues at

Indiana University. The Committee began to fund Kinsey's work in 1941, and by the mid-1940s Kinsey's research group was receiving up to half of the annual resources allocated to the Committee by the Rockefeller Foundation. Kinsey's research was the first work supported by the Committee that focused on human sexual behaviour rather than the sexual behaviour of other animals, and it would soon prove to be not only the most visible but by far the most controversial as well.

Like much of the research that has emerged from the naturalist tradition and its focus on sexuality and science, the political implications of sexuality research were ambiguous at best. Perhaps nowhere is this seen more clearly than in the work of Kinsey and his colleagues, who might well be taken as the quintessential representatives of the sexological approach. Kinsey's major studies were carried out from the 1930s to the early 1950s and published in two major volumes, *Sexual Behavior in the Human Male* in 1948 and *Sexual Behavior in the Human Female* in 1953 (Kinsey *et al.* 1948, 1953). Based on extensive survey research with 5300 male respondents and 5940 female respondents from across the USA (Gebhard and Johnson 1979), Kinsey's studies were in many ways the epistemological opposite of the clinical case studies of the psychoanalytic and psychological tradition in sex research and the observational work developed by anthropologists and ethnographers. A zoologist by training (who began his career as a specialist in the study of gall wasps), Kinsey's firm conviction was that only through amassing extensive numbers of interviews could the idiosyncratic character (and hence scientific bias) of individual cases be overcome. Indeed, the structured interview, carried out by a trained interviewer and integrated within a huge data set in order to make sustainable generalizations at the level of the population as a whole, was surely the most powerful innovation and contribution made by Kinsey and his colleagues to the study of sexuality. As Paul Robinson has pointed out, the sexual history interview was in many ways Kinsey's most brilliant creation – an investigative *tour de force* in which each fragment of sexual information accessible to memory was elicited from research subjects in less than two hours (Robinson 1976). Between 1938 and 1956, Kinsey and his colleagues, Wardell Pomeroy, Clyde Martin, and Paul Gebhard, recorded more than 18,000 such interviews – with Kinsey himself reportedly responsible for about 8000 of them.

Ironically, while the massive number of interviews gave popular weight to the Kinsey reports, the statistical bases of his studies have always been questionable due to the extended period over which data were collected using a convenience sample that was undifferentiated in terms of analysis (see, e.g., Turner *et al.* 1989). As innovative as the in-depth personal interview and the collection of detailed sexual histories would be for the history of all sex research that followed, the problems with sampling, and the naive assumption that the sheer number of interviews carried out would provide scientific legitimacy, would pose lasting problems for the acceptance of Kinsey's findings.

Yet, in spite of methodological limitations, the Kinsey studies were none the less groundbreaking in terms of their impact – particularly with regard to opening up an understanding of sexual conduct independent of heterosexual reproduction. Kinsey's understanding, on the contrary, situated both heterosexual sexuality and reproductive sexuality within a far broader repertoire of normal sexual expression:

> Biologists and psychologists who have accepted the doctrine that the only natural function of sex is reproduction have simply ignored the existence of sexual activity which is not reproductive. They have assumed that heterosexual responses are part of an innate 'instinctive' equipment, and that all other types of sexual activity represent 'perversions' of the 'normal instincts'. Such interpretations are, however, mystical.
>
> (Kinsey *et al.* 1953, p. 448)

In broadening the definition of 'normal' sexuality – and in a sense defining all forms of sexual experience (though not without some ambiguity) as 'natural' – Kinsey and his colleagues dismissed any sense of unacceptable perversion but also any kind of uniform development in terms of sexual desire and experience over the life course. On the contrary, his data confirmed the immense variability of sexual experience, with different statistical patterns emerging depending on the questions posed in analysis. This was perhaps most widely discussed in relation to homosexuality in which Kinsey developed his famous notion of a continuum, a six-point scale running from exclusively heterosexual behaviour (zero on Kinsey's scale) to exclusively homosexual behaviour (a perfect six) to describe the permutations of heterosexual, bisexual, and homosexual behaviour, while seeking to avoid the classification of different sexual identities as necessarily linked to different behavioural patterns (see Kinsey *et al.* 1948).

Kinsey's documentation of sexual diversity and variation may have been empirically questionable, marred as it was by sampling limitations. However, there can be little doubt of the repercussions that it had more broadly, through the media coverage and popular debate that quickly became associated with both volumes and in the extensive follow-up research it would stimulate over many years. As Weeks has written:

> When it became possible to say, on the basis of what is still the most thorough investigation ever done, that 37 per cent of the male sample had had sexual contact to orgasm with another male, then even if the sample was unrepresentative and the percentage figures were exaggerated, homosexual activity could no longer be seen as a morbid

symptom of a tiny, sick minority. At least amongst a significant section of American life it was a fairly common occurrence. And if this was true of homosexuality, then it was potentially true also for a wide range of other sexualities, from bestiality to paedophilia, from sado-masochism to a passion for pornography. Kinsey was fascinated by the range of variations in human sexual behaviours.

(Weeks 1986, p. 76)

Indeed, the overriding tolerance for sexual diversity that seemed to characterize Kinsey's work (and that caused many to condemn him as morally bankrupt or personally perverse), and the naturalist basis for this position, clearly place Kinsey at the height of the sexological tradition. Like other earlier writers, only perhaps more so, his work sought to provide a scientific basis that would embrace the broadest possible range of sexual expression as part of the scientific record of human behaviour, recognizing that, from a biological perspective, no form of sexual 'outlet' could be classified as 'right or wrong' (Pomeroy 1972, p. 77).

These same characteristics that typified Kinsey's work also led to significant political controversy and public outcry when his findings were published. Some of the objections were couched in scientific terms – in particular, the criticism that his statistical sampling was flawed and should be validated with a random sample (Cochran et al. 1953).[3] But the biggest uproar was caused by the fact that his findings directly contradicted social norms with regard to the sexual behaviours and experiences of both men and women. Kinsey's study reported masturbation, for example, to be frequent in a period when it was still highly stigmatized. It reported extra-marital relations to be far more frequent than had been acknowledged, without necessarily having a negative impact on preserving marriage. In a time when homosexuality was almost universally taboo, Kinsey's data suggested that homosexual feelings and behaviours were far more common than previously believed. In the book on female sexuality, published in an era when the asexuality of women was assumed by many to be the norm, Kinsey's data documented the widespread experience of female orgasm. Perhaps most controversial of all – at the time of his writings up until the present – in a society that resolutely condemned sexual relations between adults and children or minors, Kinsey's retrospective data tended to suggest that many individuals who experienced intergenerational sex as children were not seriously harmed by it (see Bullough 1994, 1998, di Mauro 1995, Robinson 1976).[4]

With the publication of the second major volume in 1953, public outcry over Kinsey's work reached a high point. Shortly thereafter, in 1954, the American Medical Association attacked Kinsey for provoking what it claimed was a wave of sex hysteria. Louis Heller, a conservative Congressman from New York, accused Kinsey of contributing to the spread of juvenile delinquency and depravity, and called for an investigation of his work, urging that his books be banned from the US mail service (see Fausto-Sterling 1992). The accumulated effect of such criticisms was to undermine both Kinsey's reputation and the funding for his research. Key staff members at the National Research Council were in favour of continuing support for Kinsey's work and made a formal request to the Rockefeller Foundation for new funds. By this time, however, Kinsey's work as well as his funding sources had caught the attention of conservative forces in the US Congress (during an extremely conservative time, when the House Un-American Activities Committee hearings and fears of communist influence on American life dominated much of the attention in Washington, DC), and both Kinsey and the Rockefeller Foundation were threatened with an investigation by the Congressional Committee to Investigate Tax Exempt Foundations, chaired by conservative Tennessee Congressman Carroll Reece (Bullough 1985, 1994, 1998, di Mauro 1995, Fausto-Sterling 1992). In February 1954, the Foundation's new President, Dean Rusk (who would later become US Secretary of State under Presidents John F. Kennedy and Lyndon B. Johnson), began reconsidering funding priorities, and the request for continued support for Kinsey's research was denied.[5]

The controversies surrounding Kinsey's work and the discontinuation of funding had an extended impact on the field of sexuality research that in some ways continues to the present day. Funding for sexuality research utilizing national samples disappeared for an extended period and it was not until well into the 1960s that a number of more focused surveys began to be conducted on more narrowly defined population groups, such as young people, focusing less on the collection of broad-based data on sexual behaviour than on specific issues perceived to be social problems, such as adolescent premarital sex, contraception, and pregnancy (see di Mauro 1995, Laumann et al. 1994b). It was only in the late 1960s and the 1970s that broader work on sex in relation to reproduction and fertility issues began to be conducted in the USA and other industrialized countries. In 1969, a national survey of sexual behaviour in Sweden, which appears to be the first modern representative sex survey using a standardized questionnaire, was carried out under the leadership of Hans Zetterberg (see Feldman 1975, Michaels and Giami 1999). A national sample of 3000 adults in the USA, funded by the US National Institute of Mental Health, was conducted in 1970, but, due to legal complications, the results were not made available until 1989 (di Mauro 1995, Klassen et al. 1989). Also in 1970, a national survey on sexual conduct, led by Pierre Simon, was carried out in France and was designed by a public opinion research institute using a standardized questionnaire with male and female versions (Simon et al. 1972). A national survey using random sampling and face-to-face interviews was carried out in Finland in 1971 and replicated in 1992

(Kontula and Haavio-Mannila 1995). For the most part, these studies differed from Kinsey's pioneering work, and not only because of their increased methodological rigor. They also signalled an important shift of emphasis from sex acts themselves, defined by Kinsey primarily in terms of orgasm, to the relational context of sex and what Alain Giami (1991) has described as 'contraceptive sexuality' – heterosexual relations in an era of increased sexual liberation heavily influenced by the widespread availability of newly developed contraceptive methods.

Finally, with the emergence of HIV and AIDS in the early 1980s came a new demand for quantitative data on sexual behaviours that might exacerbate the risk of HIV infection – first among specific populations, such as gay and bisexual men or sex workers, who were identified as potential 'high risk groups', and then increasingly among the broader population in countries such as the USA, the UK, and France. Again, bodies such as the US National Research Council and the Institute of Medicine played a key role in underscoring the urgent need for such research in order to more fully understand, monitor, and respond to the evolving epidemic.[6] Many of the more targeted studies were carried out in a relatively straightforward fashion, with funding from governmental agencies such as the National Institutes of Health (NIH) in the USA and the Medical Research Council (MRC) in the UK. However, in the conservative political climates that characterized the Reagan/Bush administrations in the USA and the Thatcher government in the UK, political controversy and conservative attacks led to the cancellation of public funding for the most high-profile general population surveys.

The 1990 National Survey of Sexual Attitudes and Lifestyles (NATSAL) in the UK was made possible through support from the Wellcome Trust (though the second wave, carried out in 2000 after the Blair government had come to power, was funded by the MRC) (see Johnson et al. 1994). The National Health and Social Life Survey (NHSLS) in the USA was subjected to acrimonious criticism on the floor of Congress, and the Division of Health and Human Services cancelled previously awarded funding based on the NIH peer review process. Ultimately the NHSLS was only made possible through the intervention of a coalition of private foundations headed by the Robert Wood Johnson Foundation (Laumann et al. 1994a, 1994b).[7] The French National Survey on Sexual Behaviour (ACSF – Analyse des Comportements Sexuels en France), on the contrary, appears to have caused relatively little controversy, and was made possible through the financial support of the French National AIDS Research Agency (ANRS – Agence Nationale de Recherches sur le Sida) (Spira et al. 1994).

Just as the wave of surveys conducted in the late 1960s and the 1970s are products of their time, the surveys carried out primarily in response to HIV and AIDS also represent a 'new model for the study of sexual behaviour understood as an epidemiological problem' (Michaels and Giami

1999, p. 410). They are marked by decreased interest in issues such as orgasm, masturbation, procreation, and contraception (other than condom use), and by a significant increase in attention to disease transmission, casual as well as regular sexual partnerships, homosexual activity, and both oral and anal sex in addition to vaginal intercourse. Yet, unlike the manifold studies of adolescent sexuality that would burst forth in the USA during the 1970s and 1980s, the HIV-related surveys did take into account diverse sexual relations. For the demographically oriented research on adolescents as well as adults, only one kind of sex existed: the heterosexual coital kind, that is, the kind that could produce a pregnancy (see Petchesky 1990, ch. 5, and below).

In reviewing the history of survey research on sexual behaviour it is particularly striking that even though quantitative surveys have been treated as a kind of gold standard for scientific method and rigor in sex research, they have varied widely in their conception and implementation. As a consequence their comparability, as well as their validity and reliability, are in many instances seriously compromised. While Kinsey may have hoped to naturalize sexuality through his exhaustive method, he could not escape the normative and moral context within which his research was developed – just as the work following in his scientific footsteps has been shaped by prevailing contextual and historical circumstances. This is made vividly clear by the huge political controversies – and the wide variability of political responses – that surrounded not only Kinsey's studies but also many of the surveys that followed him, no matter how much more sophisticated they have become in terms of methodological rigor (see Giami 1991, 1996, Michaels and Giami 1999).

Sexuality, demography, and development

The First World War was important in shifting much sex research from Europe to the USA and in providing new financial incentives for the development of a science of sexuality. Similarly, developments in the period following the Second World War shaped research agendas and epistemological approaches to sexuality in a number of important ways. As we saw in the controversies Kinsey's research ignited, the years following the end of the Second World War were marked by a growing conservatism in the USA, which had a serious (and surprisingly long-term) impact on sexuality research in that country. The period was characterized by the emerging Cold War between the USA and the Soviet Union and a shift of attention from the North Atlantic to development and modernization challenges in the countries of Africa, Asia, and Latin America. A revival of neo-Malthusian concern with population growth as a force impeding development and threatening political stability provided new impetus for the development of demography and population research as an important vehicle for extending some of the same kinds of epistemological approaches that had characterized sexology in Europe and the USA.

Just how deeply these processes were intertwined may best be seen in observing the shift in attention from sexology to demography and population research in the early 1950s when the Kinsey controversies exploded in the USA. It was during this period that the Rockefeller philanthropies withdrew their support for Kinsey and other sex researchers and moved decisively into the field of population studies and population planning. In 1952, John D. Rockefeller III played a key role in establishing the Population Council – with significant initial funding from the Rockefeller Brothers Fund – providing an organizational base for the support of research on societies outside of the USA. This initiative would become especially important in 1954 when the Rockefeller Foundation cut off its funding for US-based sex research (Bullough 1985, 1994, di Mauro 1995). The Rockefellers were hardly the only influential players to invest in issues of population and development following the war. They would be joined by a range of private and public donors, including other philanthropic institutions such as the Ford Foundation and later The John D. and Catherine T. MacArthur Foundation, the Hewlett and Packard Foundation, and others as well as governmental agencies such as the US Agency for International Development and intergovernmental agencies such as the UN Fund for Population Activities (now the UN Population Fund) and the World Bank.[8]

The whole issue of population and population control – together with a complex set of relationships among eugenics, racism, and colonialism – had long been a dark underside to the growing preoccupation with the scientific study of sexuality in Europe and the USA (see Bandarage 1997, Ewen and Ewen 2006, Petchesky 1990, Weeks 1981, 1985). Francis Galton, a cousin of Charles Darwin, founded the eugenics movement in the mid-nineteenth century. Galton was a major figure in nineteenth-century science and is credited with creating key statistical concepts such as 'correlation' and 'regression toward the mean'. He was especially well known for his studies of gifted individuals and for applying statistical methods to analyse human differences in intelligence – in particular, the *inheritance* of intelligence. He was also credited with introducing the use of questionnaires and surveys for collecting data on social relations and the now famous phrase, 'nature vs. nurture'. In 1883, Galton coined the term 'eugenics' from the Greek root meaning 'noble in heredity' to describe the study of 'the agencies under social control that may improve or impair racial qualities' (Kelves 1985, p. ix):

> He maintained that society should not leave evolution to chance but that scientists should help governments to implement policies aimed at engineering biological improvements in people. The time had come, he

believed, to interfere in the slow process of 'natural selection', which Charles Darwin had discovered.

(Quine 1996, p. 11)

The eugenics movement quickly became popular in Europe and the USA, particularly among middle-class professionals.[9] Many of the British and American writers who began to focus on sex and sex research in the late nineteenth and early twentieth centuries were influenced by, or had formal connections with, the eugenics movement. Scientists such as Karl Pearson, for example, who was one of the founders of statistics as a distinct discipline, was a key advocate for what he called 'sexualogy' and for many key eugenic ideas. While Galton focused much of his attention on elite populations, followers such as Pearson decried the high birth rates of the poor and argued that what he described as the 'higher races' must supplant the 'lower' in order for human society to progress. In the USA, eugenicists placed special emphasis on the superiority of the 'white race' over and above all others, and drew on Alfred Binet's intelligence tests to justify the superiority of both the white race and the upper classes. They called for population control using contraceptives and voluntary or involuntary sterilization in order to contain those populations they viewed as undesirable: the poor, blacks and other racial minorities, immigrants, the disabled, and the so-called 'feeble-minded'. Indeed, much of the early birth control/contraceptive movement was closely linked to the eugenics movement, and many feminist and radical political activists such as Margaret Sanger remained publicly uncritical in relation to the problematic and fundamentally racist underpinnings of eugenic thinking, even tenuously associating with the eugenics movement.[10]

Over the first half of the twentieth century, with varying degrees of sophistication, thinkers, policy makers, and activists influenced by eugenics sought to substantiate their claims through a positivist reliance on scientific methodology – and in particular on newly developed quantitative tools such as censuses, intelligence testing, and the use of statistics to address an array of social problems (Petchesky 1990). Different human populations thus became subject to measurement, and the emerging disciplines of population studies and demography took on special importance. Both in Europe and in the USA, the emergence of population studies as a field – as evidenced by the creation, in 1928, of the Union for the Scientific Investigation of Population Problems (renamed the International Union for the Scientific Study of Population (IUSSP) in 1947) and the Population Association of America in 1931 – provided the intellectual space for debating and refining eugenic ideas and for giving them the scientific legitimacy perceived as necessary in order to substantiate their political claims.[11] Indeed, analysts such as Susan Greenhalgh (1996) suggest it was partly due to its close association with such political movements as eugenics (as well as birth control, immigration restrictions, and compulsory sterilization) that demography became practically driven to develop as 'the most scientistic' of the social science disciplines:

> Lacking a home in the university, students of population in the early twentieth century lacked status, security, and access to regular funding. Thus, from the very beginning, population specialists had a particularly strong professional need to construct their field as a science in order to acquire the social status, intellectual authority, and material resources that the more institutionalized social sciences enjoyed.
>
> (Greenhalgh 1996, p. 30)

While an emphasis on hard science and mathematical technique has been a constant of demographic thinking over the past century, the political propositions that have figured so prominently in its early development have, of course, not gone unquestioned. For example, by the mid-1930s and early 1940s, with the rise of fascism in Europe, the potential consequences of many key eugenics approaches became evident. The German sterilization laws passed in 1933 eventually led to the sterilization of more than 200,000 women perceived to be 'inferiors', and the atrocities perpetuated in the Nazi gas chambers helped to discredit much of the eugenic thinking that had been evolving in the period between the First World War and the Second World War. The irony here is that the Nazis learned their sterilization techniques and the eugenic theories to back them up from the intense crusades to sterilize 'mental defectives' and others deemed 'unfit' in the USA, led by eugenicists Harry Laughlin and Madison Grant in the 1920s and 1930s. Despite the supposed discrediting of eugenics in the wake of Nazi atrocities, '[b]etween 1907 and 1968, an estimated sixty thousand forced sterilizations [took place] in the United States'; moreover, Hitler fashioned the Third Reich's Sterilization Law on the model law drafted by Laughlin and passed in the state of Virginia (Ewen and Ewen 2006, p. 299). This shameful legacy is too often forgotten, as is the sexual apartheid implicit in forced sterilization and anti-miscegenation laws as prototypes of biopolitics.

In the immediate post-war period, while the racial, gender, and class underpinnings of demographic science and its practices remained intact, its objects of analysis and geopolitical scale began to change. Having emerged from the war as the major world power, the USA turned its attention to what were now labelled 'developing countries'. Emerging nations of the so-called Third World were no longer perceived as European colonies but rather as sources for the raw materials needed by the post-war industrial boom and as candidates for the industrialization and modernization that would deliver them from Soviet socialism to capitalist democracy. At the same time, earlier fears of the 'invading hordes' would now be replaced by a new image of the 'population bomb' and claims that rapid population growth in these emerging nations was fuelling many of the evils of under-development, such as hunger and disease, and posing serious risks for their political and economic growth and stability. In spite of doubts raised by the twentieth century's cataclysmic encounter with fascism, then, it was none the less a relatively easy step for many key eugenic ideas to be trans-ferred to this new site in the battle for elite hearts and minds.

While the governments of the USA, the UK, and other world powers recognized the perils of overpopulation in the 'Third World', the problem of population control in the developing world was first addressed through private organizations and foundations. In the 1940s, for example, the publications of the Planned Parenthood Federation began to emphasize the problem of overpopulation, and in 1948, largely through the efforts of Margaret Sanger, the International Planned Parenthood Federation was founded (with funds from the Cleveland-based Brush foundation, which was linked to the US eugenics movement and based in offices in London provided by the British Eugenics Society). In 1952, as they began with-drawing support from sexuality research in the USA, the Rockefellers turned their attention to the problems of overpopulation, founding the Population Council, as described above, and focusing on 'the relationship of population to material and cultural resources of the world' as one of the most crucial problems of the post-war era (Hartmann 1995, p. 102). By 1955, the Population Council was advising the government of India on setting up family planning programmes, and shortly thereafter was provid-ing technical support to Pakistan and later Bangladesh.

By the beginning of the 1960s, the 'population dilemma' had come to be widely accepted both by private organizations as well as governments in the industrialized West. Funds began to flow from private sources such as the Ford Foundation, the Rockefeller Foundation, and the Population Council, as well as from government agencies like USAID and intergovern-mental institutions like UNFPA and the World Bank, into development organizations focusing on family planning and population control activ-ities. Investments were also channelled into universities and academic insti-tutions to advance population science particularly focused on the Third World. It was through population studies, in turn, that the systematic scientific study of sexuality – or at least those aspects of sexuality related to fertility and fertility control – would be extended from sexological research originally developed in the Northern contexts of Western Europe and the USA, to the Southern realities of countries in the developing world.

Over the course of the 1970s and the 1980s, large-scale demographic surveys became a primary way of knowing about sexuality, at least in rela-tion to reproduction, across the developing world. The most large-scale efforts included the World Fertility Surveys (WFS), internationally comparable surveys on human fertility that were carried out in 42 developing countries (and in 20 developed countries) with nationally representative samples. These surveys were implemented from the early 1970s through the early 1980s. From the late 1970s to the mid-1980s they were complemented by the Contraceptive Prevalence Surveys (CPS), focusing on family planning and contraceptive use. Beginning in the mid-1980s, and continuing up to the present, the Demographic and Health Surveys combined the qualities of the WFS and the CPS and added important questions on maternal and child health and nutrition, with nationally representative household samples and large sample sizes ranging between 5000 and 30,000 households. With primary funding support from agencies such as UNFPA and USAID, as well as the involvement of key population science associations such as IUSSP and leading population research centres in Western Europe and the USA, these large-scale surveys have been the primary source of data on sexuality and reproduction for purposes of policy making and planning – and, as we will discuss in greater detail in Chapter 6, have also incorporated important questions related to aspects of sexual health and sexually transmitted infections in the wake of HIV and AIDS.

Only a few surprises have emerged from these extensive (and expensive) studies. For instance, contrary to neo-Malthusian assumptions, fertility rates have declined in a number of developing countries as a result of transformed gender relations and increased access to education and contraception.[12] Such findings would change the policy climate and favour the population paradigm shift of the 1990s as consolidated in the ICPD Programme of Action guidelines on gender equality, women's empowerment, health, and human rights (Corrêa 1997, Petchesky 2000, 2003, Sen 1995). However, concerns with fertility and its correlation with economics have not disappeared. Since the early 2000s, a number of books and articles have been published with the aim of bringing demographics back into the picture (Birdsal et al. 2001, Bloom et al. 2003, Bongaarts 2005).[13]

The resurgence of demography's focus on fertility and reproductive relations, as opposed to sexuality and sexual practice more broadly defined, has limited the ability of population studies to adequately address the full range of sexual conduct found in diverse societies and cultures – although, it must be said, there are some remarkable examples of population studies that have broken through these narrow boundaries (see, e.g., Berquó 2000, 2006, Presser and Sen 2000). While the topical focus of traditional demographic studies has gradually broadened (particularly after HIV became a serious concern) to embrace a wider vision of sexuality, the methodological approaches and the underlying assumptions about the biomedical roots of sexual desire place serious limits on the range of interpretive frameworks that are used to make sense of sexual experience.

Sexuality has generally been understood as a universal physiological drive, rooted in our shared biology (or, at times, psychology) as human beings, and hence measurable and analysable in accord with the basic precepts of a positivist science of human behaviour (Corrêa and Parker 2004). Moreover, the presumed binary sexed structure and heterosexual destiny of this 'shared biology' – and thus what it even means to be human – has gone entirely unquestioned. Indeed, it would seem that the most enlightened findings of sexologists such as Krafft-Ebing and Kinsey on sexual diversity were swept aside in demography's singular preoccupation with fertility and curbing population growth.

Just as this conception of sexual desire has limited the possibilities for demographic analysis of sexual practices, the typical units of demographic research and analysis – the individual, the household, and the country – have generally been reproduced in the investigation of sexuality (Corrêa and Parker 2004). The limitations of focusing exclusively on the individual are evidenced even in the case of fertility surveys and analyses; as we will discuss in Chapter 5, most feminist anthropological research on reproductive decisions and fertility outcomes emphasizes the contextual and relational character of these phenomena, which can never be adequately captured by research focused only on individual women. Over the course of the 1990s, Demographic and Health Surveys began to include men in their samples in some countries. Yet this has not been enough to fundamentally reframe the units of analysis and has largely failed to incorporate social science findings that have increasingly called attention to the importance of sexual cultures and the broader sociocultural context in which sexuality is constituted or constructed.

The typical demographic focus on households has also posed a number of problems by tending to ignore the heterogeneity of households that may exist in different social systems. Particularly in the case of fertility and health research and analysis, the household has been assumed to be the main place where sex (of the procreative couple) takes place – an assumption that is easily transposed to sexuality research. Qualitative research indicates, however, that sexual interactions are not confined to a couple's bedroom – or to couples. They can occur anywhere: at home, in the streets, at the workplace, and among groups as well as in casual encounters. The concepts of networks and spatial dynamics are much more appropriate than 'fixed units' to capture sexualities at play, even when the major focus of analysis is fertility outcomes. The fact that not all 'mothers' have become pregnant in the marital bedroom is something that many demographers have not yet fully grasped (Corrêa and Parker 2004).

Finally, the country (or nation state), which is assumed to be the most important unit of demographic analysis, is also problematic, especially when the subject under examination is sexuality. Large aggregates can provide relevant insights in terms of demographic and epidemiological dynamics, but they do not lead to linear correlations with sexual practices, meanings, and trends. The demographic aggregate description of countries has a strong appeal for crystallizing the image of a 'national sexual pattern', yet this description typically oversimplifies reality and almost never fits with the lived experience of sexualities at the local level, let alone for individuals. As in the case of the household, the unit of 'the country' does not permit researchers to describe and analyse sexual flows (linked to migration, for example) that increasingly cross borders, or the kinds of cultural influences that may shape sexuality in an interconnected, global-ized world (Corrêa and Parker 2004; see also Chapters 5 and 6).

The science of sex from one turn of the century to the next

From the turn of the twentieth to the turn of the twenty-first century, the project of building a scientific study of sexuality and reproduction has been an ongoing effort in fields as disparate as medicine and psychiatry, anthropology and sociology, and public opinion research and social demography. In spite of some disciplinary differences, as well as a number of important changes that have taken place over time, research and analy-sis in this positivist tradition have generally shared a number of important commonalities. Nearly all of the work emerging from this tradition has conceived of sex as a kind of natural force that exists in opposition to civilization, culture, or society. While researchers have differed on whether or not the sex drive was a positive force warped by a negative civilization (as Ellis and Kinsey tended to see it) or a negative force in need of social control (as Freud and most of his followers tended to view it), they gener-ally agreed on the power of sexuality to define who we are as human beings (Gagnon and Parker 1995).

Alongside this 'force of nature' model, sexual sciences have also had an equally strong propensity to reduce the question of sex to some kind of underlying drive or essence – a biological or psychological imperative that ultimately determines the meaning of even the most seemingly disparate beliefs and practices. This underlying 'essentialism' of the scientific, sexo-logical project, reproduced in population studies and demographic think-ing, has continued up until the present to provide the dominant framework for the investigation and understanding of human sexuality across both time and space. It was not without a trace of irony that Foucault called this reductive notion of 'sex' 'the most speculative, most ideal, and most internal element in a deployment of sexuality organized by power in its grip on bodies and their materiality, their forces, energies, sensations, and pleasures' (1978, p. 155).

The essentialist approach has not gone unquestioned even though it continues to be the predominant paradigm within the field of sex research and is the focus for the lion's share of research activities and funding in fields ranging from biomedical to public health and much social science research. In the next chapter, on the social construction of sexuality and sexual experience, we turn to major critiques of this dominant paradigm, particularly on the part of thinkers influenced by feminism, Marxism, and sexual liberation movements.

Chapter 5

The social construction of sexual life

While essentialist ideas have continued to dominate much thinking about sexual life, they constitute a perspective that came under increasing attack during the latter part of the twentieth century. By the mid- to late 1960s, it was becoming apparent to many that the 'sexological paradigm' had started to disintegrate. Whether in structuralist thought, Marxist theory, or certain streams of psychoanalysis, the 1970s and 1980s were characterized by a new willingness to call into question the 'naturalness' of all human experience. Since much of the power of sex seemed linked to biological being and the experience of the body, sexuality was perhaps more resistant to such interrogation than many other areas of human life, but even here, important doubts began to be raised from a number of different theoretical vantage points. The primary challenge came from social theorists and researchers working on issues related to gender and sexuality and from activists, particularly from the feminist and emerging gay and lesbian movements, who questioned key elements of the sexological paradigm that they viewed as antithetical to their most important interests (Gagnon and Parker 1995).

Changing conceptual frameworks

There were at least three distinct disciplinary approaches used in interrogating the supposedly 'natural' basis of gender and sexuality. In sex research itself, the work of sociologists such as John H. Gagnon, William Simon, and Kenneth Plummer, who were heavily influenced by symbolic interactionist theory, was especially important. Psychoanalytical theory has also provided key tools and insights to challenge sex essentialism as exemplified by works of continental European writers such as Jacques Lacan, Gilles Deleuze, Félix Guatarri, and Guy Hocquenghem, and of feminists such as Juliet Mitchell, Jessica Benjamin, and Nancy Chodorow. A third, distinct set of challenges emerged in the historical analyses of Michel Foucault, Randolph Trumbach, Robert Padgug, Jeffrey Weeks, John D'Emilio, and Estelle Freedman, and in the anthropological work of writers such as Gayle Rubin, Esther Newton, Gilbert Herdt, Peter Fry, and Carole Vance.[1]

Having served as senior researchers at the Kinsey Institute, Gagnon and Simon were in a unique position to offer a telling critique of the naturalist, or essentialist, position. In work beginning as early as the mid-1960s and continuing through to the 1990s, they sought to move from the categorizing empiricism of essentialist thought to a new concern with the significance or meaning that a sexual act has for the actor (Gagnon and Simon 1973, Simon and Gagnon 1984, 1986, 1987). In so doing, they linked this subjective meaning to the wider social and cultural context in which the sexual act takes place. They argued that sexual life is subject to a 'socio-cultural molding ... surpassed by few other forms of human behavior' (Gagnon and Simon 1973, p. 26), and were thus among the foremost proponents of the notion that 'sexual meanings' are socially constituted or constructed.

In developing this position, Gagnon and Simon, as well as Plummer and others working within an interactionist perspective, drew on a theoretical tradition stretching back to the work of writers such as Alfred Schutz (1967 [orig. 1932]) and George Herbert Mead (1934). From this perspective, the subjective significance of sexual life is built up in the flow of social life in interaction with other social actors. It links the question of sex to that of social inequality through the analysis of sexual deviance and gender difference as social facts. Gagnon and Simon suggested that perhaps nothing in human life should be seen as intrinsically sexual, but that virtually anything can be given sexual significance within a determined social context. They also drew on the dramatistic perspective of writers such as Kenneth Burke (1945) and Erving Goffman (1959) in developing the notion that sexual behaviour is thus socially 'scripted' – that meaningful sexual practices are produced according to socially determined scenarios, rules, and sanctions, which make possible certain understandings of the sexual world while excluding others:

> Scripts are a metaphor for conceptualizing the production of behaviour within social life. Most of social life most of the time must operate under the guidance of an operating syntax, much as language is a precondition for speech. For behaviour to occur, something resembling scripting must occur on three distinct levels: cultural scenarios, interpersonal scripts, and intra-psychic scripts.
>
> (Simon and Gagnon 1999, p. 29)

Gagnon and Simon defined cultural scenarios as 'instructional guides' existing at the level of collective social life – systems of signs and symbols through which the requirements for the practice of specific roles are given. These scenarios, they argued, are generally too abstract to be applied in all circumstances. The possibility of a lack of congruence between the abstract scenario and the concrete situation must be resolved by the creation of interpersonal scripts – a process that transforms the social actor into a scriptwriter, adapting and shaping the materials of cultural scenarios into scripts for behaviour in specific contexts. The need to script one's behaviour, as well as to anticipate the scripted behaviour of others, is what creates a kind of 'internal rehearsal' (what Simon and Gagnon described as 'intra-psychic scripting'), the symbolic reorganization of reality in ways that allow individual desires to be linked to social meanings. Their work thus called attention to the fact that nothing is intrinsically 'sexual' and that anything can be 'sexualized' in a given social context. Lacy lingerie or black leather may indeed incite desire or become the object of fantasy in specific cultural systems, but such desires or fantasies are learned responses rather than intrinsically grounded in some kind of underlying human nature. Even solitary sexual acts and masturbatory fantasies thus become socially constructed precisely because they are typically articulated in relation to a world of images and meanings that are appropriated, through intra-psychic scripting, from the wider social universe outside the individual and his or her subjective experience.

Within this framework, an understanding of the roots of sexuality, and the challenges that need to be faced in seeking to investigate sexual experience, is radically different from perspectives developed in more naturalist or essentialist approaches to sexual life. In contrast to the deep hermeneutic of Freudian psychoanalysis or the hydraulic theory of biological urges, emphasis is placed much more directly on the experience of desire, not simply as an individual reality but as part and parcel of the constitution of the individual's social existence. As Simon and Gagnon put it, 'Desire is not reducible to an appetite, a drive, an instinct; it does not create the self, rather it is part of the process of the creation of the self' (Simon and Gagnon 1999, p. 30).[2]

While Gagnon and Simon's work on sexual scripts was pioneering and is probably the best-known example of using an interactionist approach to study sexuality, this approach has been further developed over a number of decades by a range of researchers (see Longmore 1998). Laws and Schwartz, for example, sought to apply scripting theory to explore women's sexuality (Laws and Schwartz 1977). Plummer's work on interactionism and sexual identity has drawn on interactionist theories of 'deviance' as well as Goffman's classic work on stigma (Goffman 1963) and has used them, together with social labelling theory, to analyse the construction of sexual identities and sexual stigma (Plummer 1975). Arguing that sexuality 'has no meaning other than that given to it in social situations' (Plummer 1982, p. 233), Plummer and others working along similar lines have emphasized the fundamentally contingent character of sexual meanings – as well as the fact that sexual development must be thought of as a kind of 'life-long learning process which is historically malleable' (Plummer 1982, p. 235). Plummer called attention to the stories that human beings tell in order to create sexual meaning and to the ways in which the invention of the sexual self has increasingly blurred the boundaries between private and public experience in contemporary social life (Plummer 1995, 2003). Drawing on ethnomethodology as well as interactionism, this work has also sought to explore the ways in which male and female are practically accomplished through 'doing gender', with important consequences for social stratification along the lines of gender as played out structurally in social spaces or domains of family, work, the state, and so on (Kessler and McKenna 1978, West and Zimmerman 1991).

Although work drawing on social interactionism has created an important alternative to the positivist science of sexuality that has dominated the field, it has arguably been more effective in describing sexual diversity than in theorizing about it (Weeks 1999a, p. 129). Interactionist accounts recognize the inequalities that exist between different groups and the ways in which social stratification may impact on patterns of sexual conduct, but the interactionist framework has provided relatively little insight into the variables at work in relation to structural differentials in power and authority. Thus interactionist work has not provided a theoretical grounding for political action seeking to address inequality and power in relation to sexuality. Perhaps because of this, while interactionist work has made an important contribution to research on sexual experience, interest has also focused on a number of other approaches that might provide a more far-reaching theoretical framework for challenging sexual oppression.

Although drawing inspiration from very different sources, an equally important critique of the essentialist position emerged at about the same time – the structuralist influence most closely associated with the work of Lacan in psychoanalysis (Lacan 1968, 1977, 1981; see also Mannoni 1971, Turkle 1981). Moving away from the biological emphasis present in much early psychoanalytic writing, Lacan and his followers turned increasingly to a concern with language and its role in the constitution of both the unconscious and sexual desire. They concentrated on the entry of 'society' into the mind of the child; on the child's movement from an 'imaginary order' that emphasizes his/her bond with the mother to a 'symbolic order' in which the law of the father imposes itself and gives rise to an unconscious and ultimately insatiable desire to be the other, to be the father (Lacan 1977). As Weeks has pointed out:

> In Lacan's 'recovery' of Freud, it is the law of the father, the castration fear and the pained entry into the symbolic order – the order of language – at the Oedipal moment which instigates desire.... It is the expression of a fundamental absence, which can never be fulfilled, the desire to be the other, the father, which is both alienated and insa-

tiable: alienated because the child can only express its desire by means of language which itself constitutes its submission to the father, and insatiable because it is desire for a symbolic position which is itself arbiter of the possibilities for the expression of desire. The law of the father therefore constitutes both desire and the lack on which it is predicated.

(Weeks 1999b, p. 127)

While the Lacanian formulation tended to reproduce many of the universalistic assumptions found in earlier psychoanalytic frameworks, its extension in the work of writers such as Juliet Mitchell, Jane Gallop, Elizabeth Grosz, Gilles Deleuze, Félix Guattari, and Guy Hocquenghem has also sought to more fully historicize the Oedipal situation by focusing on the particular contexts of patriarchal society and capitalist economy. In *Psychoanalysis and Feminism* (1974), for example, Mitchell drew heavily on Lacan's reading of Freud in order to focus on the production of male domination within the symbolic world of the unconscious:

In the briefest possible terms we could say that psychoanalysis is about the material reality of ideas both within, and of, man's history; thus in 'penis-envy' we are talking not about an anatomical organ, but about the ideas of it that people hold and live by within general culture, the order of human society. It is this last factor that also prescribes the reference point of psychoanalysis. The way we live as 'ideas' the necessary laws of human society is not so much conscious as *unconscious* – the particular task of psychoanalysis is to decipher how we acquire our heritage of the ideas and laws of human society within the unconscious mind, or, to put it another way, the unconscious mind *is* the way in which we acquire these laws.

(Mitchell 1974, p. xiv)

In Mitchell's reading of psychoanalysis, then, the phallus becomes the central signifier, in Lacan's sense, as a cluster of words, images, and ideas: 'the very mark of human desire' (Mitchell 1974, p. 395). But this is clearly located socially in relation to patriarchy:

'Patriarchy' is a vague term; in anthropology we are used to the greater precisions of 'patrilineal', 'patrilateral', 'patrilocal', but these omit to tell us about power and a general law. I have taken patriarchy to be the law of the father – and it is the operation of this law within the life of the individual boy and girl that Freud's work can help us to understand ... the operations of a patriarchal system that must by definition oppress women.

(Mitchell 1974, pp. xiv–xv)

This focus on the production and reproduction of patriarchal domination through the symbolic order, which can be captured by psychoanalytic interpretation, was an important step beyond Lacan and a key feminist contribution to the analysis of sexuality in the 1970s and 1980s. In the work of Mitchell and similar feminist thinkers, however, it still remained an essentially universalistic formulation linked to the overarching structures of patriarchal domination.[3] The writings of Deleuze and Guattari sought to move beyond psychoanalysis by focusing on the symbolic order of the unconscious, not in relation to patriarchy but rather in relation to capitalism.

For Deleuze and Guattari, as for Lacan, the forms of desire are produced not by nature but by social relations – but they none the less rejected psychoanalysis and the psychoanalytic notion of the Oedipus complex as a necessary stage in human development. They criticized Lacan for working within the Freudian psychoanalytic framework, arguing that this framework is trapped within the capitalist social and economic order. In their major work, *Anti-Oedipus: Capitalism and Schizophrenia* (Deleuze and Guatarri 1977 [orig. 1972]), they sought to move beyond both Marxism and psychoanalysis arguing that capitalist society trains us to believe that desire equals *lack* and therefore the only way to satisfy desire is to *consume*. Rejecting both psychoanalysis and the capitalist system that produced it, they argued, on the contrary, that rather than being produced by a 'fundamental absence', as the psychoanalytic formulation would have it, desire is in fact a *productive force* – that human beings should be understood as 'desiring machines' and that every person's machine parts can plug into and unplug from the machine parts of other people in an almost infinite variety of relationships. From their perspective, the psychoanalytic notion of the 'self' is an illusion – there is no single or unified self, but rather a fundamental fragmentation. Because capitalist society cannot live with the infinite variety of desires, interconnections, and relationships, it imposes constraints aimed at regulating and channelling desire, such as the social norms that concentrate reproduction in the nuclear family. By focusing its attention on the Oedipal relationship between parent and child, psychoanalytic theory – as much in its Freudian articulation as in Lacan's reinvention – thus reproduces the forms of domination present in capitalist society and offers no real hope, in Deleuze and Guattari's reading, of a radical critique capable of overcoming such domination.[4]

In focusing on desire as a productive force and grounding their analysis historically in relation to capitalism, Deleuze and Guattari's approach provided an alternative not only to psychoanalysis, but also to previous work on the social dimensions of sexuality. Their work placed new emphasis on links between sex, language, and power not in terms of the linguistic structures that establish the authority of the father and the subservience of the mother within contexts of patriarchal domination, but rather in regard to the channelling and control of sexual desire under capitalist systems of production. This emphasis on the social production of sexuality would, in turn, prove to be an important influence on a new wave of historical and anthropological work focusing on gender and sexuality over the course of the 1970s and 1980s.[5] The work carried out along these lines by Foucault and the writers who have followed him, in seeking to examine the 'history of sexuality' in Western civilization, has been particularly important and influential.[6] Eschewing both the interactionist and the psychoanalytic traditions, Foucault was able to step outside the central arguments that typified the examination of sex in Western societies to relativize the very terms of the debate and to analyse the naturalist understanding of sexuality as itself a cultural system:

> Sexuality must not be thought of as a kind of natural given which power tries to hold in check, or as an obscure domain which knowledge gradually tries to uncover. It is the name that can be given to a historical construct: not a furtive reality that is difficult to grasp, but a great surface network in which the stimulation of bodies, the intensification of pleasures, the incitement to discourse, the formation of special knowledges, the strengthening of controls and resistances, are linked to one another in accordance with a few major strategies of knowledge and power.
>
> (Foucault 1978, pp. 105–106)

Foucault thus focused not so much on the question of sex per se as on the question of discourse and on its relation to knowledge and power, suggesting that it is precisely through discourse, through the structures of language and ideology, that our most fundamental relation to reality is organized. With this in mind, he argued that 'sexuality' must therefore be understood not as a natural given but as an historical construct that is quite literally constituted by the discourses we have devised to talk about it (Foucault 1978).[7]

In examining this historical construct, Foucault – along with writers such as Donzelot and Weeks – turned to the 'discursive strategies' that, since at least the mid-nineteenth century, have delineated sex as a privileged object of knowledge in Western culture (Donzelot 1978, Foucault 1978, Weeks 1981). This focus on sex as an object of knowledge was correlated, in turn, to a new way of understanding power that is not simply linked to the state:

> By power, I do not mean 'Power' as a group of institutions and mechanisms that ensure the subservience of the citizens of a given state. By power, I do not mean, either, a mode of subjugation, which,

in contrast to violence, has the form of the rule. Finally, I do not have in mind a general system of domination exerted by one group over another ... these are only the terminal forms power takes. It seems to me that power must be understood in the first instance as the multiplicity of force relations, immanent in the sphere in which they operate and which constitute their own organisation; as the process which, through ceaseless struggles and confrontations transforms, strengthens, or reverses them; as the support which these force relations find in one another, thus forming a chain or a system, or on the contrary, the disfunctions and contradictions which isolate them from one another; and lastly, as the strategies in which they take effect, whose general design or institutional crystallization is embodied in the state apparatus, in the formulation of the law, in the various social hegemonies.

(Foucault 1978, pp. 92–93)

In Foucault's interpretation, the articulation of sexuality as an object of knowledge has made possible the emergence and deployment of a fundamentally new form of power in Western society – what Foucault has described as 'biopower' (Foucault 1978) – which seems to function not so much through traditional sanctions, such as the threat of violence or even death, as through the highly modern and rationalized regulation of life: 'The old power of death that symbolized sovereign power was now carefully supplanted by the administration of bodies and the calculated management of life' (Foucault 1978, pp. 139–140). Indeed, it is precisely through the various forms of knowledge elaborated around questions linked to sexuality and reproduction – in disciplines such as sexology and demography, and in the social policies, services, and sectors they have given rise to in practice – that, in Foucault's view, the operations of this new form of power were most evident.

Yet if the relations of power that quite literally constitute the sexual field appear, at one level, as a kind of seamless web or network enveloping everything in its path within determined historical junctures, this all-encompassing system of power also implies multiple points of resistance. Indeed, as Foucault stressed in his interviews and lectures as well as in his published works, 'where there is power, there is resistance' (Foucault 1978, p. 95). Yet his view of resistance was complex and unromanticized, insisting that we all always operate 'inside' power – that we participate in its 'deployment' even as we confront it – and that in this sense we simultaneously shape power even as we resist it.

This view of power and resistance, each implicated in the other, made Foucault highly sceptical of any claim concerning 'liberation' – at least to the extent that the idea of liberation would imply the existence of some kind of space outside of or apart from existing structures of power. Yet he saw the important possibilities for sexual rights movements understood in his terms as 'movements of affirmation':

> I believe that the movements labelled 'sexual liberation' ought to be understood as movements of affirmation starting with sexuality. Which means two things: they are movements that start with sexuality, with the apparatus of sexuality in the midst of which we're caught, and which make it function to the limit; but, at the same time, they are in motion relative to it, disengaging themselves and surmounting it.
>
> (Foucault 1977a, p. 155)

This formulation was clearly very different from the self-understanding of many sectors of the feminist or gay and lesbian movements that had emerged in many parts of the world during the 1960s and 1970s, but it provided an important linkage between the intellectual project of analysis aimed at deconstructing the conceptual architecture of sexuality as a discursive field and the possibilities for taking meaningful political action within this field. As in the comparable work of interactionists and psychoanalysts, sex was again linked to questions of language and power – understood to be constituted through discourse as the key point of convergence for the innumerable strategies that regulate both the life of the body and the life of the population in contemporary Western societies. In the case of Foucault and his followers, however, the lines of intersection between these phenomena were altered or transformed; rather than being subject to an externally imposed oppression or repression functioning through language and the laws which it constitutes, sexuality seems to have been positively produced not merely by discourse but by power itself as a suitable object for regulation and intervention in the modern world. Resistance became a necessary corollary to power precisely because the functioning of power necessarily implies resistance as part of its very definition.

This insight about the interconnections between power and resistance proved to be a potent source of inspiration for an ongoing examination of the relations between power and knowledge in the construction of the edifice of 'sexuality' in Western history, and thus provided perhaps the most far-reaching critique of the search for a science of sexuality. In addition to focusing attention on the role of science and sexology in constituting the sexual field as part of a broader project of Western modernity, his analysis of 'biopower' may also be applied to the role of demography in creating 'compulsory heterosexuality' – in Adrienne Rich's (2007) words – in the discourse on human development. While the familiar figures of Foucault's history (the Malthusian couple, the masturbating child, the perverse homosexual, and so on) were all fixed in Western discourse long before the emergence and development of demography as a distinct disciplinary frame, demography has none the less been crucial to the importation of these figures into the discursive tropes of contemporary development discourse. Such tropes include the fertile (or infertile) couples of population-based surveys, the unwanted pregnancies of sexually active teenagers, the epidemiological risk groups of HIV-positive homosexuals, the transmission vectors of sex workers, and so on. To the extent that demography has traditionally constructed itself as simultaneously both objective and utilitarian – as a scientific toolkit capable of providing the basis for practical interventions in the field of population – it has played a profound role in crystallizing many of the key symbolic structures and social representations employed in the service not only of gender oppression, but also of diverse forms of sexual exploitation and discrimination (see Corrêa and Parker 2004).[8]

Gender, sexuality, and the politics of difference

Foucault's work is probably best understood as analytic rather than historical, or what he himself might describe as 'the history of the present' rather than the history of the past. None the less, it exerted great influence in opening up the intellectual space for a rapidly expanding body of work in both social history and cultural anthropology. This work sought to relativize the presumed normality (or hegemony) of sexuality in contemporary Western societies, confronting these patterns with a wide array of alternative arrangements identified across both time and space. In the historical work of a growing range of researchers, the contemporary organization of sexual relations and sexual experience was juxtaposed with the very different constructions found in ancient Greece or Rome, in pre-industrial societies, in the Western world of the nineteenth or early twentieth centuries, or even in the immediate post-Second World War era in the West.[9] In much the same way, a growing number of social and cultural anthropologists began to explore the significant differences between the construction of sexuality in Western societies and the systems found in the diverse countries and cultures of sub-Saharan Africa, Asia, Latin America, and elsewhere in the so-called developing world.[10]

While the disciplinary roots of both historical and anthropological research on sexuality could clearly be found in a certain elaboration of the 'scientific/sexological' project described above in Chapter 4 – empirically documenting the range of human sexual expressions and including them in the scientific record of human diversity – the primary motivation for much of the earliest work on the social and historical construction of diverse sexualities was largely political rather than academic. The research and analysis of almost all the earliest social historians and anthropologists, who in the 1970s and early 1980s began to describe the variations of gender and sexuality historically and cross-culturally, came as much from the leftist political commitments of many of the pioneering writers as from the margins of the academy. Indeed, many of the most important early researchers worked independently or as part of progressive political collectives rather than inside universities or research institutes (see D'Emilio 1983, 1992, Katz 1976). Much of the most important historical and anthropological work carried out during this period was thus a response not only to the intellectual challenges posed by writers such as Foucault, but also to the emerging problematics of gender power and sexual diversity articulated first by the feminist movement and then increasingly by the gay and lesbian liberation movement.

In work carried out during the 1970s and 1980s, therefore, there was an important shift of emphasis as researchers sought to empirically document the social arrangements and cultural forms through which sexuality and sexual practices are differentially organized at specific points in time and space. They sought to move beyond gendered and sexualized differences, in and of themselves, to also examine the ways in which systems of hierarchy and inequality operate through both gender and sexuality in different cultural and historical contexts (Ortner and Whitehead 1981, Ross and Rapp 1983). Early work documenting the general question of inequality between the sexes sought, largely through cross-cultural comparison, to identify the social and cultural mechanisms that constitute and maintain hierarchical ideologies of gender (see, e.g., MacCormack and Strathern 1980, Reiter 1975, Rosaldo and Lamphere 1974). This led, over time, to an increasingly sophisticated analysis of concrete case studies focusing on issues of gender and reproductive relations and of the diverse organization of same-sex relations.[11] These issues, in turn, were key in the development of a more widespread recognition of what Rubin described as 'sex/gender systems': 'a set of arrangements by which a society transforms biological sexuality into products of human activity, and in which these transformed sexual needs are satisfied' (Rubin 1975, p. 159).

Human beings may have an innate biological capacity and need for sex but this fact in and of itself tells us nothing about the actual workings of sexuality. On the contrary, the focus for investigation, in Rubin's view, must be the way in which sexuality is historically produced: 'Sex as we know it – gender identity, sexual desire and fantasy, concepts of childhood – is itself a social product. We need to understand the relations of its production' (Rubin 1975, p. 166). Thus, within this formulation, the structures of sexual inequality, and even the psychological construction of desire, emerge not as a natural or biological phenomenon, but as a social product articulated within specific political and economic frameworks. The challenge for research on sexuality becomes that of developing what may be described as a 'political economy' of the sexual order – or, perhaps more broadly, a 'political economy of the body' (see, e.g., Lancaster 1995, Lancaster and di Leonardo 1997, Parker and Aggleton 1999; see also Chapter 6).

The development of work on sex/gender systems has been significantly advanced in recent decades through the application of a range of theoretical insights and methodological tools drawn from the wider field of cultural analysis and interpretive theory. Research on gender and sexuality has increasingly developed into a more all-encompassing examination of what Sherry Ortner and Harriet Whitehead described in the early 1980s as 'sexual meanings'; an analysis of the intersubjective symbolic forms and the associated structures of social organization that constitute the sexual realm in particular social and cultural contexts and invest it with subjective meaning for the concrete social actors who pass through it and live out their lives on its terms (see Ortner and Whitehead 1981).

From this point of view, the sexual universe emerges as simultaneously material and ideological – a construct that can only be fully understood when situated in relation to other social, cultural, political, and economic domains (e.g., religion, kinship, work). It is through this emphasis on sexual meanings that the whole question of sexuality is articulated with issues related to gender and reproduction, on the one hand, and the dynamics of desire, understandings of sexual pleasure, and sociocultural organization of sexual practices, on the other. Here, in the emphasis placed upon the social and cultural constitution of such meanings, the anthropological tradition, elaborated largely with reference to non-Western societies, most clearly intersects with the developments described above that have taken place in the sociological, psychological, and historical examination of sexual life in the West – the interactionism of thinkers such as Gagnon and Simon or Plummer, the psychoanalysis of Lacan and others influenced by him, such as Mitchell or Deleuze and Guattari, and the historical analyses of Foucault or Weeks. Taken together, these perspectives offered the possibility for a radically new understanding of the full range of human sexual experience – an understanding focused less on the scientific search for universal truths than on the awareness of diversity; based less on the definition of an assumed essence than on the detailed interpretation of difference.

Particularly over the course of the 1980s, this increasing emphasis on sexual meanings and on sexual diversity and difference was, in turn, linked to an important analytic distinction between gender and sexuality as key axes for the workings of power within the sexual field. Most clearly laid out by Rubin in another pioneering essay, 'Thinking sex: notes for a radical theory of the politics of sexuality' (Rubin 1984), in which she defended a clear analytical distinction between gender and sexuality rather than their unification in the notion of sex/gender systems:

> I am now arguing that it is essential to separate gender and sexuality analytically to reflect more accurately their separate social existence.

This goes against the grain of much contemporary feminist thought, which treats sexuality as a derivation of gender.

(Rubin 1984, p. 308)

Rubin recognized that an intimate link exists between these two systems, but she argued that it is important to recognize that they are not the same:

Gender affects the operation of the sexual system, and the sexual system has had gender-specific manifestations. But although sex and gender are related, they are not the same thing, and they form the basis of two distinct arenas of social practice.

(Rubin 1984, p. 308)

As Rubin continued to focus attention on the workings of gender power and gender oppression, she began outlining the characteristics of what she described as a 'sex hierarchy' that operates, at least in contemporary Western societies, as distinct from the 'gender hierarchy'. This sex hierarchy maps out the range of possible sexual practices on a kind of continuum. At one end of this continuum we find a 'good', 'natural', or 'normal' sexuality that is reproductive, monogamous, marital, non-commercial, and heterosexual and recognized as acceptable by medical, religious, and political power centres, while at the other end, at the bottom of the sex hierarchy, lie other sexual practices defined as 'evil', 'unnatural', or 'abnormal' sexual practices:

According to this system, sexuality that is 'good', 'normal', and 'natural' should ideally be heterosexual, marital, monogamous, reproductive, and non-commercial. It should be coupled, relational, within the same generation, and occur at home. It should not involve pornography, fetish objects, sex toys of any sort, or roles other than male and female. Any sex that violates these rules is 'bad', 'abnormal', or 'unnatural'. Bad sex may be homosexual, unmarried, promiscuous, non-procreative, or commercial. It may be masturbatory or take place at orgies, may be casual, may cross generational lines, and may take place in 'public', or at least in the bushes or the baths. It may involve the use of pornography, fetish objects, sex toys, or unusual roles.... [A]n imaginary line ... distinguishes these from all other erotic behaviours, which are understood to be the work of the devil, dangerous, psychopathological, infantile, or politically reprehensible.... The line appears to stand between sexual order and chaos. It expresses the fear that if anything is permitted to cross this erotic DMZ [Demilitarized Zone], the barrier against scary sex will crumble and something unspeakable will skitter across.

(Rubin 1984, pp. 280–282)

In shifting emphasis from gender to sexuality and exploring the ways in which frameworks for thinking about, investigating, and regulating sexuality have been used for purposes of oppression and domination of sexual minorities, Rubin thus played a key role in linking the analysis of sexuality, knowledge, and power developed by Foucault and his followers to a much clearer agenda for political mobilization and social change than has typically been articulated from a Foucaultian perspective. Her work suggests some of the ways in which historical and anthropological analysis might be used strategically as a point of departure not just for thinking about and knowing about sex, but for engaging in projects aimed at social and political change.[12]

Normatization, subversion, and the possibilities of queer theory

By the mid- to late 1980s, a series of seismic shocks had begun to shake the social context in which thinking on sexuality and sexual politics was developing. In countries such as the USA and the UK a conservative backlash had begun to be felt, as much in social mores as in politics, and reactionary political leaders and platforms had swept into power. Without yet having been named, or even clearly articulated, patterns of economic restructuring and processes of social, cultural, and economic integration had begun to take shape across almost all regions of the world as part of what would later come to be defined as a significant intensification of neoliberal globalization. Linked to these changes, in ways that would only begin to be fully understood over time, the HIV epidemic had emerged both North and South of the equator, creating an extended crisis within many of the sexual communities at the forefront of progressive sexual thinking and sexual politics during the 1970s and the early 1980s. The impact of HIV and AIDS, in particular, will be examined in greater detail in Chapter 6, but it is none the less important to highlight here the ways in which these interrelated changes in the broader social, cultural, political, and economic context both destabilized and provided new challenges to the important work being carried out on historical and cross-cultural differences in the construction of genders and sexualities and on the politics of sexuality.

This unsettling turmoil is especially vivid in Gayle Rubin's ethnographic and historical work during this period. For example, what began in the late 1970s as a kind of celebration of sexual rebellion and transgression on the part of the gay male S-and-M subculture in the South of Market district in San Francisco (see Rubin 1982, 1991, 2000) became by the late 1980s what Rubin described as an 'elegy' for a community that had been devastated by the HIV epidemic (Rubin 1997). Indeed, over the course of the 1980s many of the key figures in the first wave of social constructionist thought on sexuality, including Michel Foucault, died of AIDS, while many others whose work was informed in important ways by social constructionist concerns came to concentrate much of their intellectual energy on research and activism in relation to the epidemic. Some of the most insightful critical work on the social and cultural politics of HIV and AIDS – developed by writers such as Crimp (1988), Patton (1990), Treichler (1999), and Watney (1987) – has been informed by social constructionist insights and perspectives and has offered an important counter-current to the remedicalization of sexuality research and analysis that would emerge in the wake of the epidemic (see Chapter 6).

Within an increasingly polarized political climate – particularly in the USA, where what were often described as 'the culture wars' (Hunter 1992) emerged as especially intense – a new focus on the cultural articulation of both normativity and subversion in relation to gender and sexuality gave rise over the course of the 1990s to a new wave of research and analysis sometimes described as 'queer theory' (de Lauretis 1991).[13] While this relatively imprecise label is probably inadequate for truly capturing the wide range of work to which it has been applied, it was initially a useful way to gloss an overarching concern with the ways in which gendered and sexualized identities are constituted as a function of social and cultural representations. Precisely because representation pre-exists and therefore precedes identity formation, disruptions of normative representations can play a key role in seeking to transform existing relations and power structures. This insight has been a central motivation for a large body of work carried out in the 1990s and early 2000s that aimed at unsettling accepted notions of gender and sexuality – and perhaps in particular at analysing the structures of perception, knowledge, and thought that have shaped understandings of homosexuality and other forms of sexual dissidence, particularly in Western societies.

While this literature is now quite extensive, with influential contributions such as Sedgwick's *Epistemology of the Closet* (1990) and Warner's edited volume, *Fear of a Queer Planet* (1993), perhaps no one working along these lines has had as much influence as Judith Butler, an American philosopher and political theorist whose writings on gender and the body have extended social constructionist critiques in important ways.[14] Butler has drawn heavily on Foucault's work, along with structuralist and post-structuralist psychoanalysis and literary criticism, in ways that have opened up important new insights in relation to gender and sexuality. While Rubin emphasized material relations and historical practices, Butler has placed greater emphasis on the role of language and discourse in understanding the cultural construction of gendered and sexualized identities. In her first influential work, *Gender Trouble: Feminism and the Subversion of Identity* (Butler 1990a), Butler argued against the ontological coherence of categories such as sex, gender, and sexuality. She challenged the notion of binary sexes as a biological or natural phenomenon, arguing that the sexed body is itself culturally constructed within 'regulative discourses' and 'disciplinary techniques' that guide subjects into performing stylized acts that in fact produce gender and sexuality rather than the other way around. It is in this sense that Butler has described gender, as well as sex and sexuality, as 'performative': 'There is no gender identity behind the expressions of gender; ... identity is performatively constituted by the very "expressions" that are said to be its results' (Butler 1990a, p. 25).

Precisely because of this, the very notion of gender as an essential category disintegrates in the performances from which both the sexes and sexualities are produced:

> Because there is neither an 'essence' that gender expresses or externalizes nor an objective ideal to which gender aspires; because gender is not a fact, the various acts of gender create the idea of gender, and without those acts, there would be no gender at all. Gender is, thus, a construction that regularly conceals its genesis.
>
> (Butler 1990b, p. 271)

Based on this formulation, Butler has argued that traditional feminist analyses of gender have in fact unwittingly reproduced gender hierarchies by assuming that masculinity and femininity are inevitably constituted on the basis of male and female bodies – reinforcing a binary view of gender as divided into the two clearly distinct groups of men and women. Through the repeated acts of culturally constituted performance, male and female sex is thus seen to cause masculine and feminine gender. The binary nature of gender, in turn, is constitutive of heteronormative desire: the desire of one gender for the other.[15]

Butler's work has been important in destabilizing the supposed normality of heterosexuality. Because heterosexuality – like all other forms of sexuality – must be constantly produced and reproduced through the reiteration of its performance, its tenuous and precarious character is unmasked: 'That heterosexuality is always in the act of elaborating itself is evidence that it is perpetually at risk, that is, that it "knows" its own possibility of being undone' (Butler 1991, p. 23).

This idea of identity (and desire) – not as an essence anchored in bodily reality, but rather as performative and therefore free from the constraints of the body and open to multiple permutations and transformations – is perhaps more forcefully articulated in a sustained theoretical argument by Butler than by any other writer. In her 1993 work, *Bodies that Matter: On the Discursive Limits of 'Sex'*, Butler continued to raise important questions of both an epistemological and ethical nature. First, she complicated the very notion of materiality, positing that the material body is not an irreducible subtext or *tabula rasa* that gets inscribed by culture but rather always exists in a relationship of dynamic interaction with social meaning and power: 'it is clear from the start that matter has a history (indeed, more than one) and that the history of matter is in part determined by the negotiation of sexual difference' (Butler 1993, p. 29). This perspective challenged the familiar nature–culture or body–mind dualism taken for granted by many social constructionist theories, including long-standing feminist distinctions between 'sex' (the biologically sexed body as fixed, innate) and 'gender' (the social meanings attached, variously and arbitrarily, to biological, sexed bodies). In Butler's view, as in that of feminist biologist Anne Fausto-Sterling, bodies are socially and culturally embedded from the start and compelling evidence (for example, about intersex infants or the tremendous range of sexual and reproductive possibilities, or bodily strength and agility) attests to the continual and complex interactions between bodies and their environments, especially the 'regulatory norms' that prescribe which bodies matter and how they matter (Butler 1993, p. 2, Fausto-Sterling 2000, pp. 22–23).

This epistemological understanding sets up the empirical ground for a radical rethinking of the ethics of sexual normativity and sexual exclusions. In *Bodies that Matter*, Butler argued that the 'excluded sites' of sexual and gender subjectivity 'come to bound the "human" as its constitutive outside, and to haunt those boundaries as the persistent possibility of their disruption and re-articulation'. She announced as her task 'to understand how what has been foreclosed or banished from the proper domain of "sex" – where that domain is secured through a heterosexualizing imperative – might at once be produced as a troubling return ... as an enabling disruption' (Butler 1993, pp. 8, 23). Thus it becomes possible to see the subversive potential of drag (as represented by the East Harlem transvestites in the Jennie Livingston film, *Paris Is Burning*) in its disclosure that 'all gender ... is drag'. Drag queens and kings (and presumably all instances of transgender life) expose the imitative, performative impulse 'at the heart of the *heterosexual* project and its gender binarisms'; heterosexuality and gender dualism are themselves always an approximation of an impossible ideal (Butler 1993, p. 125).

In her more recent work – particularly the books *Precarious Life* (2004a) and *Undoing Gender* (2004b) – Butler explores the ethical and political implications of these epistemological insights in greater depth. She poses fundamental questions: How do we define the terms of what it means to be human? Who counts as belonging to the universe of 'humanness' and is thus entitled to respect and human rights? What are the conditions of a 'liveable' – or a 'grievable' – life? (Butler 2004a, pp. 31–33, 2004b, p. 17). Since these questions are always and everywhere bound up with sites of power, the power of recognition (or its denial), they are also profoundly political. Recognition necessarily involves regulatory practices – the production of norms (normativization) and the conferring of names, categories, diagnoses, and intelligibility on subjects. Such processes too often bring forms of exclusion or even dehumanization (such as in the medicalization and mutilation of intersex infants and the treatment of prisoners in Guantánamo).

Paradoxically, however, they also produce the very subjects they seek to define and thus, because of what Butler earlier called 'the slippage between a discursive command and its appropriated effect' (Butler 1993, p. 122), the possibility of resisting reality as it is currently constituted. Fantasy itself, in this understanding, 'is not the opposite of reality' but 'what reality forecloses'; 'it establishes the possible in excess of the real' (Butler 2004b, p. 29). In this way, fantasy and its embodiment in sexually diverse subjects have political and strategic importance:

> One of the central tasks of lesbian and gay [and transgender] international rights is to assert in clear and public terms the reality of homosexuality [and 'drag, femme, transgender, transsexual persons'], not as an inner truth, not as a sexual practice, but as one of the defining features of the social world in its very intelligibility.
>
> (Butler 2005, p. 29)

We will come back to the implications of this ethical theory for human rights in Chapter 9. For now, it is most important to emphasize that Butler's work (and that of other thinkers such as Fausto-Sterling) has been especially important in moving beyond the often overly self-referential boundaries of some queer theory work in the academy to reach out to a broader audience.

While the influence of queer theory has been most significant in literary criticism and cultural studies and much more limited in social and political theory, it has none the less provided inspiration for work that has increasingly understood sexuality in relation to power that is embedded in different levels of social life, expressed discursively and enforced through boundaries and binary divides. It has thus led to an important problematization of previously taken-for-granted sexual and gender categories, and of identities more generally (see Stein and Plummer 1994). Although largely based in relatively elite academic settings in the USA, and to a lesser extent in the UK and other Western European countries, the emergence of queer theory and queer studies has none the less offered important new insights that have been useful in rethinking over-simplistic oppositions between masculinity and femininity and homosexuality and heterosexuality, as well as in breaking down monolithic (typically white and middle-class) notions of 'gay and lesbian community' especially in the Anglo-European world (Parker 1999).[16] In particular, it has called our attention to questions of internal differences in gender power, race and ethnicity, and related social distinctions, and over time has gradually expanded beyond its elite

Western roots, opening up new understandings of sexual diversity and difference in a range of non-Western settings as well (see, e.g., Boellstorff 2005, Parker 1999, Rofel 2007).

Both building on and, in important ways, expanding the work of Butler and queer theorists, other writers during the decade of the mid-1990s to the present have explored what Currah has called 'the transgender imaginary' (Currah 2003). Transgender writers and activists such as Currah, Bornstein (1994), Stryker (1994), Feinberg (1996), Halberstam (1998), and Minter (2006) have clearly built upon Rubin's rethinking of a conceptual and lived distinction between sexuality and gender and on Butler's radical critique of binaries and exclusions in both realms. They have expanded upon queer theory's rejection of the privileging of 'gay and lesbian' in gendered sexual politics by developing the concept of the 'transgender umbrella' (see Introduction). In contrast to queer theorists, however, transgender writers and advocates have moved the recognition of the (racialized, class-based) power relations challenging the boundaries of both sex and gender to a more pragmatic and policy-oriented space. Concerned with forming communities and a social movement that confronts political and medical authorities around issues as basic to 'a liveable life' as identification on birth certificates and drivers' licenses, access to public bathrooms as well as medical services, and recognition of trans-persons as full human beings with rights, they have taken the critical study of sexuality and gender outside the academy and into the arena of political strategy and social change (see Cabral and Viturro 2006, Currah 2003, Currah *et al.* 2006, Spade 2006, Thomas 2006).

In this sense, queer theory and transgender theory represent an important extension of earlier work in history, anthropology, and sociology that focused on the social dimensions of gender and sexuality. There are many important differences that distinguish these diverse strands of what came to be known, perhaps too generically, as social constructionist theory in sexuality research. None the less, the work carried out from this perspective converged on a number of crucially important issues and changed not only the epistemological framing but the empirical research agendas for the investigation of sexuality and sexual conduct during the 1990s and the early 2000s. In opposition to the essentialist assumptions that have dominated more mainstream research on sexuality and sexual behaviour, work on the social construction of sexuality has challenged both the universalistic conceptualization of sexuality and sexual practices, on the one hand, and the privileged status of perceived objective scientific inquiry, on the other. It has clearly rejected the analysis of sex as an autonomous phenomenon – as a force of nature that the social order must somehow seek to stifle or control (Gagnon and Parker 1995).

Social construction theory developed the alternative view that sexual conduct was based not on universal, internal biological, or psychological drives but rather that it was constituted and elicited in specific contexts and circumstances, seeing the sexual realm as a highly particular product of specific social, cultural, and historical processes (Vance 1989). Although in different ways, all of the approaches that have focused on the social construction of sexuality have sought to situate the question of sex within a wider analytic framework – to focus on its relation to the structures of gender, kinship, and family life, to conceptualize it within historical transformations of economy and society, and to link it to an examination of the politics of culture itself. Ultimately, when taken together, these various currents of social constructionist thought have thus opened up an intellectual space for the analysis not so much of sex itself – understood as a discrete phenomenon or a distinct object of knowledge – but of the various processes through which the sexual realm is socially and culturally defined, delineated, and invested with meaning, together with the ways in which it is politically and economically shaped and integrated into broader systems of power and domination. It is in its understanding of sexuality as positioned at a kind of intersection of culture and power that much of its analytic force has been most clearly realized.

Chapter 6

After AIDS

Just as the early development of sexology sought to liberate sexuality from the influence of religious doctrine and religious authority, the social constructionist approach as it emerged during the 1970s and 1980s was an equally conscious attempt to resist the medicalization of sexuality that had become so deeply rooted in the early twentieth century. With the emergence of the HIV epidemic in the early 1980s, however, a rapid remedicalization of approaches to sexuality began to take place within research and as part of the broader social response to the epidemic.

Among the most immediate consequences of the growing epidemic was a massive increase in sexual behaviour research. It quickly became apparent that due to the long-term neglect of investment in research (and research infrastructure) within this field, an exceptionally limited knowledge base existed with regard to many of the key sources of information needed in order to respond to an inevitably fatal disease transmitted primarily through sexual contact. This provided a major stimulus for the investment of significant new resources, particularly in relation to HIV and AIDS, as well as other issues of relevance to sexuality and health.

Epidemiology, epistemology, and 'health behaviours'

During the early years of the HIV epidemic in the USA, one of the most frequently repeated laments of public health officials and activists alike was the lack of available data on sexual behaviour and the need to rely on findings from the initial Kinsey studies, now nearly 50 years out of date. At its most absurd, findings from the Kinsey studies, or from more recent research in the USA, were even used to speculate about behavioural frequencies in completely unrelated settings such as the countries and cultures of sub-Saharan Africa, where the epidemic was quickly perceived to be especially widespread (see Chouinard and Albert 1990, Turner et al. 1989, pp. 73–74). The urgent need to respond to the epidemic with more contemporary and more meaningful research thus provided the justification for a massive increase in research funding on sexuality and sexual behaviour among diverse population groups.

New resources became available relatively quickly, particularly through agencies such as the U.S. National Institutes of Health, but almost exclusively for the collection of behavioural data perceived to be necessary for understanding the epidemiology of HIV infection and for the development of prevention programmes and interventions. This work was, however, conceptualized almost exclusively within a biomedical framework that reproduced many of the essentialist and naturalist tendencies previously called into question in work focusing on the social, cultural, and historical construction of sexuality.

As discussed in Chapter 5, the development of social constructionist research in disciplines such as anthropology, history, and sociology during the late 1970s and early 1980s was characterized by a politically engaged critique of sexual science and of the medicalization of sexuality as a form of social and political control, particularly as it related to the sexuality of women and same-sex sexual relations. This trend would change in important and problematic ways with the emergence of AIDS and the development of biomedical and behavioural research on HIV and AIDS during the 1980s and 1990s. Driven by epidemiological concerns, research on sexuality in relation to AIDS arose first and foremost within medical institutions and frameworks. This inevitably meant it would be shaped by Western biomedical assumptions about the universality of its own categories and the essential truth and reliability of its methods of investigation (see Treichler 1999).

Since mainstream public health research and practice was largely modelled on, and organized within, broader medical frameworks[1] – a kind of extension of the biomedical enterprise from the individual body to the social body – it is perhaps not surprising that the early research response to AIDS and to HIV infection (as soon as the causal agent was identified) would lead to a remedicalization of the field of sexuality research and a wide-ranging revival of the search for scientific rigor in the investigation and analysis of sexual behaviour. Indeed, much of the research activity that emerged in response to AIDS in the mid-1980s focused not on the social construction of sexual experience, let alone its political dimensions, but on surveys of risk-related sexual behaviour and on the knowledge, attitudes, and practices that might be associated with the risk of infection. Most studies collected quantifiable data on numbers of sexual partners, specific sexual practices, sexually transmitted infections, and a range of similar issues understood to contribute to the spread of HIV. On the basis of this documentation, studies hoped to pave the way for policies and intervention programmes aimed at reducing the behavioural risk of infection (see, e.g., Carballo et al. 1989, Cleland and Ferry 1995).

Particularly in the USA, a long-standing focus on 'behavioural' research in the field of public health and the individual determinants of 'health behaviours' led to a relatively uncritical adoption of the notion of 'rational' decision-making processes driving theories of 'behavioural change' in response to perceived health threats, such as the potential for HIV infection. This meant that many of the earliest research initiatives that emerged in response to the HIV epidemic were designed to provide an empirical basis for 'behavioural interventions' (understood as a social equivalent to surgical or biomedical interventions into the physiological body) aimed at modifying behaviours thought to pose the risk of infection. It is also important to remember that the HIV epidemic first emerged in the USA during the 1980s, at the height of the 'Reagan revolution' in American politics (see also our discussion in Chapter 3 on the origin of the Moral Majority movement in US politics). Within this context, research focused on individual psychology was far more politically and ideologically acceptable than more sociological approaches. Much the same political climate was present in the UK, where the then Prime Minister Margaret Thatcher looked suspiciously upon social science research generally, as well as in many of the countries where social and behavioural research on HIV and AIDS was first initiated. In Australia, one of the few industrialized democracies with a more progressive political climate during this period, a very different approach to social research on HIV/AIDS emerged early in the history of the epidemic (see, e.g., the discussions in Altman 1986, Dowsett 1996, Kirp and Bayer 1992).[2]

Based on a range of 'cognitive-behavioural' theoretical models (e.g., Ajzen and Fishbein 1980, Bandura 1977, Becker and Joseph 1988), what came rather quickly to be described as 'intervention research' was carried out with the aim of producing behavioural change by providing target population groups with adequate knowledge and information about the risk of HIV infection. The belief was that increasing perception and awareness of risk would stimulate the rational decision-making process that would then lead to significant risk reduction. By focusing on the links between sexual behaviour and individual psychology, researchers assumed that more broad-based prevention programmes could be developed based upon intervention research findings. If individuals could be persuaded to change their behaviours in ways that would reduce the risk of HIV infection, it was thought, this would open up solutions to a range of other problems perceived to be linked to sexual conduct, such as the spread of other sexually transmitted infections, the alleged epidemic of teenage pregnancy in the inner cities of the USA, and the population explosion supposedly taking place in the developing world. The extent to which such perceptions were based more on moral panic than on empirical reality is open to debate, but most important for our purposes is the way these concerns served to justify and legitimize a turn from more critical social constructionist approaches to a renewed search for scientific 'rigor' and 'objectivity' in the investigation of sexual behaviours.

The development of this approach was most pronounced in the USA, where the size of the HIV epidemic, the availability of resources, and the presence of the individualistic behavioural research tradition in public health were also most pronounced. But similar initiatives took place throughout the 1980s and early 1990s in some other parts of the Anglo-European world, with large-scale surveys of sexual behaviour being conducted among populations believed to be especially high-risk, such as gay and bisexual men and female sex workers, and among the so-called general population in countries such as the USA, the UK, and France as well as in other developed countries (see Chapter 4).

Under the auspices of bilateral development agencies like USAID and intergovernmental institutions like the World Health Organization, similar studies were carried out in a growing number of developing countries in Africa, Asia, and Latin America – in some cases, simply by adding a set of questions on sexual behaviour to existing surveys, such as the Demographic and Health Surveys, and in some cases by developing new survey instruments and studies focused exclusively on HIV-related risk. Indeed, over the course of the late 1980s and the 1990s, sexological and social demographic approaches increasingly merged in a new wave of scientific investigation on HIV and AIDS (see Cleland and Ferry 1995, Turner *et al.* 1989). The growing number of available studies has made possible a range of cross-national comparisons, both on a regional level (see, e.g., Hubert *et al.* 1998), as well as globally. One recent comparison, for example, compiled findings from 59 countries, with representation from every major region of the world (see Wellings *et al.* 2006).

While the descriptive data emerging from such large-scale surveys has highlighted both cross-national similarities and differences in sexual behaviour, knowledge, information, and risk-related behaviour change, it has also called attention to the extent to which 'social context' shapes sexual practice and is a crucial consideration in relation to the possibilities for intervention aimed at health promotion (Wellings *et al.* 2006, p. 1724). Yet this understanding has long been one of the key insights to emerge from AIDS-related research. By the early 1990s, as behavioural research and interventions began to develop in a growing range of diverse social and cultural settings, critics began to question the relative effectiveness of both the research instruments and intervention strategies (Aggleton 1996b). The difficulties of translating or adapting research protocols for cross-cultural application quickly became apparent in the face of often radically different understandings of sexual expression and practices in different societies and cultures – and even in different subcultures within the same society. Further, the efficacy of interventions based largely on information and reasoned persuasion as a stimulus for risk reduction became evident almost immediately.

In study after study, the finding that information in and of itself is insufficient to produce risk-reducing behavioural change was repeated, and the relative limitations of individual psychology as the basis for intervention and prevention programmes (even in the USA, where such approaches had largely originated) became apparent. By the late 1980s and the early 1990s, on the basis of both empirical research findings and practical experience from around the world, it had become clear that a far more complex set of social, cultural, political, and economic factors combine in multiple ways to mediate the structure of risk in every population group or community. The dynamics of individual psychology could never be expected to explain (let alone produce or even stimulate) changes in sexual conduct without taking these broader issues into account.

Shifting paradigms: culture and structure

As the importance of broader social forces shaping the HIV epidemic came to be recognized, the limitations of traditional behavioural research approaches also became clear. Influenced by concurrent developments in relation to the social construction and production of sexual relations, research in response to HIV and AIDS began to draw on interactionist sociology and cultural anthropology as well as on some of the more radical approaches to social psychology. What all these perspectives had in common was their focus on the social and cultural structures and mean-ings that shape sexual experience in different settings. As Rafael Diaz suggested:

> There is obviously need for a 'shift of paradigm' in HIV prevention research. We need to develop models that are domain-specific (sexual-ity and drug use) and that focus on the difficulties that persons, dyads, and communities face in enacting personal intentions. More import-ant, we need models that focus on the breakdown of intentionality, and that are sensitive to the historical, cultural, situational, and con-textual variables where (so-called) risk behavior occurs. Of special importance would be an attempt to understand risk behavior not in terms of 'deficits' in individuals' knowledge, motivation, or skills, but rather as behavior that may have meaning and be quite rational within a given socio-cultural context.
>
> (Diaz 2000, p. 196)

Stimulated by such concerns, the emphasis began to shift from a focus on individual psychology to a new concern with 'intersubjective' cultural meanings related to sexuality and their shared and collective qualities as the property, not of atomized or isolated individuals, but of social persons integrated within the context of distinct, and diverse, cultures. Social science research on the HIV and related issues of sexual and reproductive health increasingly sought to draw on social constructionist insights and to go beyond the calculation of behavioural frequencies and the identification of statistical correlates of sexual risk behaviour. The objective has been to examine what sex means to the parties involved, the contexts in which it takes place, the structure and scripting of sexual encounters, and the sexual cultures (and subcultures) present and emergent within particular societies (see, e.g., Herdt and Lindenbaum 1992, Parker and Gagnon 1995). It is not surprising that much of this work first emerged in cross-cultural research and in the analysis of cultural settings in which the bio-medical categories of epidemiological analysis failed to be fully applicable (e.g., Parker 1987, de Zalduondo 1999). Increasingly, however, cultural analysis has also been developed in specific sexual cultures or subcultures in the industrialized West, offering important new insights even in settings where extensive behavioural research had already been carried out – among Latino and African-American populations in the USA (Alonso and Koreck 1989, Carrier and Magaña 1991, Cohen 1999), and gay communities and cultures in a range of Western countries (Dowsett 1996, Henriksson 1995).

During the 1990s, this emphasis on the social organization of sexual interactions, the contexts within which sexual practices occur, and the complex relations between meaning and power in the constitution of sexual experience, has led to a new focus on the investigation of diverse 'sexual cultures'. Research attention has thus increasingly shifted from sexual behaviour in and of itself to the cultural settings within which it takes place and the cultural rules that organize it. Special emphasis has been given to analysing the cultural categories and systems of classification that structure and define sexual experience in different social and cultural contexts (see Parker and Aggleton 1999).

With the focus on such issues it quickly became apparent that many of the key categories and classifications used to describe sexual life in Western biomedicine (and, more recently, in public health epidemiology) are far from universal, or a given, in all cultural settings. On the contrary, categories such as 'homosexuality', 'prostitution', and even 'masculinity' and 'femininity' may be very differently understood in diverse social and cultural settings, while any number of other significant categories may be present that fail to conform or fit neatly into the classificatory systems of Western science. By focusing more carefully on local categories and classifications, social researchers sought to move from what may be described in anthropology or linguistics as an 'outsider' perspective, to what is described as an 'insider' perspective – from the 'experience-distant' concepts of science to the 'experience-near' concepts that the members of specific cultures use to understand and interpret their own reality. In sexual life as much as in any other area, subjective meanings are ultimately built up from the intersubjective cultural systems that exist in specific social settings. Precisely because erotic meanings take form within a wider cultural context, it is possible to gain access to them through the interpretation of the symbolic systems that shape them. Without minimizing the complex psychological processes involved, it is possible to approach the erotic much as one might examine a system of religious beliefs or a particular political ideology. On the basis of such an examination, we can develop an understanding of sexual life that will be directly relevant not only to understanding the transmission of HIV but also to the task of designing effective health programmes in response to the epidemic.[3]

Nowhere has the importance of understanding the specific, or 'experience-near', concepts organizing sexual life been more clearly evident than in examining the complex relationship between sexual behaviour and sexual identity. Early on in the HIV epidemic, it became apparent that epidemiological categories related to homosexuality and heterosexuality were at best a poor reflection of the complexity and diversity of lived sexual experience, and that neither homosexual nor heterosexual behaviour was necessarily associated with a distinct sense of self or sexual identity. Indeed, even 'heterosexuality' as a category would need to be problematized in many social and cultural settings. As a result of this understanding, significant research attention focused on the different ways in which sexual interactions are structured and the diverse sexual identities organized around such interactions. In many settings, for example, notions of 'activity' and 'passivity' in sexual interactions, translated into gendered symbols of masculinity and femininity, proved to be more important in defining sexual identity than one's choice of sexual object or the sex/gender of one's partner. Biomedical models of sexual experience have often posited a necessary relationship between sexual desire, sexual behaviour, and sexual identity, but research in diverse cultural contexts quickly called this relationship into question, demonstrating an extensive range of possible variations that seemed to be present across different social and cultural settings.[4]

Although much of the research on sexual identity and HIV has focused on relations among men who have sex with men, the same kind of critical reflection has been applied to a number of other epidemiological categories, particularly in relation to perceived 'risk groups'.[5] Studies of sex work, for example, documented the fact that relations of sexual and economic exchange are far more complex and varied than was originally assumed. In many contexts the exchange of sexual services for money, gifts, or favours is a common part of sexual interaction that implies no special sexual (or, for that matter, social) identity, while in others such exchanges may be specifically organized around a distinct sense of shared identity on the part of sex workers. The social sanctions and stigma associated with female or male prostitution in some settings do not necessarily transfer to all local variants of sex-for-money exchange, and the relationship between behaviour and identity is as problematic, and as situationally variable, in relation to sex work as it is in relation to same-sex interactions.[6]

Indeed, in much recent work, even notions of gender and gender identity have increasingly been called into question. What it is to be male or female, masculine or feminine, or somewhere in between this binary, in different social and cultural contexts, may vary greatly, and gender identity is clearly not reducible to any underlying biological dichotomy. A new focus on gender relations has brought fresh attention to the social construction of masculinity and femininity and to the diversity of gender cultures in different settings, with important emphasis being given to the influence of social class and racial and ethnic identity as they intersect with and impact upon masculine, feminine, and trans identities and subjectivities.[7] Under the rules of binary sex, all biological males and females as well as intersex persons undergo a process of sexual regulation – in some cases normativization through surgical 'reassignment' – in which culturally specific notions of masculinity and femininity are transmitted across the life course (Butler 2004b). Through this process of sexual regulation individuals learn the sexual desires, feelings, roles, and practices typical of their cohorts or statuses within society, as well as the sexual alternatives their culture opens up to them (Parker *et al.* 2000a). Research in diverse settings has increasingly focused on the processes of sexual socialization and on the sexual experience of young people, not only in and of itself but also as an important window to the dynamics of sexual life – to the ways in which intersubjective sexual meanings are internalized, reproduced, and sometimes resisted in social and sexual interaction (Aggleton *et al.* 2006, Heilborn *et al.* 2006, Holland *et al.* 1998, Irvine 1994, Paiva 2000). Stereotypical conceptions of gender have been called into question, and the role of men as well as of women – and slowly but increasingly of trans- and gender-queer persons – in reproductive and sexual processes and decision making has become an important area of investigation. This made possible an important reconceptualization of the complexity of conjugal and intimate relationships, as well as a growing understanding of the multiple forms of social differentiation that structure the diversity of gender relations in different social contexts (see, e.g., Cabral and Viturro 2006, Currah 2001, 2003, Gregg 2003, Hirsch 2003, Hunter 2005).

This focus on the social construction of sexual identities has also been associated with an increasing emphasis on the organization of distinct sexual communities (Weeks and Holland 1996). Indeed, just as recent research initiatives have demonstrated that there is no necessary or intrinsic relationship between sexual behaviours and sexual identities, many studies have also demonstrated the complex (and sometimes contradictory) links between sexual identity and the formation of sexual communities (Dowsett 1996, Herdt 1992, Kennedy and Davis 1993, Levine *et al.* 1997). The different ways in which sexual communities and subcultures take shape and evolve have thus become central questions for research aimed at understanding the broader social and cultural context of sexual conduct (Murray 1992, Rubin 1997, Peacock *et al.* 2001).

Early studies of behaviour changes in response to HIV and AIDS within the gay communities of a number of Northern countries have pointed to the importance of community development and support structures as correlates for the reduction of sexual risk behaviour (Kippax *et al.* 1993). In contrast, research carried out in other social and cultural contexts, particularly in societies where the emergence of gay, lesbian, and trans communities has been more limited, has found the lack of such structures equally important in understanding limited behavioural change (Daniel and Parker 1993). These studies pointed to the importance of emerging community structures – ranging from commercial venues such as bars, discos, or saunas, to civil society organizations such as NGOs and CBOs – as part of a broader process of change through which sexual communities take shape and provide social support for changing sexual practices (Boellstorff 2005, Manalansan 2003, Parker 1999).

Awareness of fundamental differences in the organization of sexual communities has led to greater research attention to the diverse sexual subcultures that exist in many societies. In relation to men who have sex with men, the different social and sexual networks and value systems associated with same-sex interactions between lower or working-class men as opposed to men from the middle and upper classes, and the specific contexts associated with transgender experience, male prostitution, and a range of other variations, have all become a focus for study. Many of the same approaches and insights gained through the study of variations in male same-sex practices have also been applied to other groups such as sex workers, youth cultures, and the sexual subcultures of different class and ethnic groups. Research has thus turned increasingly to the study of social and sexual networks in an attempt to investigate not only the systems of meaning but also the social structural principles that organize the possibilities of sexual interaction in different communities (Laumann and Gagnon 1995, Laumann *et al.* 2004).

On the basis of such work, an important reformulation of the very notion of 'intervention' has begun to take place. It has become increasingly apparent that the idea of a 'behavioural intervention' may in fact be a misnomer, since HIV prevention interventions almost never function at the level of behaviour but rather at the level of social or collective representations. New knowledge and information about perceived sexual risk will always be interpreted within the context of pre-existing systems of meaning that necessarily mediate the ways in which such information must always be incorporated into action. Because action has increasingly come to be understood as socially constructed and fundamentally collective in nature, earlier notions of behavioural intervention have given way to more ethnographically grounded HIV education and prevention programmes that are community-based and culturally sensitive. Such programmes attempt to transform social norms and cultural values and thus to reconstitute collective meanings in ways that will ultimately promote safer sexual practices (see Altman 1994, Paiva 2000).

By the early to mid-1990s, just as cultural analysis had surfaced as an important corrective to the perceived limitations of earlier behavioural approaches, a new focus on historical and political-economic analysis of the structural factors associated with HIV infection and barriers to risk reduction also emerged as central to the evolving response to the epidemic.[8] As Paul Farmer argued in his early work on HIV and AIDS in Haiti, for example, issues such as gender power relations, forced migration patterns, and, above all, poverty have shaped the dynamics of HIV infection in settings characterized by social and economic exclusion and marginalization. The politics of stigma and discrimination, as well as the widespread displacements due to large-scale development initiatives supported by bilateral and multilateral donor agencies, become key points of origin for a chain of events ultimately linked to the rapid spread of HIV infection and the devastation caused by AIDS in local communities and among migrant and immigrant populations (see Farmer 1992).

Similar social and ecological disruption linked to uneven and unequal processes of economic development, particularly as they impact upon gender and sexuality, are apparent in other detailed studies of development policies and practices in relation to HIV-related vulnerability. For example, Decosas (1996) has examined how the construction of the Akosombo dam in the 1960s unleashed a complex chain of conditions that fostered the HIV epidemic among the Krobo in Ghana during the 1980s and 1990s. When construction on the Akosombo dam started, many Krobo men went downstream to work on the project. Many Krobo women followed, providing services at hotels and drinking spots in the construction area, including sexual-economic exchanges. When the creation of Lake Volta destroyed the land which Krobo men and women had previously farmed, many women went abroad to work as sex workers, and remittances from sex work became an important source of development in the region. Many of these women's daughters, similarly facing few employment opportunities, became sex workers as well, and both generations have high HIV incidence. In recent years, with the economic future of Ghana looking brighter, remittances from women working abroad are becoming scarce and prostitution is no longer such an attractive option for economic survival. Fewer young girls are entering sex work and HIV infection rates among younger Krobo women are approaching the lower rates in the rest of Ghana.

More broadly, international and intergovernmental development policies and practices have been linked to the disintegration of traditional social and economic structures and the accentuation of social and economic inequalities. In turn, these inequalities have contributed significantly to the pronounced impact of the epidemic, especially in sub-Saharan Africa but also in South Asia and the Caribbean and in some important sectors of the so-called developed world.[9] Indeed, poverty itself, more than any other single socioeconomic factor, has been identified as perhaps the key driving force of the epidemic, and much recent research has focused on the synergistic effects of poverty when linked to other forms of social inequality, instability, and discrimination (see, e.g., Farmer *et al.* 1996, Singer 1998).

In addition to the general conditions of poverty, the link between migration and increased HIV incidence and vulnerability has been demonstrated in a variety of contexts and locations, ranging from seasonal labourers in southern Africa to immigrant populations in the USA and mobile sex workers in many different regions.[10] Research on the impact of population movement and displacement has focused, in particular, on the causal mechanisms behind labour mobility and its connections to HIV transmission. For example, male migrant labourers often frequent female sex workers (who themselves may be migrants) or establish secondary households in the field, leading to increased incidence of STDs and HIV in locations where there are generally poor health care services. Meanwhile back at home women face severe economic and emotional demands, which they typically try to meet through agricultural and sometimes sex work. And, since men and women migrant workers move back and forth between two or more locations, HIV may spread from higher incidence to lower incidence areas.

Migration-related vulnerability to HIV can be exacerbated by the introduction of 'economic reforms' such as structural adjustment programmes (SAPs). For example, Bassett has described how the structural adjustment that Zimbabwe was forced to accept in the 1990s resulted in reductions in social expenditures, including reduced condom availability (Bassett 1993), while Turshen has developed a similar analysis of the negative consequences of World Bank-imposed economic reforms throughout the African continent in the late 1980s and 1990s (Turshen 1998). More generally, the structural adjustment programmes enforced by the World Bank and International Monetary Fund as stipulations for loans made to developing countries, especially during the 1980s, had a direct impact on the explosion of HIV incidence in Asia and Africa during the late 1980s and early 1990s. In an examination of the historical and political framework of SAPs, for example, Lurie *et al.* (1995) described how the decreasing demand for oil exportation following the 1970s oil embargo in industrialized countries created the need for loans in developing countries. Structural adjustments imposed with the loans demanded cuts in government spending, tax increases, and price increases on both imported goods and goods and services within a country. The decline of rural economies and the growth of urbanization and infrastructures resulting from SAPs forced families to split apart in search of work. Migration to urban areas with more job opportunities multiplied potential sexual contacts and eventually intensified the spread of HIV internationally.[11]

Just as increased vulnerability to HIV infection has been one of the unintended consequences of ill-fated economic development policies, it has also been linked to social upheaval associated with 'low-intensity' wars and internal political conflicts occurring in various parts of the world (e.g., Uganda, Rwanda, Haiti) in recent decades (Farmer 1995, Turshen 1995, Webb 1997). Focusing on the long-term ramifications of Uganda's civil war, Bond and Vincent (1997) have described several war-linked demographic trends relevant to the spread of HIV (see also the discussion of HIV/AIDS in Uganda in Chapter 2). These include changes in household structure, a strong association between wealth and polygamy, a growing dependence on non-agricultural activities for income, and the creation of a black-market, crop-smuggling network during the reign of Idi Amin, which inadvertently laid the groundwork for the economic and communication infrastructure that facilitated the spread of HIV. Webb (1997) has provided similar examples in the aftermath of the civil wars in Angola, Namibia, and Mozambique, where HIV incidence is higher in areas directly affected by military mobilization and conflict. In addition, Farmer's work in Haiti (1995) has shown that political instability need not rise to the level of an ongoing armed conflict to increase vulnerability to HIV. In the case of Haiti, political instability has exacerbated already high levels of poverty causing people to relocate from rural to urban areas, where a series of factors, including sexism, traditional and emergent patterns of sexual union, the prevalence of, and unavailability of treatment for, STDs, lack of timely response by public health workers, and the absence of appropriate responses, all facilitate HIV transmission.[12]

Research in this field has increased understanding of how macro-level inequalities are articulated with inequalities that exist in even the most intimate forms of social and sexual interaction. Just as detailed cross-cultural and comparative investigation of the social construction of same-sex relations provided a key test case for demonstrating the importance of cultural analysis in relation to sexuality and HIV, the investigation of gender power inequalities and forms of sexual oppression has been central to building understanding of the importance of structural factors in organizing sexual relations and HIV-related vulnerability. This has been particularly true of work focusing on women's vulnerability, especially in situations where gender power inequalities cross with economic exclusion and/or racial or ethnic discrimination.

In the 1990s, the growing interest in the role of gender and sexuality structures in promoting HIV vulnerability, particularly among heterosexually active women and men, generated a number of impressive analyses that are attentive to both cultural and political economic factors. For example, Schoepf used vignettes from the life histories of women from various socioeconomic classes in Kinshasa, Zaire, to demonstrate that HIV is transmitted not through exotic cultural practices but due to many people's normal responses to situations of everyday life, such as dealing with substantial economic hardship and uncertainty. Her work promoted a participatory and collaborative form of action research with vulnerable women as a means to help redefine the gendered social roles and socioeconomic conditions contributing to the rapid spread of HIV in many parts of the world (Schoepf 1992).[13] Kammerer et al. (1995) examined the ways in which state and capitalist penetration exposed the mountain tribes in the northern Thailand periphery to the threat of HIV. This penetration led to a breakdown of the material base of rural life and caused young people to migrate to valley towns in order to work not only as prostitutes but also as maids, waiters, and construction workers. These socioeconomic transformations have affected hillside sexuality, which until recently was structured around core values of 'shame, name, and blame'. The authors provide ethnographic descriptions of these core values in relation to HIV and how the gender power relations and customary prescriptions and prohibitions of hillside sexuality make talking about sex and taking precautions against HIV transmission difficult.

Similarly, Symonds, writing on the Hmong in northern Thailand, examined how the HIV epidemic in Thailand, and the place of the Hmong within it, can only be explained by a combination of interrelated factors: the commercial sex industry, the prevalence of injection drug use, the political economic changes that have forced the Hmong living in the highlands to rely on lowland markets, racism and discrimination against the Hmong by the Thai majority, and a sexual double standard that permits polygyny among men yet controls the sexuality of young women (Symonds 1998).

Less research focusing on structural factors has been carried out on individuals involved in same-sex relations, as compared with the quantity of work focusing on heterosexual women or young people. None the less, recent findings suggest that structures of gender inequality are typically replicated in relation to transgender and other gender nonconforming persons, who often have few options for earning a living other than sex work, and who are in many instances subject to socially sanctioned forms of physical violence. While relatively few studies have examined the structural and environmental factors that impact upon the vulnerability of men who have sex with men, it is apparent from what research does exist that men who have sex with men are present in all societies – even if they may be less visible in some – and that they are subject to the same kinds of synergistic impact of multiple forms of oppression that affect other population groups. This is particularly the case when stigma and discrimination directed against homosexuality interact with issues such as poverty, racism, and gender and age-related inequalities (see Parker *et al.* 1998). It is now clear that pervasive heterosexism intersects with other forms of inequality to create situations of extreme vulnerability in relation to gender nonconformity, transgender and male sex work, gay men from ethnic minority groups, and young men who have sex with men generally (see, e.g., Carrier *et al.* 1997, Diaz 2000, McKenna 1996, Whitehead 1997). The issue of violence has also been central in recent research in sub-Saharan Africa, suggesting that women involved in same-sex relations are frequently at risk of HIV infection through forced sexual relations with men and situational heterosexuality due to social pressures to be married or in relationships with men (Kendall 1998, Kheshwa and Wieringa 2005, Lorway 2006, Morgan and Wieringa 2005).

Ultimately, a fuller understanding of the synergy that exists between sexuality and multiple forms of social inequality and exclusion may well be one of the most important long-term results of the research carried out in recent decades on the social dimensions of HIV and AIDS. By shifting paradigms and moving from the kinds of epistemological frameworks that have dominated mainstream biomedical and epidemiological research on sexuality and sexual conduct in relation to the epidemic, critical social science research has highlighted both the cultural and the structural forces shaping its course. This has helped open the way for a fuller understanding of political and economic factors that impact not only upon HIV and AIDS, but also upon the sexual interactions and relationships that have been so intimately linked to AIDS since it emerged.

Toward a political economy of the body

Work casting the body as both a symbolic and a material product of social relations – a construct that is necessarily conditioned by a whole range of structural forces – thus provided an important paradigm shift for research on sexuality in the wake of HIV and AIDS. Work on these issues over the past ten to 15 years offers an important alternative to mainstream epidemiological and public health approaches with regard not only to HIV and AIDS but also to sexual health more broadly. It provides an important point of intersection with social constructionist thinking on the importance of sexual cultures, identities, and communities and their relation to sexual politics (see, e.g., Manderson and Jolly 1997, Parker 1999, Petchesky 2003). By focusing on the ways sexual cultures are integrated within and cross-cut by complex systems of power and domination, such approaches make possible an increasing engagement with issues of power and the relationship between culture and power, allowing research and analysis on sexuality to begin addressing broader structural factors that shape the possibilities open to sexual subjects. This work makes it increasingly possible to move beyond the theoretical limitations of exclusively cultural approaches to sexuality studies, in particular by framing social constructionism with political economy (see Altman 2001, Lancaster and di Leonardo 1997, Parker and Aggleton 2007).

Much recent research on sexuality thus seeks to reach beyond postmodernism while still embracing postmodernist problematizations of traditionally defined categories of sex, gender, race, and class. But it also moves beyond earlier mechanistic models of political economy, in which an economic base determines a cultural superstructure, in favour of a more complex, interactive model. The result is a more grounded and politically relevant social constructionist theory – or what some have described as a new 'political economy of the body' and its sexual pleasures:

> To follow the circuitries of power in culture, we need an approach that can demonstrate concrete links between gender and sexuality, where those links exist, but without collapsing distinctions between the two or naturalizing their interrelationships. That is, we need 'a political economy of the body' that neither confuses itself with the more standard political economy of an economic mode of production, nor attempts to duplicate its every move, and is unwilling to say – before the fact – where the one ends and the other begins, or even whether there is a logical demarcation at all between the two.
>
> (Lancaster 1995, p. 145)

Within this framework, research focuses on the ways in which sexual meanings and experiences are situated in historically constituted political and economic systems. It attempts to illuminate how diverse political and economic processes and policies related to issues such as economic development, housing, labour, migration and immigration, health, education, and welfare impact upon communities and cultures, shaping health and well-being as well as the possibilities for agency, self-determination, and sexual freedom (see, e.g., Padilla *et al.* 2007, Parker *et al.* 2000a, Petchesky and Judd 1998).

Because research on structural factors emerged in a number of different settings – ranging from deeply impoverished rural areas in so-called developing countries to the marginalized inner cities of supposedly developed or industrialized nations – the language used, the conceptual tools employed, and the specific focus of analysis have often varied. In spite of differences in terminology and research emphasis, however, this work focuses on the interactive or synergistic effects of social factors such as poverty and economic exploitation, gender power, sexual oppression, racism, and social exclusion in creating forms of 'structural violence' that determine the social vulnerability of groups and individuals (Farmer *et al.* 1996, Parker *et al.* 2000b, Singer 1998). It examines the ways in which these forms of structural violence are historically and politically situated and the contexts in which sexual subjectivity and struggles for sexual freedoms emerge. Issues such as whom one may have sex with, in what ways, under what circumstances, and with what specific outcomes, are never simply random; they are shaped not only by cultural rules and regulations but also by social, political, and economic relations that determine the possibilities (and obligations) of sexual contact. These relations, in turn, condition the possibilities for negotiation in sexual interactions, for the occurrence of sexual violence, for patterns of contraceptive use, for sexual negotiation, for HIV-related risk reduction strategies, and so on (Parker 2001).

By emphasizing the body as a concrete product of social relations, this recent work provides an important way of reframing research on sexuality, sexual cultures, and sexual communities. In some of the most dynamic current work these concerns have also led researchers to focus new attention on the diverse social movements related to sexuality, sexual health, and sexual rights – including the feminist and lesbian and gay movements, but also movements for sex worker rights, for transgender identity and autonomy, the sexual rights of young people, and a range of related issues (see, e.g., Adam *et al.* 1998, Martinot and James 2001, Petchesky and Judd 1998, Petchesky 2003).

Sexuality, silence, and invisibility

In recent decades, then, we have seen major developments in social research on sexuality – work that has provided an important conceptual architecture for promoting sexual health and expanding the boundaries of sexual politics. A far-reaching critique of essentialist assumptions concerning the nature of sexual life has developed, along with the articulation of an increasingly sophisticated alternative framework that places the social and cultural dimensions of sexual experience within a perspective sensitive to historical processes and political and economic forces. Research in this field has greatly expanded, particularly following the emergence of the HIV epidemic, with new sources of funding, new programmes in training and capacity building, and a growing number of institutional centres and professional associations focusing on these issues. This increasingly multi-dimensional understanding taking shape in sex research, emphasizing structures and inequalities, is in keeping with a concurrent shift in the field of human rights languages and procedures to address sexual matters within an intersectional frame – which we will discuss further in Part 3.

In spite of these important advances, however, many significant challenges remain. In light of the issues prioritized thus far, what questions have we failed to ask? What answers have eluded us because of the kinds of questions that we *have* asked? What kinds of issues do we need to focus on in the future in order to continue moving this field forward? While

answers to these queries can only be tentative at best, we want to emphasize a number of points in the hope of opening up future discussion and
debate.

First, it may be that the strong emphasis which social constructionist
work has placed on issues of culture – and, as a surrogate for culture, language and discourse – has unintentionally diverted attention from the
importance of certain kinds of 'silence'. Indeed, it may even have produced
at least some kinds of silence that would not have been the case had other
theoretical perspectives and methodological approaches been adopted. It is
striking that in much recent sexuality research, particularly in relation to
some streams of cultural studies, sex itself seems to be increasingly absent
– the actual sexual practices that at some level are the point of departure
for the development of sexuality research as a field seem to have disappeared (perhaps in a kind of inverse relationship to the development of
theoretical frames and methodological tools).

One could ask whether the growing legitimacy of sexuality research as a
field – with its own institutional centres, the attention of funding agencies,
and so on – might not have taken place at the expense of a certain kind of
'sanitization' of the subject matter. Sexuality research may have become
increasingly legitimate over time (particularly in the wake of the HIV epidemic, but also as a result of movements for gender equity and sexual
freedom) but at the price of losing a certain kind of transgressive power
that characterized some of the most important early work in this field.
With that, perhaps, it may also have sacrificed some of its potential as a
source of resistance and of meaningful social, political, and cultural
critique of the power of hegemonic mainstream sexual moralities.

In spite of the fact that we have come to understand sexuality as
socially and culturally constructed, much of what actually takes place in
sexual exchanges happens in relative silence and beyond the observation of
even the most intrusive scientific sexologists. However, as some of the
most detailed observational and ethnographic work has demonstrated,
even in many of the most public expressions of sexual conduct – such as
the exchanges that take place in public venues like video arcades, cinemas,
or saunas – what we find is often an elaborate dance of meanings and
identities, bodies and pleasures, which typically takes place in almost total
silence, with a very different set of signifiers than those examined in much
of the most theoretically sophisticated contemporary sexuality research
(see, e.g., Leap 1999, Terto Jr. 1989).

Attention to culture and voice has been important in seeking to articu-
late an epistemological approach to sexuality research that might offer an
alternative to the positivist epistemologies of sexology (and demography).
But this focus may also have drawn attention away from issues that ought
rightfully to be at the centre of concern – away from sex itself, perhaps, as
well as from the kinds of 'discursive silence' (Lützen 1995) that may be

crucial in thinking about social and cultural change and about the grass-roots politics of social and sexual transformation. The fact that something may yet have to be articulated does not mean that it is not taking place. It may well be here, in relation to the still unarticulated processes of social and sexual change, that research on sexuality fails to offer the insights we so desperately need in order to build the political movements that will be necessary if we are to mount effective struggles for sexual plurality and freedom.

We want to link this recognition back to some of the key questions of political economy discussed above as well as forward to the questions of rights that will be the focus of Part 3 of this volume. Power, in this field as in others, has the capacity to throw some issues into sharp relief (inequalities, for example) or to trigger change (through resistance, for example), but it also has the potential to silence, and by silencing, to 'invisibilize' as well. This is particularly significant when it comes to understanding new forms of sexuality, emerging modes of sexual expression, and ways of sexual relating (e.g., the power of new technologies such as the Internet, or the invisibilization of sexual identities and experiences that occur in night spaces, or in the darkness of the cinema, and so on). Indeed, invisibility may well be the other side of silence, and we would be well advised not to ignore their interactions and the intersections between them.

It is thus crucial to recognize that many important challenges still exist in seeking to move from the production of meaningful knowledge to the implementation of truly liberating practices in relation to sexual health and well-being. The growing richness of our understanding of sexual cultures must ultimately be linked to a sexual politics – to an ongoing struggle for sexual freedom (and what we will describe in Part 3 as erotic justice) – that is capable of recognizing the full diversity of sexualities in today's world and the ongoing forms of oppression and exclusion that are still characterized more by their silences and their invisibility than by the freedoms to which we ultimately hope our work will contribute.

What might a notion of pleasure mean, for example, for impoverished women struggling to escape domestic violence in their daily lives? What constitutes a notion of sexual freedom for female or transgender sex workers in the most marginalized and excluded settings? Or for the poor youth of the peri-urban communities surrounding modern metropolitan urban centres in countries and cultures around the world? How can we begin to address these forms of exclusion, through both research and practice, in ways that will be meaningful for those in the front lines of such on-the-ground struggles? These are just some of the questions that we will only begin to answer if we are willing to listen to the silences and open our eyes to the invisibilities that are still so much a part of sexual life for so many people around the world (see Parker *et al.* 2007).

The answers to such questions can only be found, we argue, to the extent that we are able to reconceive the relationship between sexual health and sexual politics. The road to such a reconception, we are convinced, lies through further refinement of the emerging framework of sexual rights. This refinement cannot be approached exclusively as an academic challenge, but rather as a non-negotiable requirement to countervail the multiple and powerful forces currently engaged in eroding recognition of, and respect for, sexual plurality, diversity, and freedom gradually constructed over the past 30 years. It is to this challenge that we turn in Part 3.

Part 3

The promises and limits of sexual rights

Chapter 7

On the indispensability and insufficiency of human rights

> This, then, is the truth of the discourse of universal human rights: the Wall separating those covered by the umbrella of Human Rights and those excluded from its protective cover. Any reference to universal human rights as an 'unfinished project' to be gradually extended to all people is here a vain ideological chimera – and, faced with this prospect, do we, in the West, have any right to condemn the excluded when they use any means, inclusive of terror, to fight their exclusion?
>
> (Žižek 2002, p. 150)

From the outset, we have tried to locate our discussion of contemporary sexuality as it intersects with public health and policy in a larger frame of politics – global capitalism, militarism, neocolonial and race-ethnic conflicts, and the gender hierarchies that persist everywhere. At this point in time it is a depressing context, one in which every promise of liberal and emancipatory aspiration from the nineteenth and twentieth centuries seems to have crashed into a bleak landscape of violence, social division, and unrestrained military power that Žižek (2002) calls (after the popular 1999 film *The Matrix*) 'the desert of the real'. Amidst this wreckage, will we also soon find human rights, including the fledgling concept of sexual rights and the UN mechanisms intended to codify and sustain these? Ironically, the convergence of globalization with the 'war on terror' that characterizes the current historical period has brought accelerated global exchanges (of capital, goods, people, ideas, information, and viruses) and a multitude of walls that separate off the abject, the less-than-human: the US offshore torture sites at Abu Ghraib and Guantánamo and their secret counterparts (the CIA sites of 'rendition'); the Israeli wall and its copies on the US–Mexico border; resurgent trade and aid barriers; and all the social and cultural walls that segregate ethnic, economic, and sexual outcasts within defined borders. For the growing throngs of the excluded, Žižek implies, human rights are little more than a cruel joke.

Any hope of escaping postmodern pessimism without retreating into the grandiose illusions of the past must take into account the ethical limitations and philosophical and political blinders of the liberal humanist tradition that bred human rights. We thus approach a discussion of human rights discourse and practice as it applies to sexuality and health with a great deal of caution, but not despair. Critics from Left and Right have faulted assertions of 'fundamental human rights' on all kinds of grounds: their individualism and bourgeois Western origins; their attempt to impose a false standard of universality and to ignore cultural and historical differences; their hypocritical political use by governments (particularly the USA) to bully or taint adversaries and bolster friends (or themselves); their racist and neocolonial uses to inferiorize 'other' cultures and societies; and their frequent lack of effective enforcement mechanisms. We will address each of these criticisms but will also argue that human rights offer the most viable rhetorical structure currently available to civil society groups for making social and erotic justice claims and seeking redress or accountability.

Derrida has written, 'we must (il faut) more than ever stand on the side of human rights', but they 'are never sufficient' (in Borradori 2003, p. 132). It is worth exploring this paradox of indispensability and insufficiency. On the side of indispensability, human rights are ethically superior to other frameworks – such as utilitarianism and social contract theory – insofar as they subordinate cost–benefit analyses and crude self-interest to principles of social, economic, gender, and racial justice. What justice means, according to Martha Nussbaum (1999), is that 'society owes people ... a basic level of support for nutrition, health, shelter, education, and physical safety', as well as 'effective guarantees of the major liberties of expression, conscience, and political participation' in order for them to realize their 'basic human capacities', across all gender, racial, ethnic, sexual, religious, and other differences (p. 20).

The problem with those approaches to social justice that attempt to substitute for human rights, such as the capabilities and the global public goods frameworks, is their reliance on the beneficence of unnamed, impersonal forces – whether they be donors, the state, an abstract 'society', or, more tenuously still, the market.[1] In other words, these frameworks lack adequate recognition of power relations and the political – including democratic mechanisms and procedures for making and scrutinizing decisions about priorities and for mobilizing the claims and struggles of social movements in countering corporate, conservative, and state power. One of the achievements of such movements during the past two decades has been the injection of concepts of gender, racial, and sexual justice into human rights discourse and documents, particularly through the work of feminist and lesbian, gay, transgender and queer human rights activists within the UN conferences of the 1990s and the UN treaty bodies. A wide array of regional and transnational groups and coalitions has brought both the principle of indivisibility (that political and civil rights are inseparable from economic, social, cultural, and environmental rights) and the social dimension of individual needs into international perspective. Their work demonstrates that human rights are an evolving, living body of ideas, not a static set of norms (see Cook 1995, Girard 2007, Petchesky 2003, and Chapter 8 below).

Effective and genuinely democratic community participation – especially participation of women and economically, racially, and sexually marginalized groups – in monitoring sexual and reproductive health policies and services will happen neither as an accident of the market nor as a beneficent gift of charitable donors.[2] Such participation can only come through the efforts of robust, politically conscious social movements. In turn, the logic of such movements arises out of radical oppositional ideologies and practices, not 'consultations' or 'partnerships' with the managing institutions of global capitalism. A human rights framework provides both the norms upon which movements can base social justice claims and systems of public regulation and accountability they can use as forums to publicize those claims and shame corporate and government violators – even when, in practice, enforcement is weak. Market-based and cost-effectiveness approaches fail in this regard because they are ethically closed systems; that is, they measure value only by private preferences or by price, with the lowest costs having the highest value (Schrecker 1998). Welfare state and philanthropic approaches fail as well, insofar as they treat the recipients of aid or services as passive victims or clients rather than as rights-bearing agents and equal participants in decision making.

The language we use here matters. When we call the people who rely on reproductive and sexual health services 'consumers' or 'users', we reinforce the marketization of health care rather than challenging it. Individual health 'consumers' may be subjects of marketing research to find out about their product preferences or may be surveyed for their evaluation of provider practices. However, this is very different from a model of health provision that treats the recipient of services as a citizen with rights, that encourages her 'to feel that she has "the right to have rights and to create rights" [and] to regard herself as the "agent and subject" of her own actions' (Paiva 2003, p. 199). And it is not at all the same as communities mobilized on the basis of claims for social justice and human rights, and organized to participate directly in the design and evaluation of services and setting priorities for budgets and programmes. We agree with Pheng Cheah that, for contemporary social movements, rights are a necessary and irrepressible mode of expression and always, inevitably bound up in politics:

> [T]he irreducible contamination of the subject of human rights indicates that we can no longer theorize the normativity of rights claims in terms of the rational universality of a pure, atemporal and context-

independent human dignity ... separated from economics or politics....
Yet, [rights] are the only way for the disenfranchised to mobilize.

(Cheah 1997, p. 261)

Of course, such participation has its costs; as Cheah observes, it 'contaminates' civil society advocates with the stain of politics. For example, to become legitimate, effective actors within the UN system, transnational feminist, AIDS, and LGBTQ groups have had to learn, and in many ways internalize, the rules and procedures of that system. Whether in special sessions of the General Assembly or meetings of the Human Rights Council, they have had to rely on, and compete among themselves for, resources and recognition from various international donors, including not only governments and private foundations but also the World Bank and other intergovernmental agencies. Even counter-hegemonic movements asserting human rights demands in the streets – against the WTO or sexually repressive national laws; in favour of a moratorium on debt or treatment access for HIV and AIDS – do so in response to institutional frameworks and agendas set by those in power, including multinational corporations. But acknowledging that we act, and even achieve our identities as actors, within existing power regimes has a liberating dimension. Misnaming this process 'co-optation' reduces all power to a zero-sum game and misconstrues the nature of power, as well as underestimating the potential of even marginalized actors to effect change.

Regarding the supposed Western bourgeois origins of rights, at least two arguments come to mind. First, origins are irrelevant in assessing the ethical validity of social justice claims (which human rights embody). But more importantly, the fact that such claims are so various, recurrent, and scattered across cultures, societies, and historical times belies the assumption that they have any single provenance. Eisenstein (2004) shows that with regard to principles of democracy, it is simply inaccurate to associate those principles exclusively with the European West, when American Indian, Bengali, and African thinkers and societies have developed their own, more pluralistic ideas of democracy. If it is '[impossible to locate] a pure voice of the subject of oppression or a genuinely popular voice, and therefore, ... any vision of human rights claiming an all-encompassing universal validity', this means it is possible to let countless human rights flowers bloom diversely, across the globe. If the collective subjects of human rights do not exist a priori but are themselves constituted by the very process of articulating and demanding enforcement of human rights, this performative nature of rights means that such subjects are continually engaged in becoming and transforming (Cheah 1997, p. 256).

In sum, we need a human rights approach to empower people to make social, racial, and gender justice claims and to provide mechanisms for holding governments, private corporations, and international agencies accountable. Such an approach implies duties, not charity; standards for evaluating programmes and services from the standpoint of the needs and well-being of those they were designed to benefit; and mechanisms of accountability for enforcing those standards. Such mechanisms may be institutionalized within formal democratic processes of the state (for example, the citizens' health councils in Brazil or the poor people's and women's budgeting projects in South Africa and elsewhere); they may consist of group appeals and shadow reports by NGO monitors to human rights treaty bodies of the UN; or they may be more informal mobilizations by civil society, such as the coalition of hundreds of AIDS activists, women's groups, youth groups, sex workers, and others that denounced the failures of the UN General Assembly Special Session on AIDS in 2006.[3] Without the rhetorical structure of human rights, however, such translation of bodily claims into social action would be unthinkable.

In attempting to incorporate sexuality and sexual diversity into a rights framework, a lively debate has ensued over the past decade, mainly within national contexts, regarding sexual citizenship. From different vantage points, sexuality and queer theorists in the UK, USA, and Latin America have explored and expanded this concept in an effort to 'queer citizenship' or 'queer the state' (Bell and Binnie 2000, p. 11, Cooper 1995, Duggan 1995, Richardson 2000, Seidman 1998, Weeks 1999b). Adding a fourth category to T.H. Marshall's classic trilogy of civil, political, and social citizenship, their aim is 'to bring in the erotic and embodied dimensions excluded in many discussions of citizenship' and, in the process, to dismantle the conventional split between 'public' and 'private' spheres (Bell and Binnie 2000, p. 20, Grabham 2007). In Cooper's terms, this means challenging attempts, including by gays and lesbians, to 'reprivatize' sexuality, examining instead 'the ways in which institutionalized terrains such as the criminal justice process, welfare provision, and education are themselves sexualized' (Cooper 1995, p. 54). Such an approach has implications for so-called sexual minorities as well as for all those touched in one way or another by state regulatory powers and democratic liberatory potentials. As Bell and Binnie put it, 'all citizenship is sexual citizenship, in that the foundational tenets of being a citizen are all inflected by sexualities' (2000, p. 10).

The literature we have been referring to is not uncritical of the neoliberal and state-centric biases of sexual citizenship discourses. Signalling the heteronormative meanings built into the very concept of citizenship, Richardson argues that 'relationship-based rights claims by lesbian and gay movements ... [reinforce] both the desirability and necessity of sexual coupledom, privileged over other forms of relationships, as a basis for many kinds of rights entitlements'. 'Rather than uncritically accepting the discourse of citizenship,' she urges, 'we need to acknowledge that such discourses have reproduced a particular version of the responsible/good citizen focused on the values and norms associated with the heterosexual, nuclear family' (2000, p. 269, Bell and Binnie 2000, p. 30). This immediately brings to mind debates over marriage equity and the image of the 'good gay' couple (invariably middle class and mainstream) taking their 'good' children to soccer practice. More profoundly, the very language of 'sexual minorities' invokes a Western liberal tradition of democratization that envisions the 'unfinished project' which Žižek (2002) calls into question: completing modernity's forward march by progressively widening its circle. Rafael de la Dehesa aptly describes this position as:

> A central narrative of progress associated with liberal modernity, the universalization of citizenship. As sectors of civil society progressively gain access to the public sphere, the story goes – through, for instance, the extension of political rights to women, former slaves, illiterates, or other disenfranchised groups – the construction of citizenship becomes increasingly universalized and abstracted from the contingency of particular identities, if only formally.
>
> (de la Dehesa 2007, p. 182)

But what is the alternative to inclusion in the liberal state on liberal terms? Critical writers on sexual citizenship, such as Bell and Binnie (2000), offer us the model of radical opposition movements like ACT-UP (AIDS Coalition to Unleash Power) that '[try] to remain outside of the logic of the liberal state'; that '[pull] together a set of radical, transgressive strategies of refusal (refusal to act "appropriately", refusal to follow familiar campaigning routes, refusal to buy into liberal-statist grammars of rights and welfare) to build a subaltern counterpublic' (p. 21). But is refusal equivalent to revolution? ACT-UP's recent retreat into a single-minded treatment access agenda suggests that it may be just as difficult to develop a socially transformative strategy from outside as from within the state.

An unusually creative deployment of the sexual citizenship framework is set out in de la Dehesa's (2007) book, *Sexual Modernities: Queering the Public Sphere in Latin America*, a study of contemporary gay, lesbian, and transgender movements in Mexico and Brazil and their political contexts. De la Dehesa steers a nuanced course between the uncritical liberal paradigm of equal access and non-discrimination (add-in-the-queer-folks-and-stir) and a postmodern pessimism that views even the most liberal democratic institutions as irredeemably normalizing. On the one hand, writing of the Brazilian gay movement in the time of transition (and one could observe the same concerning the Brazilian feminist movement), de la Dehesa shows how it was powerfully pulled by the universalist language of 'full citizenship', anti-discrimination, and equal access to the public sphere. Shifts in legislative debates from 'sexual preference' to 'sexual orientation', and from 'homosexual liberation' to 'homosexual rights', he argues, 'in effect constituted a fixed and clearly bounded, rights-bearing community meriting representation through a legitimizing scientific frame' (de la Dehesa 2007, pp. 180–186).

Yet, echoing appeals by Currah (2003) and Spade (2006) in the USA for a pragmatic approach that addresses the immediate needs of transgender people, de la Dehesa recognizes important ways in which the liberal paradigm of inclusion has 'not only expanded a discursive repertoire available to activists but also provided the symbolic weight of precedent for specific claims'. For example, bills in Mexico and Brazil to permit transsexuals to change their names and gender on official documents, or the campaign for 'Brazil without Homophobia', have '[stretched] the boundaries of citizenship and subjectivization' and thus created a more pluralized, or what Zillah Eisenstein calls 'polyversal', understanding of 'nation' (de la Dehesa 2007, pp. 277, 280, 282, Eisenstein 2004).

Of course, the tension between short-term reform and long-term transformation is a problem that has haunted every progressive social movement; on some levels, we cannot escape it. But to privilege the status of 'citizen', or to adopt a discourse of rights uncritically, is to deny the exclusions and boundaries built into those concepts. From its origins in ancient Greek politics to present-day liberal democracies, the idea of citizenship was intrinsically about drawing boundaries – between citizens and others (strangers, aliens, barbarians); between public and private spaces; between categories of virtue and categories of deviance; and between 'majorities' and 'minorities'. For Aristotle, a citizen was by definition someone capable both of ruling and being ruled, which in no way could include women, slaves, or resident aliens. Today, the 'war on terror' seems to have trumped the much-vaunted era of globalization, with its free movement of goods, capital, people, ideas, and images across borders. Instead we see the proliferation of steel and electronic fences and surveillance technologies, and an unprecedented number of refugees and internally displaced persons – those abjected from the safety of citizenship through armed violence and disasters, both natural and man-made. 'Citizenship' becomes irrelevant if you are a dark-skinned Muslim in the West, or a woman accused of honour crimes by her community, or a transgender or intersex person almost anywhere.

Useful concepts for adapting a human rights framework to the current barrage of social exclusions are those of 'discipline' and 'biopolitics' we inherit from Foucault.[4] This is particularly true when we combine Foucault's insights with the more recent ones of Italian political philosopher Giorgio Agamben and his understandings of 'states of exception' and 'bare life'. We can then apply that set of analytical lenses to the sites of exclusion – prisons, refugee camps, migrant detention centres, torture chambers – that now erupt across the globe, gathering together the less-than-human, less-than-citizens of the 'war on terror' regime. In *The*

History of Sexuality, Volume I, Foucault links the origin of biopolitics directly to class divisions:

> [T]here had to be established a whole technology of control which made it possible to keep [the] body and sexuality [of the underclass, the proletariat], finally conceded to them, under surveillance (schooling, the politics of housing, public hygiene, institutions of relief and insurance, the general medicalization of the population, in short, an entire administrative and technical machinery made it possible to safely import the deployment of sexuality into the exploited class).
>
> (Foucault 1978, p. 126)

In his Collège de France lectures of the same period, Foucault distinguishes between two forms of biopower: *Discipline*, or 'techniques of power that were essentially centred on the body, on the individual body' (we might think of surgical mutilation of intersex infants, controls on masturbation, or psychotherapy for homosexuals or 'promiscuous' women and youth); and *Biopolitics* or technologies of power that are applied to 'man-as-species' or to regulate entire populations – their mortality, morbidity, numbers, and movement. 'Both technologies,' he elaborates, 'are obviously technologies of the body, but one is a technology in which the body is individualized as an organism endowed with capacities, while the other is a technology in which bodies are replaced by general biological processes' (Foucault 2003, p. 249). In the 1975 to 1976 lectures he expands the framework of biopolitics to encompass class divisions as well as colonialism, 'colonizing genocide', and racisms of all kinds:

> What in fact is racism? It is primarily a way of introducing a break into the domain of life that is under power's control: the break between what must live and what must die ... the distinction among races, the hierarchy of races, the fact that certain races are described as good and that others, in contrast, are described as inferior: all this is a way of fragmenting the field of the biological that power controls. It is a way of separating out the groups that exist within a population.
>
> (Foucault 2003, pp. 254–255)

Genocide is the logical outcome: 'the death of the other, the death of the bad race, of the inferior race (or the degenerate, or the abnormal) is something that will make life in general healthier; healthier and purer' (2003, p. 255). Clearly Foucault means to link the ways in which biopolitics produce racisms and contain the racialized to the forms of sexual regulation that medicalize and normalize the 'deviant' sexual types from which 'society must be defended'.

Agamben's political theory adds a spatial dimension to the biopolitical framework. Going considerably beyond Foucault, Agamben defines 'states of exception' as juridical situations in which what used to be called emergency powers, or a temporary imposition of martial law suspending ordinary constitutional norms and civil rights (usually in time of war, threat of armed attack, or civil unrest), becomes indefinite if not permanent. In this state, sovereignty is defined by the capacity to determine when and where the state of exception exists, and 'the camp' – the stripped-down conditions of 'bare life' – becomes the everyday condition of life for millions of people across the globe (Agamben 1998, p. 171, 2005). Of course the paradigm for Agamben, as for Foucault, is the Nazi concentration camps, but the analysis applies just as well to today's proliferating sites of involuntary confinement, from detention points for suspects in the 'war on terror', to camps for refugees and internally displaced persons, to prisons with physical walls as well as those with legal and civil barriers that constitute the limbo in which undocumented migrants, trafficked persons, and sex workers find themselves – especially in the USA, UK, EU, and Australia. 'The camp' is thus both 'a permanent spatial arrangement ... outside the normal order' and a moral and ontological situation (Agamben 1998, p. 169). Despite its variations, those who reside in it are all excluded from the circle of persons recognized as citizens, or, indeed, fully human beings. The rhetoric of citizenship is problematic precisely because it ignores the masses of militarized and globalized bodies confined to states of exception, whether through the ravages of war or those of capitalist development. And, let us be perfectly clear, included here also are those whose very humanity is called into question because they fail to conform to normative standards of gender or sexual truth – gays and lesbians, transgender and intersex people, sex workers, queer and 'promiscuous' youth.

Feminist political theorists have analysed in detail the ways in which gendered structures and institutions thoroughly contaminate European modernity's conceptions of citizenship as a status of 'equality' (Brown 1988, Okin 1979, Pateman 1988). But these feminist frames are too narrow to encompass today's multiple exclusions. We need an understanding of gender as integral, context-specific, and inclusive of men, transgender and intersex persons, as well as women, in order to correct the partially true but limited refrain of feminized victimhood – the poor-women-and-children mantra. Men of all ages are among the burgeoning number of human beings thrown into sites of exclusion, even though women and children may be the majority in many refugee and internally displaced person (IDP) camps. Border policing and surveillance techniques take aim at those deemed sexual and gender outlaws as well as the more predictable political, religious, and racialized targets of the 'war on terror'. Contributions to the scholarly anthology *Queer Migrations* document a century and a half of a 'federal immigration control regime [in the USA] that sought to ensure a "proper" sexual and gender order' by excluding Asian women (assumed to be prostitutes), cross-dressers, or anyone of 'suspicious' sexual or gender identity, and, more recently, those infected with HIV (Luibhéid and Cantú 2005; see also Herdt 1997, Luibhéid 2002). If anything, 9/11 provided an excuse to intensify these more traditional forms of policing borders based on racial, gender, and heteronormative stereotypes. The *Observer* newspaper in the UK reported in July 2007 that the European Commission had finalized an agreement with the US Department of Homeland Security on a new passenger-name-record system that will allow US officials to access detailed biographical information about passengers entering international airports, including not only ethnicity, religion, and political views but also sexual health and orientation (Doward 2007).

Those who transgress conventional gender and sexual binaries are almost automatically caught in states of exception, in blatant disregard of their bodies and lives. Acknowledging the wide continuum of chromosomal and morphological variation that exists between the poles of 'male' and 'female', Butler also comments on 'the arbitrariness and falsity of gender dimorphism as a prerequisite of human development'. She reminds us of the many 'humans ... who live and breathe in the interstices of this binary relation' and how they affirm 'that it is not exhaustive; it is not necessary' (Butler 2005, p. 65; see also Fausto-Sterling 2000). Transsexuals and intersex persons who seek to 'reverse' their genetic or anatomical gender through elective 'reassignment' surgery, when this is their desire, deserve our support from the point of view of human rights, as do gays and lesbians who wish to marry. But at the same time we should not lose sight of the political irony that even in the most homophobic societies such 'reversals', insofar as they reinforce the traditional binary (Grabham 2007), may win reinstatement to full citizenship, while those who remain in the interstices of gender ambiguity languish as aliens.

We have to confront not only the disciplinary and regulatory side of the human rights framework – of which sexual rights and sexual citizenship are a part – but also the ways in which that framework contains what Thomas has called 'the presumption of a sharp and necessary distinction between lives that are human and lives that are not' (Thomas 2006, p. 314). That presumption, which constitutes the bedrock of much of Western liberal political theory with its endless debates about the meaning of 'human nature', has left a legacy of unremitting violence and racism. In turn, racisms are always and everywhere saturated with anxieties about gender, sexuality, and the bestial. These links – between gender hierarchies, sexuality, animality, and racial otherness – surface time and again throughout modernity as the justifying rhetoric for colonial conquest, slavery, female subordination, lynching, racist incarceration, and genocide.

Concerning the racialized and gendered exclusions wrought by colonialism and slavery, consider the following: Jordan (1968) cites numerous seventeenth- and eighteenth-century English colonial tracts that create a triad of affinity between 'orangoutangs' and apes, 'libidinous' tendencies, and African 'Negroes' (both male and female). Ewen and Ewen (2006) and Schiebinger (1993) document 200 years of scientific racism, with its classifications and bodily taxonomies aimed at defining different races as different species – for example, the notorious display and dissection of the 'Hottentot' (Khoisan) Saartjie Bartman in early nineteenth-century Britain and France. Ewen and Ewen quote from the report of Georges Cuvier, 'Europe's leading naturalist', describing Bartman as having 'a human skull more similar to monkeys' and buttocks like 'the backsides of mandrill baboons' (Ewen and Ewen 2006, pp. 83–87). Gould quotes Cesare Lombroso, the founder of criminal anthropology, arguing at the group's 1886 international conference 'that the feet of prostitutes are often prehensile as in apes' (Gould 1981, p. 129). Indeed, the bestial, throughout the constructions of race and racism, has remained a potent signifier of the sexual. Thus classification systems intended to distinguish the human from the less-than-human, whether trans-species or transgender, have always fulfilled a dual function: displacement of (lustful, non-procreative) sexuality on to the racialized other (entire peoples, entire continents), and concentration of intelligibility and rationality in the white, heterosexual, European male. Sexual outlaws and outcasts become trapped within this same perverse logic.

We are not suggesting abandoning the language of human rights, sexual rights, or even sexual citizenship, only that we use that language very carefully, very self-critically, and always with an eye to deconstructing its implicit exclusions. We need to be aware of the underlying structure of group constitution as always, and inevitably, exclusionary. As Butler reminds us, recognition is 'a site of power by which the human is differentially produced', and thus every act of recognition (for example, granting of sexual rights) becomes a way of excluding some for the sake of establishing the human-ness of others (Butler 2005, p. 2). In this sense, citizenship is the paradigm of all identity politics, grounded in nationalism and the production of strangers.

In the end, human rights by themselves are necessary but insufficient to meet the demands of justice. Derrida (1992) associates justice with 'an aporia', a 'non-road', and 'an experience of the impossible'. It is something that is willed, desired, called for, never reducible to 'a rule' or a simple calculation of equivalency (that which is 'due', the order of law or exchange of penalty for wrong). Justice is 'incalculable' and therefore, in some sense, irrational (i.e., unsusceptible to strict cost–benefit analysis) (pp. 16, 25). Human rights alone can never fulfil justice – least of all for those who reside in the most abjected, marginalized situations or 'states of exception' – because, for one thing, human rights remain bound to texts, formal procedures, and rules. Moreover, human rights discourse is stubbornly immersed in what Ratna Kapur has called 'the tragedy of victimization rhetoric' – a variation of the helplessness and passivity that humanitarian relief and imperial policing projects typically attribute to the displaced and excluded (Kapur 2005). We need human rights, but we also need models that surpass formalism and utilize the power and local knowledge of the presumed victims of rights abuses.

An understanding of human rights as relational, evolving, and specific to historical and spatial contexts is very different from the notion of an 'unfinished project', which implies a Hegelian or Habermasian idea of linear progress. In fact, it sees rights more as a discursive process rather than a continuous project, one that distinct social groups, operating out of particular situations and constraints, are constantly reinventing. Here, already, is a useful response to one of the most frequent objections to rights frameworks voiced by leftists, some feminists, and postcolonialists, as well as religious conservatives and communitarians – their alleged individualism. Diverse critics argue that rights imply a false notion of individual autonomy that ignores community and kinship obligations and attachments.[5] Historically, however, and up until the present moment, rights have been advanced and achieved (albeit tenuously) almost always by, and on behalf of, social groups contesting hallowed definitions of tradition, nature, God's will, or who counts as 'citizens'. Whether in the name of the enslaved, the colonized, women, indigenous peoples, religious minorities, or sexual minorities, rights have been a group matter practically everywhere (Connell and Dowsett 1999, Young 1990).

To be sure, there is nothing fixed or steady about rights as achievements; the struggles have to be fought over and over again, justice won in new times and places by new generations and constituencies who give those rights different local and temporal meanings. Gays and lesbians in the USA 'won' the right to marriage equality in the highest court of one state, Massachusetts, only to see it slammed down in New York – considered the most liberal state – only two years later. African Americans, Afro-Brazilians, Dalits in India, Tutsis in Rwanda, Pakistanis in Britain, and Turks in Germany have all fought against local racisms in their different ways, reflecting their particular contexts. Women have joined together to contest gender violence and exclusion but focusing on the issues that affect them differently based on class, race/ethnicity, culture, and geography (Eisenstein 2004). Gay men, lesbians, bisexuals, transsexuals, transgenders, gender-queer and intersex people suffer common forms of injustice and non-recognition at the same time as they experience very different ones, along with differences of race, and class. Yet this very fluidity and instability is itself evidence against a unitary, liberal narrative about rights.

Rethinking human rights as a discursive field in which the terms of power and authority are continually shifting, depending 'on the constellation of forces at a given conjuncture' (Cheah 1997, p. 266), means that the process of defining, with greater and greater specificity, who is responsible for rights violations and where and how restitution should be made is part of an ongoing political struggle. We cannot escape politics. Moreover, to the extent that the historical conjuncture within which we operate (globalized, racialized, gendered, imperialistic capitalism – now complicated by the 'war on terror') is always in flux, 'no single actor' – neither the US government nor Pfizer Incorporated nor the World Bank – totally controls it. If our ideas and 'points of resistance' (sexual and reproductive rights, gender and racial equality, sustainable development) are continually being 'reinscribed into the text of global capitalism', those same ideas and resistance points, framed as human rights, also have the power to change how we think about existing historical conditions and power relations (Cheah 1997, p. 265). The advent of 'sexual rights' on the international scene surely marks one of these important historical shifts.

Chapter 8

Inventing and contesting sexual rights within the UN

In 2004, Paul Hunt, the UN Special Rapporteur on the Right to Health, issued a groundbreaking report that provoked the ire of more than a few country delegates to the Human Rights Commission (which, in early 2006, became the Human Rights Council). In that report Hunt states, 'sexuality is a characteristic of all human beings. It is a fundamental aspect of an individual's identity. It helps to define who a person is.' This means that fundamental human rights principles and norms must incorporate a 'recognition of sexual rights as human rights', including 'the right of all persons to express their sexual orientation, with due regard for the well-being and rights of others, without fear of persecution, denial of liberty or social interference' (Hunt 2004, p. 15).

If this definition, as Hunt himself suggests, is still far from complete, the fact that he felt able to assert it in an official UN document signifies a new and lively presence of sexual rights talk in international debates about the meanings and content of human rights, specifically in the domains of population and development, women's rights, gender equality, health, and HIV. In part, this 'coming out' of sexual rights in UN discussions is an effect of the HIV epidemic and the need for governments, however reluctantly, to recognize the realities of sexual behaviour and relations in everyday life (Altman 1995, 2001). But it also reflects an ongoing process of negotiation within the context of the UN conferences of the 1990s and their follow-up meetings in 1999 to 2006, where transnational feminist, LGBTQ, and AIDS activists and youth groups have carved out a new normative and conceptual terrain for human rights activism: the rights of the body and bodily integrity.

Although open debates about bodily integrity rights, including sexual rights, have surfaced within UN forums only since the early 1990s, the principles from which they derive are long-standing and contained in all the major human rights instruments – the Universal Declaration of Human Rights (UDHR), covenants on civil and political and on economic, social, and cultural rights, Convention on the Elimination of All Forms of Discrimination Against Women (CEDAW/Women's Convention), Convention on the Rights of the Child, and others. These principles consist of the right to life, to security of the person, to gender equality, and to the enjoyment of the highest attainable standard of physical and mental health, as well as to freedom from torture, degradation, and abuse. But the 1990s conferences took these abstract rights to a new level of specificity, galvanized by women's and lesbian and gay groups, and people struggling with and against HIV. These forces created a whole new constellation of norms, strategies, and institutional sites that had not been deployed previously in human rights activism – a new human rights discourse around the body and its needs for security, health, and pleasure. While our focus here is on sexual rights and sexuality, it is important to understand that sexual rights travel as part of a larger gang along with health rights and reproductive rights. The members of this gang form a conceptual unity, even though there are important differences among them and sometimes among the advocacy groups that identify most strongly with one or another aspect:

- Reproductive health, rights, and access to services, including access to adequate contraceptive information and supplies, full antenatal care and trained attendants as well as emergency obstetric services in pregnancy and childbirth, and access to safe, legal abortion and post-abortion care.
- Access to good-quality, affordable health care, especially preventive care, and to treatment, prevention, palliative care, and essential life-saving medicines for those suffering from, or at risk of, HIV and other preventable infectious diseases.
- Rights of sexual expression, enjoyment, and well-being without discrimination based on sexual or gender orientation, age, race, ethnicity, marital or HIV status, including respect for the dignity, humanity, and full citizenship of sex workers.
- Freedom from sexual, reproductive, and other bodily violence and abuses, including harmful practices such as forced marriage, honour killings, female genital mutilation, and sexual trafficking, regardless of whether these are imposed by family members, employers, medical personnel, state officials, or military (including national, international/UN, regional, and non-state) combatants.[1]

An objection frequently aimed at such human rights principles has to do with the absence of reliable instruments and mechanisms of enforcement, especially at the international level. This absence is seen as weakening the legitimacy of rights claims and contributing to their status as at best moral imperatives rather than legally binding rules.[2] But this view is incorrect. In the first place, many human rights principles – including the right to the highest attainable standard of physical and mental health – do in fact constitute binding norms of international law that national authorities and courts are obligated to enforce even if they do so only on rare occasions. Second, the absence of effective enforcement powers for civil and political rights (to say nothing of economic, social, and cultural rights) on the part of relevant international agencies like the United Nations Human Rights Council is a political matter related to transforming and democratizing global governance. It is not a reflection of the coherence and legitimacy of the norms themselves, nor does it negate the politically vital and potentially democratizing process of creating and debating norms – that is, the contestation over human rights as discourse.

In an incisive and detailed study, Françoise Girard charts two principal domains in which 'the United Nations has been the site of an overt struggle over sexuality' – whether to talk about it, 'to assert certain rights in connection with [it], or to name explicitly those aspects that give rise to discrimination' (Girard 2007, p. 312). Utilizing oral histories and archival materials and drawing on Foucault's theories of sexuality and biopower, Girard documents the step-by-step internal process whereby two incendiary phrases – 'sexual rights' and 'sexual orientation' – have been kicked around like a soccer ball at several key UN conferences and yet never made it through the goal posts. We will not try to recapitulate the story of political forces, tireless strategic manoeuvring, and Foucauldian 'reverse discourses' that Girard tells but rather to extract some of the highlights with regard to the invention and historical development of sexual rights as a discursive terrain in international politics.

First is the fact that the 'S' word enters UN parlance at all and when, where, and why it does. There is nothing surprising, argues Girard, about this eruption of sexual discourse in UN debates, given that the UN is 'one of the foremost international venues for the creation of norms and discourses'. Yet the reality is that nowhere in any international instrument relevant to human rights prior to 1993 does one find a single mention of 'sexuality' or 'sexual' (with the exception of brief references to sexual exploitation and abuse in the 1989 Convention on the Rights of the Child), which suggests a new historical juncture (Girard 2007, pp. 317–318, Petchesky 2000, p. 82). The UDHR and the covenants say a great deal about personal rights – to marry and form a family, to be respected in one's privacy and home, to educate one's children – but nothing about expressing, or being secure in, one's sexuality. Likewise, the Women's Convention (1981) and the Nairobi Forward-Looking Strategies (1985) refer to sexual equality and women's right to control their fertility, but not to sexual freedom or the rights of lesbians or trans women. Until recently, then, most human rights discourse acknowledged sexual life at best implicitly, and even then confined within the bounds of heterosexual marriage and reproduction.

Confirming other studies and amplifying them with interviews with activists, Girard rightly attributes the entrance of sexual debate and efforts (still largely unsuccessful) to codify sexual rights within the UN to feminist transnational movements. Since the 1970s and 1980s, feminists from the North and South, within national, regional, and transnational organizations, had been developing a set of political ideas and practices concerning the sexual freedom, safety, and bodily integrity of women and girls.[3] Undoubtedly this political vision was a limited one, linked as it was first of all to 'women' and, second, largely either to sexual and other forms of (male) violence against women or to reproductive freedom – in other words, implicitly to heteronormative contexts. While 'lesbians in the feminist movement and lesbian and gay groups began raising the issue of discrimination based on sexual orientation in various international forums' (Girard 2007, p. 318) and had been doing so in national and local arenas for years, it could be argued that the heterosexist and reproductive bias of many women's health and human rights groups prior to the mid-1990s contributed to the failure of a more inclusive view of sexual rights to make it through the UN goal posts. As Girard puts it:

> With issues like abusive family planning practices and unsafe abortion pre-eminent in the activism of the transnational women's health movement [during the 1980s to early 1990s], sexuality and reproduction remained linked in the thinking of many activists and academics, with sexuality often subsumed under reproduction and heteronormativity going largely unchallenged.
>
> (Girard 2007, p. 322)

Among other problems, a sub-current of tensions between lesbian and heterosexual feminist activists underlay this narrow framing. Girard quotes Mexican activist and scholar Gloria Careaga, a member of the Mexican delegation to the Beijing Fourth World Conference on Women:

> There was a lot of confusion about concepts. Most heterosexual women's health activists thought sexual rights was about lesbian, gay, bisexual, and transgender rights, while lesbians thought it was about women's rights, about sexuality. Lesbians felt that the responsibility of defending sexual rights was left to them.
>
> (Girard 2007, p. 323)

Neither our intention nor Girard's is to blame the women's groups at the International Conference on Population and Development in Cairo or the Fourth World Conference on Women in Beijing for the final outcome of the documents produced in those meetings and their erasure of any reference to 'sexual rights' or 'sexual orientation'. Women's Caucus members lobbied strenuously in both conference processes for the insertion of these phrases into various critical sections of the drafts and managed to enlist a number of government delegations, especially from the USA (then under the Clinton administration), Canada, and the Nordic countries. Yet transnational feminist thinking about sexual rights, and particularly about the wide range of genders and sexualities beyond the traditional binaries, remained conceptually undeveloped at this stage. Along with the absence of strong coalitions joining feminist, lesbian, gay, transgender, queer, HIV and AIDS, and human rights NGOs, this conceptual void left women's groups unprepared for the theoretical sophistication and vigorous presence of the Holy See and its Islamist and Christian right-wing allies who now haunted the halls of the UN and, increasingly, the world at large (see Chapter 1).[4] As a result, until the Special Rapporteur's report – which is neither binding nor intergovernmental, but only advisory – the actual words 'sexual rights' would not appear in any official UN document.

This is not to say that the concept of sexual rights (apart from the words) made no headway in the 1990s conferences; quite the contrary. First, we cannot underestimate the importance of transnational feminist campaigns for women's human rights and against violence against women during the decade preceding the Cairo and Beijing conferences in introducing the word 'sexual' into UN language and opening up space for recognition of reproductive, sexual, and bodily integrity rights of all kinds. The fact that these campaigns were focused on negative rights of ending violence and abuse made them strategically effective; even the most conservative patriarchal voices claim to oppose violence and abuse against women and children, and so find such appeals difficult to resist. Negative rights – those that involve prohibitions of egregious harm, whether by government agents or private parties – are often seen as more conservative than affirmative rights, since their achievement requires fewer material resources or structural changes and, in the case of violence against women, they tend to reinforce patriarchal stereotypes about the inherent fragility and helplessness of women (Kapur 2002, Miller 2004, Petchesky 2000). While we agree with this view, the history of UN debates none the less shows that formal recognition of sexual wrongs is not only crucial in itself but is also a necessary step toward the incorporation of sexuality as a basic domain of human ethics and affirmative rights. Negative and affirmative rights are inseparable.

Such recognition debuted in the Programme of Action of the Vienna World Conference on Human Rights in 1993 and the General Assembly's Declaration on the Elimination of Violence against Women of that same year. These documents express the consensus of the world's governments that 'gender-based violence and all forms of sexual harassment and exploitation', including trafficking in women, 'systematic rape, sexual slavery, and forced pregnancy', constitute violations of human rights. Along with the establishment of a UN special rapporteur on violence against women they were the fruit of organizing by women's NGOs, especially the public tribunals convened by the Centre for Women's Global Leadership, where women broke the silence about rape in armed conflict and prisons, forced prostitution, marital rape, and discrimination against lesbians. These public testimonies and the international agreements that followed 'put violence against women, and in particular sexual violence, on the map as a global human rights problem' (Miller 2004, p. 25). They also laid the groundwork for the jurisprudence of the international tribunals on the former Yugoslavia in The Hague and on Rwanda in Arusha, Tanzania, and the International Criminal Court Statute. With the tireless international Women's Caucus for Gender Justice driving them, these institutions codified rape, sexual trafficking and slavery, forced pregnancy, and sterilization in situations of armed conflict as war crimes, crimes against humanity, and, in certain circumstances, genocide; they thereby transformed international criminal law and the laws of war.[5]

Most importantly for our purposes, the 'anti-violence' provisions opened the door to more affirmative language about sexual rights in subsequent conference documents. The 1994 Cairo Programme of Action, in paragraph 7.2, contains a definition of 'sexual health' requiring 'that people are able to have a satisfying and safe sex life' as well as the right to decide 'if, when, and how often' to reproduce. Following the official WHO definition, paragraph 7.1 defines the purpose of sexual health as 'the enhancement of life and personal relations, and not merely counselling and care related to reproduction and sexually transmitted diseases'. Thus, although the Cairo document makes no explicit reference to sexual rights for gays, lesbians, trans-persons, unmarried persons, or anyone else for that matter, neither does it expressly limit the principle of self-determination, safety, and satisfaction in sexual life to heterosexuals, married persons, or adults. As Ignazio Saiz writes with reference to Cairo, 'Sexuality, previously on the UN agenda only as something to be circumscribed and regulated in the interest of public health, order, or morality, was for the first time implicitly recognized as a fundamental and positive aspect of human development' (Saiz 2004, p. 50).

In other sections, the Cairo Programme of Action urges governments to provide adolescents with a full array of sexual and reproductive health services and education 'to enable them to deal in a positive and responsible way with their sexuality'. It offers condoms as well as 'voluntary abstinence' as the means for men to 'share responsibility with women in matters of sexuality and reproduction'. And, most controversially, it includes references to 'family forms' in the plural ('various forms of the family') in place of the more conservative singular ('the family') preferred by the Vatican and some Islamic countries. Reflecting the ongoing battle over 'the social role of women as mothers and wives and the recognition of same-sex families' (Girard 2007, p. 325), this shift in language marks a rare and momentary victory.[6] These provisions led the way to paragraph

96 in the Beijing Platform for Action, considered by many to signal a major breakthrough in the struggle for recognition of sexual rights as human rights:

> The human rights of women include their right to have control over and decide freely and responsibly on matters related to their sexuality, including sexual and reproductive health, free of coercion, discrimination and violence. Equal relationships between women and men in matters of sexual relations and reproduction, including full respect for the integrity of the person, require mutual respect, consent and shared responsibility for sexual behaviour and its consequences.

One can read these modest gains as either the glass half empty or the glass half full. Girard emphasizes the Vatican view of 'sexual health as condoning immoral sexual behaviour, particularly extramarital sexual relations', as 'instrumental in keeping sexual health subordinated to reproductive health and thus within the heterosexual (and presumably married) realm' (2007, p. 328). Most references to sexuality within the Cairo Programme of Action, she argues, remain within the frame of heterosexuality, disease, or violence. And certainly the text of paragraph 96 gives a mixed and ambiguous message, as important for its silences as for its newly crafted statement of women's sexual rights. On the one hand, for the first time in UN discourse women are acknowledged as sexual as well as reproductive beings, with the right to decide freely about their sexuality without any explicit qualification regarding age, marital status, or sexual orientation. On the other hand, the text as adopted is steeped in heteronormativity and, even within that frame, emphasizes protection more than pleasure, responsibility more than freedom. Further, the original draft referred not to 'the human rights of women' but to 'the sexual rights of women' but, in the final draft, 'sexual rights' disappears, and various attempts by women's and lesbian and gay groups (through cooperative government delegations from Canada and the EU) to insert 'sexual orientation' into the document fell by the wayside.[7] Girard documents in particular the heroic effort by the US-based International Gay and Lesbian Human Rights Coalition in gathering some 6000 signatures on a petition advocating a far more radical feminist text than the compromise position that became paragraph 96. The petition urged governments to:

> recognize the right to determine one's sexual identity; the right to control one's body, particularly in establishing intimate relationships; and the right to choose if, when and with whom to bear or raise children as fundamental components of the human rights of all women regardless of sexual orientation.
>
> (quoted in Girard 2007, p. 331)

A significant point about the IGLHRC petition was that it represented a culturally and geographically diverse coalition of groups spanning the global South as well as the North, thus showing that sexual diversity was not just 'a Western or Northern issue' (Girard 2007, p. 331; see also Fried and Landsberg-Lewis 2000, p. 119). Barbara Klugman, a member of the South African delegations to both the Cairo and Beijing conferences, has emphasized how much the skewed geography of the HIV epidemic contributed to a realignment of forces within UN debates. The pandemic underlay a shift in government attitudes, especially in southern Africa and the Caribbean, and helped to fuel limited successes for transnational women's and lesbian and gay human rights groups. Thus, she argues, despite the absence of explicit references to 'sexual rights' or 'sexual orientation' in the Beijing document:

> Ultimately, sexual rights took prominence in Beijing as a topic of serious negotiation because so many non-Western groups supported the language. The African position in support of sexual rights, the willingness of many delegates from other southern countries at the Conference (particularly from the Caribbean) to speak explicitly for this position, and the presence of an organized lobby for sexual rights made up of NGOs from both North and South ... undermined the fundamentalist argument that sexual rights was a Western construct irrelevant to developing countries.
>
> (Klugman 2000, p. 152)

The historic nature of the IGLHRC petition and its cross-cultural breadth bring to mind our earlier discussion of human rights as an ongoing process rather than a terminal project – a never-ending dance of strategic manoeuvres and counter-manoeuvres, discourses and reverse discourses. Certainly, as Girard's narrative makes clear, paragraph 96 represents the best possible language that women's and LGBTQ groups could achieve in the particular historical moment and in the context of a series of trade-offs among governments (sexual rights for reproductive rights in the Cairo negotiations, sexual orientation for a watered-down, heteronormative sexual rights in the Beijing process).[8] In the global context of hyperconservatism and moral posturing ushered in by the Bush administration and the events of 11 September 2001, women's groups at the Cairo and Beijing five- and ten-year follow-up meetings were able to do no more than hold the line on the modest language won in the 1990s – and this defence was in itself an achievement of sorts. Yet, in the long term, the most significant human rights gains of the UN-centred process are not texts but rather the shifts in power relations and gradual building of oppositional alliances that unfold through that process.

A case in point is the growing coalition of human rights, LGBTQ, and feminist NGOs working for years to influence the thinking and practices of the human rights treaty bodies, especially the former Human Rights Commission. Based on extensive lobbying and consultation with women's and human rights NGOs, the treaty bodies have rendered dozens of comments and reports recognizing the obligations of states to respect sexual and reproductive rights, including calling for the repeal of laws in many countries that criminalize homosexuality (CRR 2002, ICJ 2004, Saiz 2004). Saiz documents an impressive array of opinions by different treaty bodies that condemn discrimination, hate crimes, arbitrary detentions, torture, and degradation against sexual minorities and affirm 'measures to protect refugees fleeing persecution on grounds of sexual orientation'.[9] The Committee on Economic, Social and Cultural Rights (CESCR) has included non-discrimination based on sexual orientation as part of the right to health and other economic and social rights. While it has thus far declined to apply the right to marry and found a family to any but heterosexuals, it has recognized partnership rights to pension benefits for gay and lesbian partners. Most remarkably, the Committee on the Rights of the Child (CRC) in 2002 affirmed the rights of gay youth and transsexuals 'to the appropriate information, support and necessary protection to enable them to live their sexual orientation' (Saiz 2004, pp. 51–54).[10] Recently, four special rapporteurs and the Committee on Torture issued reports strongly condemning the treatment of prisoners in the Guantánamo Bay detention centre, in part based on principles of sexual and health rights (see Chapter 10).

Of course, opinions by the treaty bodies and special rapporteurs condemning state laws and policies have no enforcement power and are not legally binding. Even so, they provoke vigorous disputes. In the highly politicized arena of the then Human Rights Commission in Geneva, the Brazilian delegation attempted for three years running to propose a resolution on 'Human Rights and Sexual Orientation', but each year the resolution ended up being postponed and finally was withdrawn by Brazil itself (see Chapter 1). That Brazil took on this role to begin with is not surprising, given its strong record of support for sexual rights and non-discrimination based on sexual orientation in key UN conferences and its national policies declaring access to ARV treatment a human right and promoting 'Brazil without homophobia' (Girard 2007, Petchesky 2003).[11] Yet the Brazilian delegates in Geneva expressed great surprise at the 'fierce opposition from governments' which their proposal encountered, with not only the USA and its allies in the Vatican and the Organization of Islamic Conference leading the attack but also some reluctance from within the EU (Saiz 2004, pp. 50, 57, Girard 2007, p. 342). According to Egyptian human rights activist Hossam Bahgat, the resolution met 'a significant backlash in 2004 and 2005' (quoted in Girard 2007, p. 352). In the end, the politics of sex collided with the politics of trade when Brazil withdrew its resolution (Pazello 2005; see also Chapter 1).

But here too we can see the glass half full and understand an evolving and dynamic process, the outcome of which has been the maturation of a more sophisticated and diverse coalition of civil society groups advancing sexual rights. Leading international feminist human rights advocates from New Zealand and the USA credit the Beijing conference and the unexpectedly wide impact of paragraph 96, beyond its literal words, for increasing attention to sexual orientation in the recommendations of the UN treaty bodies and the work of the special rapporteurs since 1998. A human rights and LGBTQ activist from Canada, who participated in every session of the HRC where sexual orientation was raised as well as the most recent meetings of the new Human Rights Council, emphasizes the 'significant mobilizing effect' of the entire experience and looks optimistically at the numerous openings for sexual orientation and sexual rights to further penetrate the work of that body. A member of the Brazilian delegation to the CHR who has worked within the UN for many years says optimistically, 'Everyone knows that, one day, we will pass this resolution. It's only a matter of time.'[12] In addition, as if to affirm his optimism, as already mentioned (see Chapter 1), 54 member states of the Human Rights Council, led by Norway but also including the USA, issued a statement in December 2006 condemning human rights violations aimed at people because of their sexual orientation or gender identity and calling on the UN treaty bodies, particularly the Human Rights Council, to address these violations urgently (ARC 2006).

More than anything, the campaign to secure a human rights resolution on sexual orientation – one that addresses gender orientation and identity as well – has been the fulcrum around which an increasingly diverse and more broadly representative coalition has evolved. The substantive achievements of this coalition, though incremental, have been significant. A compilation of 'References to Sexual Orientation, Gender Identity and Related Issues in Reports Submitted to the [Human Rights] Council' as of March 2007 shows serious attention to blatant abuses of the rights to life, health, sexual freedom, bodily integrity, and privacy of gays, lesbians, transgender and intersex persons as well as heterosexual women, among a wide range of UN special procedures and rapporteurs (ARC 2007a).[13] The special procedures have now signalled 'discrimination on the ground of sexual orientation' and 'discrimination on the grounds of HIV/AIDS status' as top priorities in their list of gaps in human rights protection (ARC 2007b). And, most impressive, the Yogyakarta Principles on the Application of International Human Rights Law in Relation to Sexual Orientation and Gender Identity, launched in March 2007 and developed by a diverse group of international human rights experts and activists (many of whom belong to the coalition just discussed), is achieving major visibility in the UN treaty bodies and among the special procedures.[14]

Without diminishing the historic importance of these documents – like those of the 1990s that preceded them – we want to emphasize once again that the political journey to create and deploy them is what counts in the long run. Rights of sexual and gender orientation have become an irrepressible and newly dynamic site of transnational civil society mobilization bringing together feminist, sexual and reproductive health, lesbian and gay, transgender, intersex, and human rights groups – from Latin America and the Caribbean, the Middle East, Africa, Asia and the Pacific, Europe, and North America. These groups have worked closely and strategized across many differences and, through considerable conflicts, gradually building a reservoir of unity and trust to engage in future and more inclusive struggles. Process is everything, discourse merely its imprint.

Chapter 9

Transnational debates
Sexuality, power, and new subjectivities

A vigorous and impassioned sexual rights debate at the level of the UN would never have gained the momentum it did without the contribution of a broad array of new global political actors, including, as already mentioned above, feminist and gay and lesbian movements, transgender and intersex rights groups, sex workers, people living with HIV, and youth organizations spanning diverse sexualities and gender identities, who often originate in local conditions quite separate from 'the West'. While many of these organizations share common political values that converge around notions of sexual and bodily aspirations, their agendas vary and sometimes even conflict depending on the groups and cultural/political contexts involved. In this chapter we examine four sites of ongoing contention and debate within sexual rights thinking and advocacy that illustrate the complex weave of shared concerns and political divisions currently constructing the domain of 'sexual rights'. These examples call into question certain unexamined assumptions that pervade feminist and, more broadly, sex-gender identity politics and force us to rethink our understanding of the subjects of human rights and their positioning within fields of power relations.

Delinking sexual health and rights from reproduction

> Since many expressions of sexuality are non-reproductive, it is misguided to subsume sexual rights, including the right to sexual health, under reproductive rights and reproductive health.
>
> (Hunt 2004)

The insight that sexuality and reproduction are separate domains of human (and some non-human) activity is as old as women's aspirations to be defined as 'citizens' and not confined as procreators, and underlies campaigns for birth control in countries across the globe beginning in the mid-nineteenth century. Rubin's groundbreaking essay, 'Thinking sex' (1984), marked an important deepening of this idea which reflected the emergence of diverse sexual identities and movements during that period, particularly in response to punitive public policies with regard to gay, lesbian, and other queer lifestyles. Rubin mapped a long history of public hysteria about sexuality and the resultant production of what she termed 'hierarchies of sexual value', codified through religious, psychiatric, and cultural as well as political authorities. Recognizing that sexuality is entirely 'a human product' mediated by cultural meanings, Rubin understood that these hierarchies and their contents vary tremendously with historical and cultural contexts. Yet she provided a snapshot of 'the sexual value system', with all its restrictions and taboos, which is relevant for a depressingly wide variety of times and places (see Chapter 5, and Rubin 1984, pp. 280–281).

Parker, elaborating on Rubin's analysis in the Brazilian context, notes how the role of 'the police in urban centres' reinforces the work of

> priests, hygienists, and doctors in seeking to regulate sexual conduct.... Sex solely for pleasure, sexual promiscuity, prostitution, and homosexuality have all been the object not merely of stigma, but often of outright repression aimed at minimizing the threat that they pose to normal sexuality.
>
> (Parker 1991, p. 96)

Numerous commentators since Rubin have built on these insights about the regulatory power of the dogma that 'natural', 'normal', 'good' sex is necessarily linked to reproduction and heteronormative, conjugal coupling and critiqued the ways this linkage persists even among feminists and reproductive rights advocates (Amuchastegui and Aggleton 2007, Connell and Dowsett 1999, Corrêa 1997, Miller 2000). Amuchastegui and Aggleton, writing about the sexual ideas and values of young men in contemporary Mexico, remind us that the separation between sexuality and reproduction has had a long-standing manifestation that persists in many traditional cultures: pleasure for men, procreation for women (2007, p. 78, n. 4). This traditional gendering of the division between sexual rights and reproduction makes it all the more urgent to deconstruct the separateness of pleasure and desire from reproduction and to disconnect this separation from the ways it has been mapped on to the bodies of men versus women.

Notwithstanding these efforts to rethink sexuality as a domain distinct from reproduction and, to some extent, even from gender (see below), the seamless elision between 'reproductive health and rights' and 'sexual health and rights' has had a stubborn and too often unexamined staying power that appears prominently in the Cairo Programme of Action and the mobilizing discourses that grew up around it.[1] In this context, the older debate about the relationship between sexuality and reproduction has taken on a new variant in the debate over the commonly used acronym 'SRHR' (Sexual and Reproductive Health and Rights).[2] We agree with Paul Hunt and others who argue that this elision is a flimsy and mechanical construction containing a fragile union between two binaries, each of which is, in itself, misleading:

- A heteronormatively framed 'reproductive rights' mainly concerned with 'women's' control over, and health within, their pregnancies and childbearing in relation to 'men', who are generally perceived as obstacles to that control (whether as husbands, partners, medical providers, religious leaders, or political and judicial authorities).
- A conception of sexual rights that grew simultaneously out of the gay and lesbian rights movements and the HIV/AIDS pandemic, with its agenda to examine sexual behaviour still framed within arbitrarily defined sexual 'risk categories' rather than actual practices (Connell and Dowsett 1999, Treichler 1988).

Simply linking these two analytically questionable clusters is much akin to a marriage of convenience or an arranged marriage between two very different clans; the parents assume the liaison makes sense in terms of the combination of family assets, but what does it have to do with the offspring's desires? Or yet, more poignantly, is this simplified articulation an evasion of the conflicts and confusions at play in each family's household?

Within the first binary construction – 'reproductive rights' assumed to be a women's issue vis-à-vis recalcitrant men – the facile grafting on of 'sexual and' has been mainly a process of accretion, with sexuality education, sexual violence, and HIV/AIDS/STI prevention and treatment now joining contraception, abortion, and maternal and child health in the catalogue of issues and services.[3] To the extent that most advocates and researchers in the reproductive health field consider sexual desires and power at all, it is still predominantly within contexts of heterosexual (or sometimes parent–child) relations. The objective is still overwhelmingly the avoidance of unwanted pregnancy, disease, and abuse rather than the proliferation of pleasures and modes of being sexual. As Dowsett has written:

> sexuality is often reduced to a component of gender. Indeed, sexuality is often subsumed within the emotional and relational domain of gendered families and culturally prevailing forms of heterosexuality. As a consequence, for example, sexuality ... is reduced to a mechanism (or vector) in demography's reproductive health and global population concerns.

(Dowsett 2003, p. 24)

Likewise, Miller has argued forcefully against 'a conflation (or submersion) of sexual rights with reproductive rights that inadvertently erases entire sets of people' (such as diverse age groups, 'nonconforming sexual identities', and kinship arrangements). Such a conflation not only excludes but also obscures 'the distinctive nature of sexual rights themselves' (Miller 2000, pp. 70, 86–87). Miller calls for a framework that would both '[link and delink] sexual rights to reproductive rights'. It would 'at a minimum require removing prohibitions against non-procreative sex', both protecting against private or state coercion and violence in sexual matters while also empowering the capacity 'to say "yes", free of limiting stereotypes and with knowledge of the implications for one's safety and contentment' (2000, pp. 93–94).

The analyses by Dowsett and Miller reorient us to see sexuality as the broad, inclusive category within which reproductive health, HIV and AIDS, and possibly even gender and its diverse expressions, are all permutations or subcategories. But this raises a further complication, since, within the sexuality or sexual rights side of the equation, scholars and activists have just begun to probe the very complex intersections, distinctions – and sometimes tensions – among homosexual, heterosexual, bisexual, transsexual, and intersex, and how gender crosses over and through all these in the unstable 'transgender' tent.[4] Peter Jackson (2007), studying the enormous variety of sexual identities in Thailand, takes issue with what he considers the Eurocentric 'discourses of sexuality' originating with Foucault and advanced by Sedgwick. In particular Jackson challenges 'the categorical separation of gender and sexuality that has underpinned the establishment of queer studies as a separate inquiry from feminism'. In contrast, following Halperin's work on ancient and medieval sexualities (2002), Jackson documents the complex interweaving of a dazzling array of sexual and gender meanings and categories among mid-twentieth-century Thai subcultures. Such empirical investigations, he suggests, 'still lack a general theory' that would account for 'the diversity of ways in which gender identity and sexual identity may be articulated in forming subjectivities which are simultaneously gendered and sexualized' (Jackson 2007, pp. 343, 352).

In light of this complexity, it is perhaps necessary to encourage a trial separation of 'RR' and 'SR' to provide the necessary time and space to do the hard work of analysing their differences as well as their interlinkages. It might be useful if reproductive rights advocates began to look seriously at the variety of ways in which diverse sexualities and reproduction can be both intertwined and delinked and to acknowledge that both sexual and gender diversities raise new kinds of challenges for reproductive locations, aspirations, and politics. Likewise, sexual rights advocates might begin to examine the reproductive potentials of non-normative sexual and gender identities at the same time as they continue to explore the transgressive (as well as accommodative) potentials of every variation in the sex-gender rainbow. They would also do well to recognize that the reproductive realm is not exempt from transgressive practices, the most evident example being the widespread recourse to abortion in contexts where it is criminalized.[5] We might imagine these analytical tasks, which are deeply ethical and political, as a series of questions including, but not confined to:

- If reproductive rights include the right not to reproduce, then does this not include all forms of non-procreative sex; so why should any one form have the status of normativity or moral virtue? That is, if we refuse the principle that only procreative sex is 'good', or that it has a higher place than any other form, are we willing to reject all sexual hierarchies? (Rubin 1984; see also Jakobson and Pellegrini 2003).
- What would it mean to talk about 'reproductive and sexual health services' in a way that is not framed within the dominant gender binary logic? Would it mean adding to the usual list for women (pregnancy counselling, prenatal, and obstetric care; contraceptive and abortion services; sexuality education; HIV/AIDS/STI counselling, prevention and treatment; infertility treatment), urological services, transsexual surgeries and hormonal treatments, and HIV/AIDS services that are truly open to everyone, including sexual 'deviants', sex workers, and all youth? Would it also mean supporting the choice of transgender people as well as lesbians to be pregnant and to bear and raise children, with full access to obstetric and gynaecological care and services, and with complete respect for who they are?[6]
- If reproduction is about kinship and childrearing as well as pregnancy and childbearing, then what would it mean to support the reproductive rights of gay men, trans- and intersex people, and sex workers – for example, to adopt and raise children and to receive family, child care, and child health insurance benefits within non-traditional households and kin networks? Do transgender, intersex, and sex worker lives – especially in societies where increasing numbers of households are not formed around heterosexual married couples – open the possibility of attaching social benefits and kinship rights to persons rather than to marriage? (Butler 2005, Duggan 1995, Jakobsen and Pellegrini 2003).

Engaging such questions should move us toward greater inclusivity in how we conceptualize both reproductive and erotic justice. The facile SRHR acronym relieves us of responsibility for thinking through what this inclusive vision would mean and, specifically, who counts as full human beings in the discourse of human rights; or, as Butler has framed it, 'what makes a life livable' and 'whose lives count as lives' in our moral universe (Butler 2005, p. 17). Moreover, in the feminist project of liberating individual lives and desires from the strictures of patriarchal, heteronormative family codes, it sidesteps affirmation of alternative kinship arrangements. Among the most marginalized lives in the broad array of sexual and reproductive identities are those of sex workers. None the less, the struggle for recognition and dignity for sex workers represents one of the most dynamic, albeit contested, sites where activists are integrating an affirmative approach to sexuality and kinship with economic, social, and political rights.

Sex work, sex trafficking, and 'victimization rhetoric'

Sex worker organizations have emerged as a vocal presence in many countries over the past decade, especially in South and Southeast Asia and some countries in Latin America. For example, the Sonagachi project (see Chapter 2, n. 24), an HIV programme for sex workers in Kolkata's red-light district, run by the sex workers themselves, provides bank loans, schooling for children, literacy training for adults, reproductive health care, and cheap condoms. The result is 60,000 members who have pledged to use condoms regularly and an HIV prevalence rate of only 5 per cent (Mukerjee 2006). Elsewhere in India, a study of sex workers in Kerala recorded countless violations of their sexual and reproductive rights by government officials and agencies, police, men in the streets, and even some well-meaning NGOs (Jayasree 2004). More than half of the sex workers interviewed had been married and got into sex work mainly due to abusive or violent husbands, abandonment, and lack of skills or viable employment alternatives. Many were homeless due to eviction or ostracism by families and relatives. All complained of severe health, safety, and hygiene problems in shelters and on the streets, and 80 per cent suffered from physical and mental illness, mainly HIV and other sexually transmitted infections. More than 95 per cent had experienced violence from police or street thugs, including being chased out of their villages and having their heads shaved, stigmatized as carriers of HIV. Many others, denied their parental rights as 'immoral' mothers, were separated from their children or barred from visiting them in child care centres.

The Kerala study shows how difficult it is to detach the denial of basic reproductive and sexual health services from the disabling and unjust environment surrounding sex work. Since the mid-1990s, organizing among sex workers in India, Malaysia, Thailand, Brazil, and elsewhere has meant that many are well informed about HIV-related risks, safer sex, and condom use. But how do you use a condom when the police might raid at any time and seize it as evidence, or when the client refuses to pay if you do? Jayasree argues 'that HIV prevention is possible only if an enabling environment is created for sex workers, in which they can live as free citizens' (as borne out by the success of the Sonagachi project). This means not only decriminalizing sex work and assuring sex workers the right to a livelihood and freedom from violence but also changing popular perceptions to 'delink' sex workers 'from the problem of sexual morality' (Jayasree 2004, pp. 63–64). It means affirming the equal right of sex workers to bodily pleasure, self-determination, and full citizenship, and it means admitting that, with improved conditions, many sex workers might actually enjoy the work they do. Jayasree describes the 'Festival of Pleasure' organized by the National Network of Sex Worker Organisations in Kerala in 2003:

> Its theme was a safe environment for body and mind, for sex workers to attain the full potential of life. It launched a campaign for the decriminalisation of sex work, acceptance of sex workers' rights, and the right to safe and pleasurable sex. Sex workers want an equal opportunity to choose how to live their own lives, in a world without violence and in harmony with their environment.
>
> (Jayasree 2004, p. 66)

The holistic approach to erotic and social justice advanced by the national network stands in sharp contrast to the politics of more established feminist groups – in India as well as the West – that focus on women as perpetual victims of violence. Miller explains the strategic logic of the emphasis placed on violence and sexual abuse by the global feminist movements leading up to, during, and after the Beijing women's conference. Focusing on sexual violence seemed to make its gendered nature more evident 'to key human rights bodies and actors': 'To build a political force that could not be resisted, advocates had to emphasize and make visible what was different about the experiences of women; they had to make these experiences too horrendous to ignore.' Yet a preoccupation with sexual violence against women has regressive if unintended consequences. Spotlighting horrific personal testimonies and analogizing women's subordination to torture tends to reinforce the traditional patriarchal view of women as helpless victims who must be 'protected' or 'rescued' by the state (or imperial invaders) (Miller 2004, pp. 18, 25).

Kapur expands this critique of viewing women exclusively as 'victim subjects' by connecting two notions it encompasses: 'gender essentialism' and 'cultural essentialism'. 'Women in the postcolonial world are portrayed as victims of their culture', thus reinforcing both stereotypes of women as victims and those of Asian, African, or Middle Eastern cultures as inferior (Kapur 2005, p. 99). This plays into the hands of powerful political forces seeking legitimacy for patrolling borders and waging war under the cover of protecting women – as seen, for example, in Bush's justification for invading Afghanistan in 2001 in order to rescue Afghan women from the Taliban, or in his speeches before the UN General Assembly linking 'sexual slavery of girls and women' to the 'moral' objectives of the 'war against terror' (Miller 2004, p. 17, Eisenstein 2004, 2007). However, the same dynamic can occur within domestic politics. Kapur argues that Indian feminists echo their Western counterparts by re-invoking Indian women's victim status and that this image, of the Indian woman as 'chaste and vulnerable to exploitation', also replicates 'the discourse on the purity of the nation and the preservation of Indian womanhood' propagated by earlier generations of nationalists in the colonial era and by the Hindu Right (specifically regarding Hindu womanhood) today (see Chapters 2 and 3). Feminist victim politics thus 'reinforce the law-and-order agenda of the Hindu Right, their paternalistic approach to women's issues, and their communalizing agenda' (Kapur 2005, pp. 124–126). Such politics also obscure the active presence of multiple gendered and sexual subjects on the national and global political stage:

> What is to be done with Malleswari, who won the bronze medal (the only medal for India) at the Sydney Olympics in 2000 in women's weightlifting? Or with Lara Datta, who won the Miss Universe Pageant in 2000 and has no reluctance to speak explicitly about sex, safe sexual practices, and the issue of AIDS? Or the sex workers who state, 'We want bread. We also want roses!' Where do we locate these women in a politics that operates along the strict binaries of victim/agent, East/West, First World/Third World, or the West and the Rest?
>
> (Kapur 2005, p. 127)

The neo-colonial discourse of the 'victim subject' is particularly evident in the politics of sex trafficking – a favourite 'human rights' cause of the Bush administration and the Christian right in the USA (Girard 2004). A punitive, criminalizing approach that conflates all forms of commercialized sex work with sex trafficking has become a staple of US policy, reflecting the strong influence of 'abolitionist' feminists (e.g., the Coalition against Trafficking of Women) who view any sort of commercial sex as violence against women. This approach (focusing on 'demand') mandates prosecution and policing methods rather than social and economic justice, ignoring the conditions of poverty and lack of livelihoods that make people vulnerable to trafficking and refusing to provide health or other social services to trafficked persons. It also serves the 'antiterrorism' agenda of controlling migration, sealing borders, and constricting human mobility (Girard 2004, Kapur 2005, Miller 2004).[7] The criminalization/abolitionist approach contrasts sharply with the view of many sex worker advocates in South and Southeast Asia, South Africa, the Americas, and elsewhere, who urge that sex workers be treated like 'any other set of migrant workers' or like the marginal and casualized workers they often are, who need improved conditions, safety, access to health services, and freedom from harassment and abuse as a matter of human right and dignity (Kempadoo 1998, Saunders 2004, pp. 185–187; see also Chapter 2).

We do not subscribe to an ultra-liberal position that views all commercial sex as 'just work'; although the line between coercion and consent is not always easy to discern, situations of extreme power imbalance, social exclusion, and physical violence are fairly reliable markers of non-consent. Documented cases of young women (and, less frequently, men) defrauded into sex work by promises of 'legitimate' jobs and then kept in virtual servitude; employment of minors in the trade (almost always from among the poor, sometimes sold by their parents); funnelling of trans-people into commercial sex by default because all other avenues of livelihood are blocked to them – these unjust scenarios warrant the application of existing regulatory and protective action, both national and international (see Garcia and Parker 2006, Kempadoo 1998, Miller 2004). But even here the use of criminal methods will never substitute for, and may often impede, investment of public resources in the social conditions needed to address poverty and vulnerability – schools, vocational training, jobs, infrastructure, child care, and strict enforcement of anti-discrimination laws on the grounds of sexual and gender orientation.

Yet the abolitionist view has become incorporated into the language and enforcement policies of the US Trafficking Victims Protection Act and the US government's Global AIDS Act of 2003. Both acts prohibit the channelling of funds to 'any group or organization that does not have a policy explicitly opposing prostitution and sex trafficking' or that 'advocates or supports the legalization of prostitution' (Saunders 2004, p. 186, United States 108th Congress 2003). The purposes are multiple: to endow US foreign policy with 'moral' and allegedly pro-woman credentials; to police migrant workers and cross-border migrations of all kinds by waving the flag of sexual exploitation; and, not least, to isolate and disempower sex workers as political actors. That it has had limited success in doing so becomes evident in the responses of local groups – and especially sex worker groups – to PEPFAR (see Chapter 2), and particularly to the infamous 'prostitution pledge' requiring recipients of PEPFAR funds to promise that no US funds received will 'be used to promote or advocate legalization or practice of prostitution' or 'to provide assistance to any group ... that does not have a position explicitly opposing prostitution'.[8] As mentioned earlier, when the Indian organization Sangram – long involved in HIV prevention and sex worker rights advocacy – refused to sign the pledge, USAID officials accused it of being implicated in sex trafficking. Yet the critical point is that Sangram not only defied US government power and refused to sign the pledge but also sent out an Internet message protesting against being falsely maligned. Furthermore, in Brazil the National Commission on AIDS, which incorporates a wide range of civil society organizations (including sex workers' associations), was instrumental in the decision of the Ministry of Health to refuse an AIDS grant of $40 million from USAID rather than sign the prostitution pledge (Boseley and Goldenberg 2005).[9] Such acts defy assumptions about passive victimhood and policies that fail to distinguish between voluntary sex workers and the victims of trafficking.

HIV and AIDS and the struggle for treatment access – the limits of distributive justice

US foreign policy, particularly – but not entirely – under the Bush administration, has violated the human rights of people living with HIV through its 'moral' restrictions concerning condom use and sex work. It has also infringed the human right to health as a result of its intimate linkages with pharmaceutical companies and constant manipulation of international trade in essential medicines. Although the open collision between sexual rights and health rights on the one hand and global trade rules on the other has not yet been fully mapped and addressed within the sexual politics field, its effects are deeply sexualized, gendered, and racialized. According to recent UNAIDS data, women now comprise 50 per cent of those infected with HIV worldwide and are the fastest growing group among those newly infected. In addition, in sub-Saharan Africa, which has 70 per cent of the nearly 40 million people in the world now living with HIV, women comprise up to two-thirds of adults and 75 per cent of young people (ages 15–24) who are seropositive.[10] The reasons for this gender disparity have everything to do with the power differentials that govern heterosexual relations; far from being a protection, marriage, with all its presumptions of male sexual licence, may be even more dangerous for young women than staying single. In countries such as South Africa and Kenya, women's and girls' vulnerability to infection correlates with high rates of sexual violence, a pattern of older men having sexual relations with or sexually violating much younger women, and the difficulties women have in negotiating condom use (Klugman 2000, UNAIDS 2006). The 2006 acquittal of former South African deputy president Jacob Zuma on charges of raping the 31-year-old, HIV-positive daughter of a friend is just one tragic example of this pattern.[11]

We highlight this sexual and gendered backdrop in order to make clear two troubling facts: current US trade policies pose a hidden war against women (especially poor African women) that must be addressed, and prevailing strategies for doing so have worked unwittingly to narrow and desexualize AIDS activism (see Chapter 6). History is significant here. The campaign for treatment access – arguably the first occasion for transnational movement around AIDS, and the most successful – originated concurrently with the anti-globalization movement, which has challenged

US and global capitalist hegemony in trade and macroeconomic policies generally. One of the leading organizations in that campaign, Health GAP, was founded at the International Conference on AIDS in Geneva in 1998, which had the theme 'Closing the Gap'. The synergy between the movements for global (economic) justice and for treatment access was also in evidence at the International Conference on AIDS in Vancouver in 1996, which called for 'universal access' and increasing awareness among global justice activists of the unfairness of WTO patent rules and their deadly consequences for the poorest and most afflicted in Africa, Asia, and the Caribbean.

The coordinated efforts of this movement – led by groups such as TAC (Treatment Action Campaign) in South Africa, the Health GAP Coalition, ACT UP, Oxfam, and Médecins sans Frontières – managed in a very short time to mobilize a militant and effective campaign to promote access to essential medicines for HIV/AIDS and other life-threatening diseases as a human right. A number of developing countries have also become actors in this critical arena. In 2000 the Brazilian government threatened to break the patents for key anti-retroviral medications (ARVs), and in South Africa the highest court stood up to the attempts by the Pharmaceutical Research and Manufacturers Association of America, in conjunction with the US trade representative, to impose rigid patent rules that would exclude cheaper generic drugs. In India and, later, Thailand, manufacturers who were not yet bound by restrictive patents laws, began producing lower cost ARVs for both the domestic and international markets.[12]

These developments helped bring about a historic occurrence at the 2001 WTO annual ministerial meeting in Doha, Qatar. There a bloc of Southern countries drafted and secured the passage of a declaration affirming that 'the TRIPS Agreement does not and should not prevent Members from taking measures to protect public health ... and, in particular, to promote access to medicines for all'.[13] Such measures would include the issuing of compulsory licences or parallel imports to make possible the local manufacture or importation of cheap generic drugs to address the AIDS crisis. The Doha Declaration happened in the shadow of 11 September 2001, as the 'war on terror' was being launched. The Bush administration did not oppose the declaration outright; it simply set about undermining it unilaterally. For instance, when PEPFAR stated that 60 per cent of the funds allocated should go to free treatment, this was correctly seen as a major breakthrough. But this gesture of 'compassionate conservatism' subtly eroded the global agenda in respect of intellectual property rights, since the USA administration began to pay pharmaceutical companies for non-generic drugs that would be freely distributed. In parallel, the USA used the bribe-and-bully methods it has used in all its foreign policy dealings, but with particular vigour in its pursuit of bilateral free trade agreements (FTAs).

The US trade and patents regime, known as TRIPS Plus, requires signatory countries to waive their rights to produce or import cheaper generic drugs for their citizens, and to extend the patents of US drug makers beyond the current 20-year limit – or lose billions of dollars in trade with the USA (Oxfam 2006a). While other rich countries with major PHARMA interests (particularly in the EU) have not engaged in a TRIPS Plus agenda, their passivity vis-à-vis the US effort has in effect constituted a green light (Oxfam 2006b).

Thailand, where in 2006 the USA tried to impose the Faustian bargain it calls 'free', offers a recent example of what TRIPS Plus means in practice. More than a million men, women, and children have been infected by HIV in Thailand, half a million have died, and around 20,000 new infections still occur each year. Earlier in the Thai epidemic, the most rapid transmission was among sex workers, mainly women. Today the disease is growing in the population more generally and especially among men who have sex with men, with half of all new infections among adult women infected by partners or spouses. Yet the HIV picture in Thailand, while serious, is also hopeful due to a public health offensive that combines aggressive outreach, prevention, and condom distribution strategies (for example, putting condoms in bars and clubs where sexual transactions are set up or occur) with a growing treatment access programme. Through its government pharmaceutical organization (similar to Brazil's state-owned drug production facilities) Thailand produces high-quality generic versions of expensive commercial HIV drugs and drugs to treat deadly opportunistic infections. This programme of access to inexpensive generics has made it possible to treat 80,000 HIV-positive people who otherwise would have died, and there are plans to include more in the near future.

In November 2006, the provisional Thai government issued a compulsory licence on Efavirenz, an important HIV drug under patent to the US-based drug giant Merck. It did so in the face of legal threats from Merck and pressure from the US trade representative, demanding that Thailand forfeit its rights to use TRIPS flexibilities in support of its people's lives and health, in exchange for trade preferences.[14] Then, in May 2007, as a result of strong advocacy efforts by NGOs working with intellectual property rights, the Brazilian government also issued a compulsory licensing of the same drug. Last but not least, in August 2007, following a major campaign by civil society groups, the Madras High Court in India rejected the bid by Novartis to extend its patent on an effective and lucrative cancer drug, arguing the drug had not been sufficiently changed to warrant a new patent (Gentleman 2007, Oxfam 2007).

The pharmaceutical companies say their patents and the huge profits they reap from them benefit the public, even in poor countries. Protecting their intellectual property, they say, is what makes it possible for them to conduct research and development on better, safer drugs – and the US government backs them up. But it is well known that pharmaceutical companies spend the biggest share of their revenues on marketing, advertising, and administration, while their research and development is for higher priced versions of existing medicines or products (think Viagra and Vioxx) that will sell in their major markets in North America and Europe. Most of the initial research on HIV-related medications was funded not by the private sector but by government.[15] Thus the alleged public benefit from corporate patents is a sham. 'Free trade' means little more than freedom for profit, freedom of companies to ignore international norms, freedom to cause people to die.

Popular movements for health rights in countries such as Brazil, South Africa, and Thailand have vigorously opposed such lethal policies and have urged their governments not to comply – and in so doing, they have scored some impressive victories. These debates have potentially far-reaching consequences, to the extent that they highlight the importance of understanding the connections between broad, macroeconomic facts, human development, and health-related rights. Yet there is also a troubling side to these important advances, insofar as the preoccupation with treatment and its macroeconomic dimensions has contributed to sanitizing and desexualizing the politics of AIDS under the fig leaf of distribution. In response to these harsh effects of globalization, World Bank and UNDP economists have sought to reconcile market systems with principles of social inclusion while avoiding the sexual controversies of our times.[16] They have done so through technocratic approaches such as biomedical quick fixes – with the recent emphasis on circumcision being perhaps the most obvious example[17] – that ignore the deeply gendered, racialized, and sexual matrices in which HIV and AIDS are embedded, as well as the novel concept known as 'global public goods' and the social, economic, and cultural enabling conditions necessary to curb the pandemic.[18]

In a prevailing context where markets normally determine choices and values, and any ethos of collective good appears to have been lost, it is useful to have a language for seeking common ends that is intelligible to economists – the chief arbiters of value in the regime of global capitalism. The very naming of 'global public goods' came from neo-Keynesian economists like Stiglitz who understand that markets are imperfect and inefficient and 'goods that are essentially public in nature' do exist (Stiglitz 2002, p. 222). However, the concept is still steeped in basic assumptions of neo-classical and neo-liberal economic theory, such as the abstract concept of utility, that collide with social and erotic justice (Camargo and Mattos 2007). Like neo-liberal economics more generally, it provides neither intrinsic standards nor democratic procedures for defining priorities, for distinguishing between a 'piece of cake' and a supply of condoms. Nor does it specify how such decisions might be made with the participation of those most affected or the accountability of powerful institutions and private donors.[19]

Any economic framework by definition is confined to the justice of distribution; it is useless to address the justice of recognition, those rights related to cultural identity and personal expression, which are generally unquantifiable and unexchangeable (Fraser 1997). How can we apply the notion of global public goods to principles such as the right to sexual self-expression and freedom from abuse or discrimination based on sexual and gender orientation? Tensions between these two very different strategies for addressing the epidemic – one stressing distribution of commodities and biomedical interventions, the other stressing sexual rights, diversity, and pleasure – have been very much in evidence at the World AIDS conferences almost from their onset. At the 2006 Toronto International AIDS Conference, a few members of the programme committee had to mount an intense struggle to get sex workers and their advocates into the official proceedings at all, and the monitoring of official spaces was tightly controlled (Richard Parker and Veriano Terto, personal communication).[20] In contrast, Thai, Cambodian, and Indian sex workers were a dynamic presence, overshadowing even treatment access groups, in the Global Village. But why should treatment and prevention, social and economic rights and sexual rights, be forced yet again into false dichotomies? We need a politics in the fight against HIV that reintegrates economic justice – access to goods and services – with erotic justice – the affirmation of bodies, pleasure, and desire.

Reassessing 'discrimination' and 'equality'

The principle of non-discrimination is so embedded in human rights discourse, so intuitively part of constructing the meaning of 'wrongs' in order to locate their appropriate subject categories, that it has become a part of every modern human rights document since the 1948 UDHR.[21] The UNCHR has unequivocally stated that 'non-discrimination provisions in international human rights texts should be interpreted to cover health status, including HIV/AIDS' (quoted in Maluwa et al. 2002, p. 8). With regard to both reproductive and sexual rights (for women), language emphasizing non-discrimination and equality threads through the Cairo Programme of Action and the Beijing Platform for Action (see text of Para. 96). The first, and still one of the most important, expressions of sexual orientation as a human right was rendered by the UN's Human Rights Committee in Toonen v. Australia (March 1994), which 'found that Tasmanian laws criminalizing all sexual relations between men were in breach of the International Covenant on Civil and Political Rights (ICCPR)', and that the Covenant's non-discrimination provisions specifying the term 'sex' must be understood as including 'sexual orientation' (Saiz 2004, p. 49).[22]

The stalled Brazilian resolution on sexual orientation also grounded its 'deep concern' and appeal for universality in the discourse of non-discrimination.[23]

In a lucid analysis of the relation between stigma and discrimination in the treatment of persons infected by, or even just perceived as 'at risk' for, HIV/AIDS, Maluwa et al. utilize the non-discrimination principle in a way that is both illuminating and unquestioning of its underlying epistemological assumptions:

> Within the context of HIV/AIDS, prejudiced thoughts frequently lead to actions or inactions that are harmful or that deny a person services or entitlements. Such responses may, for example, prevent a person living with HIV or AIDS from receiving health care or, alternatively, may terminate employment based on a person's HIV status. This is the definition of discrimination: when, in the absence of objective justification, a distinction is made against a person that results in that person's being treated unfairly and unjustly on the basis of their belonging or being perceived to belong, to a particular group.
>
> (Maluwa et al. 2002, p. 6)

These authors cite numerous, dramatic instances of denials by national governments and officials of very basic rights – to employment, to freedom of movement, to marriage, to treatment and health care access – based solely on HIV status. Sometimes such instances grow out of putting efficiency over humanity (the quarantining and isolation of HIV-positive prisoners); at other times, out of prejudicial and stigmatizing attitudes (the refusal of visas to HIV-positive people). In either case, the argument seems compelling that 'Stigma, discrimination, and human rights violations form a vicious, regenerative circle. Conversely, condoning human rights violations can create, legitimize, and reinforce stigma that can, if left to fester, lead to discriminatory action and further human rights violations' (2002, p. 7). Thus Maluwa and colleagues call for 'a multi-pronged response' that will address 'cultural and social values' as well as mobilizing communities 'for advocacy and change' and utilizing 'legal and structural interventions that together support a rights-based approach' (2002, pp. 11–13).

But what happens to the language of non-discrimination and equality when subject categories themselves become destabilized? Non-discrimination and equality clauses in human rights instruments derive their force from the dependability of 'fixed, universally applicable categorization', but Saiz (2004) raises the challenge to human rights approaches when it becomes difficult or impossible to '[name] the categories to be protected' (pp. 63–64).[24] This may be less daunting in the case of persons who are diagnosed as HIV-positive, though the volatility and stigmatization of diverse 'risk groups', as Maluwa et al. show, reveal this category to be one continually subjected to normative construction and reconstruction. But certainly the naming of gender and sexual subjects defies their being frozen into conventional binaries ('men' and 'women', 'heterosexual' and 'homosexual') that exclude the broad 'horizon of possibility' for queerness that many people, across diverse cultures and regions, actually live and imagine (Saiz 2004, pp. 62–63). What Currah and Minter have called 'the transgender umbrella' encompasses a vast array of 'gender outlaws', including female-to-male and male-to-female transsexuals, drag kings and queens, cross-dressers, female masculine and male feminine hybrids who do not choose to undergo surgical or chemical modification, intersex persons, and others who form a wide continuum of gendered and sexed possibilities.[25] Can 'non-discrimination' embrace a broad enough understanding of sexual rights to guarantee the freedom to be who one is, whatever that is, to seek pleasures across so many erotic possibilities, and to share a home and raise children in a variety of family forms?

In view of 'the increasingly vocal claims of transgender persons in many countries' (Dowsett 2003, p. 23), including sex worker organizations with members who are diversely sexual and gendered, it is untenable to any longer speak with confidence of 'women-only' or 'men-only' spaces or to believe that 'men who have sex with men' reflects people's actual experience of sexual or gender identities or cultural patterns. Ironically, as we explored in Chapter 1, the Vatican and conservative Islamic intellectuals seem to have had a much clearer perception of this problem than did many feminist and human rights groups over a decade ago, caught up as they were in an older form of identity politics. In its assault on the term 'gender' during the Beijing Conference process, the Vatican revealed an understanding of not only the potential fluidity of gender meanings and identities but also the ways in which gender ambiguity simultaneously challenges heteronormativity and its reliance on a fixed gender binary. The purpose of this assault was not only to 're-biologize sexual difference' (Butler 2005, p. 185, Girard 2007, pp. 335–336) but also to desexualize both gender and sexuality.

However, the fluidity and multiplicity of sexual and gender categories present a problem for conservative religious institutions as well as for liberal conceptions of human rights and sexual rights as belonging to clearly identifiable categories of the human. This is precisely the dilemma of the deconstructed postmodern subject and the challenge that Foucaultian concepts of power and discourse present to the assumptions of the liberal imaginary about fixed, stable subjects. If we 'claim an identity as homosexual [or woman, or transsexual]', it means we 'claim a place in a system of social regulation' (Connell and Dowsett 1999, p. 186). If we resist that identity, on the other hand, we destabilize the very foundation of the social movements we have been building for two generations (Garcia and Parker 2006, Riley 1988).

One of the biggest challenges for social movements of the past decade has been to establish a space for self-creating subjects of rights without reverting either to the fragmentation of narrow identity categories or to the exclusions and erasures of universal categories. Rather than seeing the instability of subject positions as presenting a hopeless catch-22 for human and sexual rights, we may return to the energizing analysis of cultural critics such as Cheah and Butler, who see the very construction of subjects and norms within power relations as a source of dynamism rather than fixity. Butler applies to gender Foucault's understanding of sexuality as performative rather than intrinsic, as constituted through disciplines and practices rather than contained as internal characteristics or properties. Both she and Jakobsen and Pellegrini (2003) aim for an ethics that '[makes] a variety of [sexual and gender] subject positions more inhabitable, more survivable, than they currently are' (p. 128). Butler's work has consistently critiqued the exclusionary tendencies of identity politics and eloquently reclaimed the 'humanity of the Other' for transgender and intersex people as well as military detainees labelled 'terrorists'. She insists 'that the necessity of keeping our notion of the "human" open to a future articulation is essential to the project of a critical international human rights discourse and politics' (Butler 2005, p. 22). It is significant that Butler, like Cheah, reaffirms the necessity in postmodernity of a 'human rights discourse and politics' – but one that is open to the constantly changing meanings and boundaries of the 'human'. In the following chapter, we shall examine the limitations of a human rights discourse, including for sexual politics, and the need to develop frameworks of justice that universalize *and* particularize, but also go beyond, the human.

Chapter 10

At the outer limits of human rights

Voids in the liberal paradigm

In previous chapters we have explored some recent criticisms of a rights-based framework, reviewed the development and substance of the concept of sexual rights, and argued for the viability of human rights and sexual rights approaches to health and social justice, despite their many deficiencies. In this concluding chapter we want to examine some deeper and perhaps intractable challenges to human rights, where its liberal trappings create exclusions or conceptual blind spots, including the very limitations of the category of the human. These dilemmas become all the more troubling in this time of intense militarization and ethnic and imperial conflict.

States of exception: rights of the body in times of war

Both consumerist and victimization discourses are problematic in characterizing the subjects of rights, denying, as they do, decisional agency and the possibility of being an active participant in challenging and transforming existing policies. But the rhetoric of 'citizenship' more commonly associated with human rights is also problematic (see critique in Chapter 7). Insofar as it refers to a world organized around nation states and their citizens, that rhetoric ignores or deliberately excludes the huge numbers of marginalized, globalized, and militarized bodies, approximately half of whom are women and girls. By the end of 2006 there were nearly 33 million refugees, asylum seekers, stateless persons, and internally displaced persons receiving humanitarian assistance worldwide, the majority in Africa, Asia, and the Middle East. This was an increase of 56 per cent over the available statistics for 2005, largely reflecting the escalation of armed conflict in Iraq, from which millions were fleeing across the borders to neighbouring states; and a steep rise in internal displacements due to conflicts there and in Lebanon, Sri Lanka, and Timor-Leste (UNHCR 2007b, USCRI 2006).[1] The wholesale concentration of internal and cross-border refugees in camps remains 'a standardized, generalizable technology of power in the management of displacement' (de Alwis 2004, p. 219, Laurie and Petchesky 2007). The excluded or abjected – those defined outside the privileged circle of 'citizens' and often, even 'humans' – include internal and transnational migrants and refugees, indigenous peoples, prison and detention camp populations, 'enemy combatants' and those designated (or imagined) as terrorists, alongside countless civilians obliterated by the ravages of war. Moreover, they include a wide range of sexual outcasts, outlaws, and exiles. These liminal, floating beings, like the wretched in Dante's inferno, have fallen into the condition of 'bare life'.

In the lowest circles of the worldly Hell that characterizes the early years of the twenty-first century we find armed conflict zones. At this writing, eight 'major wars' (defined by the UN as inflicting at least 1000 deaths a year on the battlefield) were underway along with about two dozen smaller conflicts in Asia, Africa, the Middle East, and Latin America that have been raging for decades and continue with no end in sight.[2] While the total number of armed conflicts has declined since the early 1990s, a report by the UN High Commission on Refugees points out that the post-9/11 global 'war on terror' has 'been used to justify new or intensified military offensives', particularly in Aceh, Afghanistan, Chechnya, Georgia, Iraq, Pakistan, and Palestine (UNCHR 2005). Besides acting as a green light to repressive regimes, the US-led 'war on terror' has made the situation of people forcibly displaced by local violence more precarious, as they face closed borders, deportations, and the extremes of human insecurity. The more than one million who fled Israeli bombs in Lebanon in the summer of 2006, and the more than 1000 killed in the process of fleeing, bore witness to the real state of terror that has become daily life for so many in the Middle East (HRW 2007e). This is not to mention the worldwide small arms and drug trades that make neighbourhoods in Rio de Janeiro, Los Angeles, and Bogotá sometimes as embattled as those in Baghdad.

Estimates suggest that three-quarters of those killed or wounded in armed conflicts are civilians – women, children, men; young and old.[3] In Iraq, a recent study by an American–Iraqi team of public health researchers from the Bloomberg School of Public Health at Johns Hopkins University in the USA has offered the most solidly evidence-based estimates of 'the human cost of the war'. Based on a population survey drawn from randomly selected clusters of households nationwide, the study estimated over 600,000 'excess deaths' (that is, the 'number of persons dying above what would normally have been expected had the war not occurred') from violent causes for the period 2002 to 2006, and an additional 53,000 from 'non-violent causes', most likely deterioration of health services and the environment (Burnham et al. 2006, pp. 1, 6). The web database of documented civilian deaths, Iraq Body Count (2007), registered 71,510 to 78,081 deaths for the period up until July 2007. These numbers, while small in comparison to civilian deaths during the Vietnam War or in the Democratic Republic of the Congo more recently, none the less '[dwarf] the median number of 18,000 deaths for all civil wars since 1945' (Sambanis 2006).

The gendered profile of casualties in today's wars is complex. According to the Johns Hopkins study, the overwhelming preponderance of the estimated 600,000 violent deaths in Iraq was among men of all ages, the majority in the 15 to 44-year age bracket, many of whom belonged to, or were targeted by, warring insurgent and rival sectarian groups (Burnham et al. 2006, p. 9). But other evidence suggests that the majority of those killed by 'coalition forces' (the USA and UK primarily) have been civilian women and children.[4] Among children (under 15) in Iraq, violent deaths (and, one supposes, 'excess' deaths from non-violent causes) have been gender neutral. But if we widen the definition of 'human cost' to include displacements and assaults as well as deaths and morbidities, the particular impacts on women and girls are more visible. UNHCR (2007a) estimates that, as of mid-2007, over 4.2 million Iraqis had fled their homes, more than two million to neighbouring states (mainly Syria and Jordan), with 2000 to 3000 continuing to leave each day. The remaining 2.2 million, 71 per cent of them women and children, have been internally displaced, with the numbers doubling between February 2006 and July 2007 and particularly since the US troop 'surge' began in February 2007, according to the Iraqi Red Crescent Association and the UN's International Organization for Migration (Glanz and Farrell 2007). People flee their homes because of 'direct threats to their lives', forcible removal, and fears of ongoing attacks and bombings. The result has been ethnic segregation, with a 'draining' of mixed areas and a concentration of Shi'ites, Sunnis, and Kurds in separate enclaves, as well as a major cholera epidemic in the north. So, the US government could boast in 2007 a slight decline in 'sectarian violence' thanks to the effects of forced ethnic separation while, in fact, intra-sectarian violence and health catastrophes continued to mount (Glanz and Grady 2007).

In Sudan's Darfur region, an estimated 200,000 people have been killed and some 2.2 million more displaced from their villages into refugee camps with few health or sanitary facilities and pitifully low food rations (Gettleman 2007). Women and girls caught in armed conflict zones and in camps for refugees and internally displaced persons (IDP) may face a significantly heightened risk of maternal mortality, sex trafficking, sexual abuse, and HIV[5] (Girard and Waldman 2000, McGinn and Purdin 2004, UNFPA 2006). Reports of aid workers in Syria claim that thousands of Iraqi women refugees, many of them single or heads of households, are turning to sex work out of economic desperation (Zoepf 2007). The Norwegian Refugee Council estimates 'that up to one-third of the internally displaced do not have regular access to clean drinking water and adequate sanitation facilities', making them more vulnerable 'to malnutrition and diseases than the non-displaced population' (NRC 2006, p. 23). Imagine what the lack of sanitary facilities and supplies means, especially for women and girls: no toilets or toilet paper or sanitary protection; waiting all day until dark to relieve oneself; wearing dirty rags during menstruation; the related reproductive tract infections, fistulae, pain, festering, and possible infertility; the abjection, the rejection, and the shame (Mukherjee 2002). Hunger is universal, but sanitation is profoundly gendered.

Conditions in Iraq make it impossible to obtain accurate, up-to-date figures on maternal mortality, but UNFPA warned at the beginning of the war that shortages of doctors and supplies, hospital closures, and health facilities swamped with war casualties would put pregnant women at grave risk (UNFPA 2003). Since then, reports confirm that doctors in the few functioning hospitals are too overwhelmed with the dying and wounded to offer adequate care to women undergoing childbirth, to say nothing of those who have been raped. Moreover, since the US-led invasion, some 12,000 doctors have fled the country and another 2000 have been killed, women obstetricians receive regular death threats, and the routine violence and harassment women face in public force pregnant women to stay at home rather than seek prenatal or obstetric care (Trejos 2007). Even if they take the risk, pregnant women and their doctors are often unable to navigate the dangerous roads to get to a clinic – when there is a clinic available (Ciezadlo 2005). Thanks to the failed Iraq reconstruction programme, with its rampant corruption and lax oversight, 'a $243 million program led by the United States Army Corps of Engineers to build 150 health-care clinics in Iraq has in some cases produced little more than empty shells of crumbling concrete and shattered bricks cemented together into uneven walls'. Of the 150 clinics projected, a mere 20 – with staggering structural defects – had actually materialized (Glanz 2007, p. 10).

Gender also constructs the caretaking and emotional burdens imposed by conditions of armed violence that never show up in public health and mortality statistics but are always evident in the faces of war that stare out at us from news photos. The international feminist solidarity group, MADRE, testifies, based on its broad field experience:

> Civilian attacks overwhelmingly affect women. That's because women are primarily responsible for meeting people's basic needs for food, shelter, and health care, whether there's a crisis or not. When bombs destroy homes, hospitals, bridges, and food markets, women must intensify their work to meet their families' needs. During war, people's needs also intensify, and a sharp rise in trauma, disability, disease, and homelessness compound women's responsibilities. Women also face

increased violence from within their own families [and from rival armed groups and invaders] in times of war.

(MADRE 2006)

Reports abound of physical and sexual violence and other forms of exploitation aimed at women and children (male and female) in refugee and IDP camps in Kenya, Chad, Uganda, Democratic Republic of Congo, Somalia, Darfur, Burundi, Colombia, and elsewhere. Describing conditions in southern Sudan, Macklin writes:

Women fear rape by militias, rape by men who distribute aid in exchange for sex, and rape by husbands who demand that they replace dying children by producing still more children who will grow up to wage the national struggle – that is, if the women survive their pregnancies and the children survive to adolescence.

(Macklin 2004, p. 82)

At a recent meeting of the UN Security Council, Under-Secretary-General for Peacekeeping Jean-Marie Guehenno reported:

In Afghanistan, attacks on school establishments put the lives of girls at risk when they attempt to exercise their basic rights to education.... Women and girls are raped when they go out to fetch firewood in Darfur.... In the eastern Congo [the Democratic Republic of the Congo], over 12,000 rapes of women and girls have been reported in the last six months alone.

Other UN officials spoke of similarly routine sexual violence and abuse against women and girls in Sudan, Somalia, Liberia, parts of West Africa, East Timor, Cambodia, Kosovo, and Bosnia, and often UN peacekeepers themselves are the perpetrators (Lederer 2006).

Yet we need to avoid the usual gender stereotypes of women as victims and men and boys as perpetrators. Far from being passive victims, women are organizing community-based networks and successful firewood patrols in Darfur (Marsh *et al.* 2006, Patrick 2007). They are defying the rigid spatial and hierarchical rules of aid organizations to create their own, more congenial, configurations of outdoor and indoor space and to muster resources in refugee and IDP camps (de Alwis 2004, Harrell-Bond 2002); and they are demonstrating community resilience and surviving against horrific odds in situations of acute armed crisis, such as in Lebanon (Nuwayhid *et al.* 2006). For their part, men and boys in situations of armed and ethnic conflict are often forced into the distorted forms of masculinity brought about by militarism and war, conscripted into becoming 'military men' even when they are still just children, and thus subjected to continual risk of death and brutalization (Phillips 2001). Limited but growing evidence suggests that boys within camps and militarized displacement settings – like men detained as 'enemy combatants' in the prisons of the 'war on terror' – are subject to sexual abuse and violence, and to intra-male age hierarchies that degrade and subordinate them just as ruthlessly as they do women and girls.

At the epicentre of the nightmare of today's wars lie Abu Ghraib and its echo chambers in Guantánamo, Bagram, and all the undisclosed sites of the US Central Intelligence Agency's rendition of so-called 'enemy combatants'.[6] These torture places may be likened to the lowest circle of Hell in Dante's inferno, not because more people suffer there, but because they present in microcosm the complex tangle of masculinism, misogyny, homophobia, and racism that lies at the heart of all militarist and imperialist projects. There is no need to belabour the now iconic images of sexual and cultural degradation of Muslim men transported without charge and for indefinite periods to those sinister places. We merely offer some reflections on what we can learn about the perversions of sexuality and bodily rights in war from the dark recesses of Abu Ghraib and the infamous interrogation techniques that had become systematic by late 2002.

First, it is important to recognize that women have been both victims and agents of sexual humiliation and torture. US women political leaders, prison commanders, interrogators, and rank-and-file guards participated in sexual torture at Abu Ghraib and Guantánamo; Hindu women in Gujarat goaded men in their communities to rape and mutilate Muslim women; Rwandan Hutu officials, also women, ordered similar atrocities. These are all well-documented cases that force us to rethink long-held feminist assumptions about who are the perpetrators and who the victims of sexual abuses and violations of bodily integrity in conflict zones.[7] This does not mean that war and its atrocities are gender neutral; rather that the reality is more complicated and the gender specificity more subtle than often assumed. The complicity of women in sexualized and racialized violence and the victimization of men illustrate what years of gender and queer studies have taught us: gender is always malleable, a floating signifier in which female bodies can be the vectors of patriarchal norms and phallic campaigns, and male bodies can be the targets.

Enloe associates Abu Ghraib and Guantánamo with not only 'masculinization' but also 'militarized feminization' in support of the military's 'institutional culture of sexism' (2007, p. 94). Eisenstein goes deeper, showing the 'gender confusion' of war and its use of women as 'gender and sexual decoys'. Condoleezza Rice (Bush's Secretary of State), Janis Karpinski (who later questioned her role as Abu Ghraib commander and got demoted for it), Lynddie England (the young soldier prosecuted for her role in Abu Ghraib and pictured pulling a man on a leash) became not only 'militarized and masculinized' agents of war for the Bush regime, but also signifiers of 'imperial democracy'. As 'gender decoys', they 'allow the fantasy that women are more equal, are found anywhere with no impediments to their choices and their lives' (Eisenstein 2007, p. 37). As such, they help obscure the realities of continued gender subordination and war – especially the ways its methods routinely include acts of sexual and racist aggression meant to bestialize and dehumanize the ethnic 'Other'.

Second, the bending of gender through sexual penetration and humiliation is always deeply intersected with racial and ethnic 'Othering' (Eisenstein 2007, Puar 2004). Domination, like liberation, starts from the body, and cultures of war and ethnic and male supremacy harbour a deep belief in the profanity of women's bodies. Thus the feminization and homophobization of the male enemy's body – through raping prisoners or forcing them to sodomize or urinate on one another or crawl naked like dogs or wear hoods that resemble burqas – become imperatives of military conquest. Masculinity, or manhood, is as much a part of the stakes of war as are oil, gas, and land (Enloe 2000). We are not suggesting that sexual degradation is worse than other techniques in the modern arsenal of torture, only that it is one element with a quite specific purpose: to cast the 'enemy' – here, the alleged 'terrorist' – as not only less than human but also less than masculine, to shatter his manhood.[8] In the current context of globalized Islamophobia, the notion that Muslim men will be particularly susceptible to sexualized degradation becomes an extension of Orientalist thinking and practice, but with an interesting twist. Not only is the white Christian male the subjugator and master, the white Christian female, as dominatrix, now becomes his handmaiden in torture, evoking the female superheroes of Western and Japanese video games.

Third, there is nothing new about the sexualization of ethnic and armed conflict or racialized power relations. Abu Ghraib has its prototypes in countless colonial conquests, US slavery, the lynching and castration of African-Americans, Nazi concentration camps, the Korean War, Algerian War, Vietnam, Pinochet's Chile, Israeli checkpoints, Palestinian security headquarters, the wars in Rwanda and Bosnia, and on and on.[9] Dubravka Zarkov (2001) cites a UN report on the wars in the former Yugoslavia in the 1990s that documented frequent incidents of male combatants, from all three major ethnic groups, being beaten across the genitals, forced to be naked, raped, and castrated, though the international media reported nothing of this. 'Sexual humiliation of a man from another ethnicity,' Zarkov writes, 'is … proof not only that he is a lesser man, but also that his ethnicity is a lesser ethnicity. Emasculation annihilates the power of the ethnic "Other" by annihilating the power of its men's masculinity' (2001, p. 78). It is also the mirror image of how raping and impregnating the female ethnic Other annihilates her womanhood, her men's manhood, and the reproductive capacity of their group by 'planting the seed' of the conqueror (Eisenstein 1996).

But there is a difference. In these earlier conquests and conflicts, the violation of women was more visible, eventually (thanks to feminist activists) becoming classified as a war crime and crime against humanity under the ICC Statute. The rapes and sexual humiliation of men were the unspoken underside, hidden from the media's eye. As Zarkov (2001) observes, 'Rapes of women [in Bosnia] were newsworthy; rapes of men were not' – or rather, were not seen because they so transgressed the dominant cultural narratives of masculinity (p. 72). What is different about the US-led 'war on terror' is the shifting balance in the relation between silence and exposure; the whole world knows about the victimization of Muslim men in Abu Ghraib and Guantánamo, but the systematic raping, brutalization, and torture of Muslim women to which we will return remains cloaked in secrecy. Why is this? Because the US imperial command, acting as the good global father that rescues Muslim women from their 'backward' men, cannot allow its soldiers' wrongs or its own complicity in religious extremism to be exposed before the ICC or any kind of international public scrutiny. Without weapons of mass destruction or links to Al Qaeda, the rationale behind US occupation and 'regime change' in Iraq depends heavily on a triple gendered trope: imperial male liberator, emasculated 'enemy', and feminized victim, whether Afghani women under the Taliban or all of Iraq under Saddam Hussein.

By 2006, it had become apparent to most of the world that the Bush government's stated goal of bringing 'democracy' to Iraq was a sham – a tragic farce of world historical proportions. But still hidden from the eyes of the public and the mainstream media was 'the relationship between Iraq's civil war and its "gender war"' (Susskind 2007, p. 18) – specifically, the ways in which US policies in Iraq were saturated in gender-based and sexual violence. In a compelling report for MADRE, 'Promising democracy, imposing theocracy', Yifat Susskind lays bare the complicated political, military, and criminal actions through which the US war on Iraq, far from bringing democracy and 'freedoms' to its citizens, has unleashed a reign of misogynist and homophobic terror. Consistent with its historic policies throughout the Persian Gulf, Middle East, and Afghanistan, the USA has strategically allied with and empowered Islamist militia groups, including the most fundamentalist.[10] In Iraq, contrary to its public rhetoric about securing democracy and liberating women, the Bush administration has put into power Shi'ite politicians and parties – such as that led by Grand Ayatollah Sayyid Ali Sistani – and armed, trained, and funded Shi'ite militia groups seeking to establish an Islamist state that subjugates women and persecutes gays, lesbians, and transgenders. At the legal level, the USA and its ambassador have supported a new family law and constitution that would enshrine 'established provisions of Islam' and make Islamic clerics their ultimate interpreters, especially in the settlement of marriage and family matters. This has amounted to a cynical trade-off of women's rights for alliances with Islamist parties and clans (Susskind 2007, p. 5).[11]

The more immediate consequence of this appeasement policy, however, has been a systematic 'campaign of gender-based violence' on Iraqi streets – fully tolerated, if not condoned, by US-led coalition forces, and intended to shore up and signify the new theocratic regime. Both the MADRE report and an earlier one by Marjorie Lasky (2006) for the NGO, CODEPINK, describe the escalating insecurity under US occupation and its disproportionate impact on women and girls, as the country slid rapidly into civil war. These reports make clear that whole societies are imprisoned in the lowest circle of Hell, and as in the official prisons, the conditions are sharply gendered. With the growing power of Shi'ite militias and local tribal groups, due to the countrywide breakdown in security and order, has come a new regimen of Taliban-like moral policing and a wave of harassment, attacks, and public executions of women and girls for violations of behaviour and dress codes.[12] The Organization of Women's Freedom in Iraq estimates 'that at least 30 women are executed monthly for honour-related reasons' (Ramdas 2006). As a result, women and girls are afraid to leave their homes; along with loss of access to food, safe water, electricity, and jobs, Iraqi women find their physical mobility greatly restricted. Iraqi men who are kidnapped and tortured feel 'like women', unable to protect their families and also afraid to leave home (Semple 2006).

Yanar Mohammed, director of the Organization of Women's Freedom in Iraq, explains how enforcing veiling by threat of death becomes a sign that militias have taken control of a neighbourhood or district, an emblem of political and military power: 'The veil on women is like a flag now', she says (quoted in Susskind 2007, p. 8). Moreover, it is clear that 'certain groups of women have been specifically targeted' for beatings, kidnapping, rape, and assassination, including the well educated (doctors, teachers, journalists, academics, and students) and all those who openly defend women's human rights, attempt to advance women socially and politically, or simply represent the more secular era of women's relative equality that preceded the occupation.[13] In turn, these attacks and the rise in 'honour killings' provide a pretext for further confining women and girls: '[I]n 2006, the Iraqi Interior Ministry [supported by the USA] issued a series of notices warning women not to leave their homes alone and echoing the directives of religious leaders who urge men to prevent women family members from holding jobs.' Thus a vicious circle is created whereby politically induced, gender-based violence justifies Islamist restrictions on women's mobility in public spaces, which then reinforce further violence and entrenchment of Islamist and misogynist rule. Moreover, the terrorizing of women shuts down the kinds of public demonstrations that women's groups led early in the occupation, effectively silencing women as a political force (Susskind 2007, pp. 9–10).

Even less known, and completely ignored by the mainstream media, are the homophobic dimensions of US-supported Islamist politics in Iraq. Both Susskind (2007) and a recent *New York Times* article report a campaign targeting gay Iraqis under US occupation for torture and extrajudicial killing (Buckley 2007). Homophobic attacks have been carried out not only by the Sunni insurgent groups the USA claims to oppose (one such group boycotted the 2005 elections, among other reasons, 'to prevent Iraq from "becoming homosexual"') but also by the Shi'ites it backs. According to the *Observer* in London (6 August 2006), 'There is growing evidence that Shia militias have been killing men suspected of being gay and children who have been sold to criminal gangs to be sexually abused.' Grand Ayatollah Ali Sistani – much touted in the US press as an alleged 'moderate' – has issued a number of *fatwas* urging that homosexual relations be subjected to the death penalty; one issued in 2005, though rescinded a year later, called for gay men and lesbians to be killed in the 'worst, most severe way' (Buckley 2007). The *fatwas* may have triggered a 'witch-hunt' by the Badr Brigade (the militia supporting Nuri al-Maliki, Iraq's US-backed Prime Minister) to prosecute and kill those accused of sexual deviancy. Moreover, homophobia has become a weapon in a media campaign to support the 'war on terror' inside Iraq. The country's most popular television show, *Terrorists in the Hands of Justice* – aired six nights a week on the Iraqiya network and funded by the Pentagon and US tax dollars – features 'live confessions from alleged insurgents' of homosexuality, paedophilia, rape, 'gay orgies', and the like (Susskind 2007, p. 20). The US-sponsored Iraqi media has become the pornographic mirror image of Abu Ghraib.

Central to this climate of gendered and sexualized violence are the atrocities committed by US forces and military contractors. Reporting from Mahmudiyah, a town south of Baghdad where a 15-year-old Iraqi girl was raped and, along with her father, mother, and nine-year-old sister, murdered by US soldiers, Haifa Zangana tells the *Guardian*, 'Today, four years into the Anglo-American occupation, the whole of Iraq has become Abu Ghraib, with our streets as prison corridors and homes as cells' (Zangana 2006). Numerous incidents of wanton killings, rapes, and abuse of Iraqi civilians in their own homes by their supposed 'liberators' – like the Mahmudiyah incident and the murder of 24 men, women, and children in Haditha in 2006 – take place under the pretext of rooting out insurgents (Wong 2006). The Associated Press calls it a 'pattern of troops failing to understand and follow the rules'. A feminist analysis of this 'pattern' reveals instead a pervasive culture of racist masculinism that denigrates 'enemy' women and feminizes 'enemy' men, as well as a systematic climate of impunity that encourages soldiers to 'shoot first, ask questions later' (von Zielbauer 2007b).

There is no doubt that the untold hundreds of women imprisoned, detained, and tortured by US occupation forces have been subjected to widespread sexual humiliation. 'Women detainees have been forced to remove their headscarves, dragged by their hair, made to eat from dirty toilets, and urinated on', as well as raped, stripped naked, and separated from nursing infants (Susskind 2007, pp. 21–22, Ciezadlo 2004). The *Guardian*, Al Jazeera, Iraqi lawyers, and General Taguba's report on Abu Ghraib prison cite photographs and testimony released to members of the US Congress giving direct evidence of such abuses, but unlike the photos of sexual abuses of men in Abu Ghraib, those of women were kept from public dissemination.[14] Susskind (2007) cites reports by the International Committee of the Red Cross, *Newsweek*, and the Organization of Women's Freedom in Iraq, detailing how wives and daughters of male detainees have been raped or threatened 'with rape in front of their male relatives in order to coerce the men into confessions' (p. 22). In a perverse double jeopardy, women and girls who return from Abu Ghraib and other detention centres, some of them pregnant, are assumed to have been 'defiled' (raped) and thus become the victims of honour killings by family members, or suicide, urged on by the tribal and militia leaders whose dominance US military intervention has secured.

Killings and rapes of civilians, like torture and 'harsh methods of interrogation' in US-run prisons, are war crimes and crimes against humanity under the Geneva Conventions and all the laws of war. None the less, despite evidence that these crimes stem directly from policies approved or condoned at the highest levels of the US chain of command, only the lowest enlisted personnel have been prosecuted[15] (*New York Times* 2007, von Zielbauer 2007a, 2007b). A moment of accountability did occur in June 2006, when the US Supreme Court, in the case of *Hamdan* v. *Rumsfeld*, ruled that the detention of prisoners in Guantánamo without charge or trial, subjecting them to cruel and degrading treatment and coercive interrogation methods, and plans to try them before special military tribunals without any of 'the judicial guarantees which are recognized as indispensable by civilized peoples', were in direct violation of both US and international law, specifically the Geneva Conventions (Greenhouse 2006).

It soon became clear that politics, not human rights, would decide the matter as the administration officials sought congressional allies to shape new legislation more friendly to its view of 'enemy combatants' as exceptions, and construction continued apace 'on a hulking, $24 million concrete structure' to house more alleged terrorist captives at Guantánamo (Golden 2006).[16] Yet to date, 'only ten of the more than seven hundred men who have been imprisoned at Guantánamo have been formally charged with any wrongdoing' (Mayer 2006, p. 44). At least three detainees have killed themselves, confirming that indefinite confinement and inhumane treatment on no specific charges can drive people to suicide (Risen and Golden 2006). What is striking here is how typically the abjected, the *homo sacer*, the Other, achieve public recognition as human only in death – after s/he is massacred, dragged from her/his bed, raped and murdered, or commits suicide.[17]

On the humanism of the 'other': sexual outcasts

> And that is the great thing I hold against pseudo-humanism: that for too long it has diminished the rights of man, that its concept of those rights has been – and still is – narrow and fragmentary, incomplete and biased and, all things considered, sordidly racist.
>
> (Césaire 1972/2000, p. 37)

For at least three decades, feminist, postmodernist, and postcolonial social theory and criticism have worked to dismantle the universal subject inherited from the European Enlightenment and entrenched in the epistemological bedrock of human rights. Earlier, in the 1950s, Aimé Césaire and his protégé, Frantz Fanon, rejected as fraudulent a humanism that pretended to include all ('the people') but under whose cloak lay white, Western, property-owning, colonizing masculinity. Instead of a single humanity or humanness – what seventeenth- and eighteenth-century political philosophers tried to define as a transcendent 'human nature' – postmodern thought has insisted on a wide array of situated subjectivities based on class, caste, race, ethnicity, gender, geography, and also sexuality. Multiple voices have demanded 'the need to translate universal claims into the specific, concrete terms of sexed subjectivities that are also concrete' (Cabral 2005). But even these attempts to parse the many ways of being human, 'doing gender', or living sex may continue to inscribe certain exclusions through underlying norms or assumptions about what kinds of bodies count as human bodies. As Butler suggests,

> The terms by which we are recognized as human are socially articulated and changeable. And sometimes the very terms that confer 'humanness' on some individuals are those that deprive certain other individuals of the possibility of achieving that status, producing a differential between the human and the less-than-human. These norms have far-reaching consequences for how we understand the model of the human entitled to rights or included in the participatory sphere of political deliberation.
>
> (2004b, p. 2)

Butler tells the story of David Reimer, a genetic male who, during childhood, had his penis accidentally mutilated in a medical procedure. The famed sexologist, Dr John Money, recommended – and Reimer's parents acceded – that he be surgically transformed and raised as a girl to 'correct' the error. Despite the attempt to impose a 'natural' sex on the child by reconstructing his anatomy (implanting a vagina), he continued to feel himself 'really male'. Butler, quoting from his case history, highlights Reimer's acute ethical awareness that there was something 'pretty shallow' about people who thought that the only way he could 'have a productive life' or 'be loved' was because of what was 'between my legs'. By '[refusing] to be reduced to the body part he has acquired' he has asserted 'the human in its anonymity ... the anonymous – and critical – condition of the human as it speaks itself at the limits of what we think we know'. David Reimer committed suicide at the age of 38; whether because of the impossible strictures of sex normativity the 'real' world imposed or the doubly mutilating surgery that sought to 'normalize' him, his life as a human being became, in Butler's terms, 'unliveable' (Butler 2004a, pp. 71–72, 74).[18] Butler's reference to 'the anonymous condition of the human' seems to recover the universal, 'pure, atemporal and context-independent human dignity' that Cheah (1997) warns postmodernity has shattered. Yet Butler is struggling with the dilemma that all progressive activists and human rights proponents face. Without some idea of the 'human' that contains the principles both of individual selves and personhood and of bodily integrity and autonomy, the fate of David Reimer, like that of the detainees who committed suicide in Guantánamo, would seem to become inconsequential and the concept of justice itself meaningless (Corrêa and Petchesky 1994).

While we need to avoid the Enlightenment's illusion of linear progress, we cannot escape the ways in which temporality and history shape how we think. Butler recognizes 'the historicity of the term ... "human"' and its contamination with racism, gender, and sexual dogmatism. This is the history that caused Césaire and Fanon to disavow humanism since its 'contemporary articulation is so fully racialized that no black man [or woman] could qualify as human' (Butler 2004b, p. 13). At the same time, like Malcolm X in the USA, both Césaire and Fanon used the critique of humanism to expand the meaning of humanness. Similar issues arise with regard to contemporary sexual outcasts. Even Freud saw normative heterosexuality as 'a serious injustice' and the rigidities of contemporary civilization's sexual codes as leaving the 'sexual life of civilized man ... severely impaired' (Freud 1962, pp. 51–52). Cabral (2005) raises the dilemma posed for intersex activists in the fact that current ideas of sexual citizenship, or sexual rights as human rights, still 'work on a standard conception of corporality' that contains an unexamined cultural assumption of 'dimorphic, binary sexual difference as a *value*'. That is, the 'subjects of rights' are still understood to be male and female (or homosexual and heterosexual) – a binary deeply embedded in human rights discourse:

> [O]n the one hand, the human rights discourse appears as a privileged instrument to which intersex children's claims for decisional auto-

nomy and personal integrity might be addressed. On the other hand, for as long as sexed humanity remains caged in a standard assumed to be valuable and desirable *tout court*, human rights humanism will be insufficient (in the best of cases) or an argumentative trap (in the worst), able to justify what intersex activism and political theory condemn as *inhuman forms of humanization*.

(Cabral 2005, p. 7)

So what would it mean if we took the poor, black Brazilian *travesti*'s body as the principal site of 'the human'? Or that of the transgender migrant sex worker? Or the intersex body?[19] Is this what Cabral (2005) means when he invokes 'a radicalized humanism' or 'a post-humanism' that would challenge 'even the regulatory ideals we have learned to call nature'? And how would this complicate our notions of citizenship, to say nothing of the subjects of human rights?

Sexual and gender outcasts and outlaws are not a unified or consistent group, hence the designation 'queer'.[20] Transgenders, 'tranny boys', 'female guys', intersex persons, and so many other self-named sexual subjects dissolve traditional gender and sexual binaries; transsexuals seeking transition through surgical, chemical, or merely cosmetic means, to a clear 'opposite gender' identity, wish to reinscribe and reappropriate these binaries. Heterosexual women may seek to avoid traditional definitions of their sexual servicing and reproductive roles, and be thwarted by abstinence-only policies and men's refusal to wear condoms; or they may wish to have children and be thwarted (until the development and marketing of effective microbicides) by the risk and fear of HIV infection. Sex workers may wish to work with dignity, respect, and access to social and health services – that is, full citizenship rights – or they may feel exploited, in constant danger, and desperate for alternatives. Young people seeking private space for sexual experience and pleasure, with a variety of partners or even just one, may see themselves as political freedom fighters or as following their hearts and 'expressing their independence' to families who would kill them or force them to kill themselves.[21] Marginalized sexual subjects are a messy lot, and continue to live and die in a hostile world. The recent wave of brutal murders of lesbians in South Africa (HRW 2007f) – one of the few countries in the world with a national constitution that recognizes freedom of sexual orientation – reminds us in the starkest terms of the limited capacity of formal rights to assure the 'humanness' of all.[22]

The complexity that actual sexed, gendered, and racialized bodies live recalls once again the disciplinary and regulatory side of the human rights framework. If we accept Foucault's conception of power as a set of regulatory norms and apparatuses that 'circumscribe in advance what will and will not count as truth', including what counts as a person, a body, a gender, a citizen, a human, then what is the point of talking about justice or human rights? Are we not all, as Žižek and the Wachowski brothers (directors of the 1999 film *The Matrix*) would have it, caught up in 'The Matrix' and our notions of autonomy or the possibility of refusal a colossal illusion (Butler 2004b, pp. 57–58, Žižek 2002, p. 96)? If every act of recognizing the full humanness of some previously marginalized group also excludes others, then is not every instance of human rights claiming also a resignification of difference and exclusion – the committing of an injustice?[23] One current example is the 'marriage equity' movement for same-sex couples: in claiming the 'human (or civil) right' to marry, like 'normal' couples, gay male and lesbian marriage seekers simultaneously reinscribe state-sanctioned marriage as the exclusive site of a host of social benefits and privileges, thereby excluding from those benefits and privileges all who will never be, or do not wish to be, part of a conjugal couple (Butler 2004b, Duggan 2004). In contrast, Cabral and Viturro (2006) want to redefine 'sexual citizenship' as a form of 'decisional autonomy' of individual persons '[undiminished] by inequalities based on characteristics associated with sex, gender, and reproductive capacity' (p. 262). Sexual citizenship, in other words, still stands or falls on the possibility of individual human agency. But insofar as 'the human' is always already gendered, then, assuredly, both human rights and human agency 'are never enough'.

Toward a transgender and transhumanist ethics

It is useful to examine more deeply the ways in which transgender and intersex ethics open up new space in negotiating the troubled waters of 'humanness' and 'humanism'. Echoing Cabral's description of the dilemma intersex people face, Thomas poses two alternative ethical paths: inclusion in the human versus transhumanism. He reminds us that a world in which binary gender and 'normative human identity' are everywhere grafted on to each other puts transpeople 'in an impossible double bind':

> Recognizing the need to become more fully human, the transgender person realizes she or he must break free of the constricting bonds of 'normal' gender. However, in renouncing normative gender, she or he must forfeit any right to recognition and respect as a 'normal' human being ... we might say that the transgendered [*sic*] person must either choose, or risk being forced, to 'stand on the side' of the inhuman.
> (Thomas 2006, p. 317)

Thomas' solution to this dilemma goes further than either Butler or Cabral but, one could argue, not far enough in articulating what a transhumanist ethics might look like. He suggests that we have only two choices: reverting to liberalism's 'unfinished project' of gradual, successive inclusions or celebrating the status of exclusion – that is, 'the idea of a human right to *inhumanity*' (hence the 'transgender rights as *in*human rights' of his title) – as a kind of privileged location. The rash of transphobic hate crimes Thomas recites, or the agony of David Reimer, to say nothing of the history and persistence of racisms, make clear the limits of the former option. Along with its claims to 'progress', a tradition based on 'the presumption of a sharp and necessary distinction between lives that are human and lives that are not' (Thomas 2006, p. 314) has left a legacy of unremitting violence. This presumption constitutes the bedrock of much of Western liberal political theory from the seventeenth century up until now, with the debates among Hobbes, Locke, Rousseau, Condillac, Wollstonecraft, Marx, and others concerning the essence of 'human nature' in contradistinction to animals. It crosses over into right-wing conservative ethics, with Vatican and Christian evangelical attempts to claim '*human* life' for foetuses, embryos, stem cells, and brain-dead people. It seems to us that Butler's gloss on Levinas' 'humanism of the Other' is still clinging to the 'unfinished (liberal) project' insofar as it poses a restoration of humanism to the inhuman.[24]

Alternatively, Thomas proposes that '"standing on the side" of the inhuman' would necessitate a 'kind of "cultural work" at the level of collective political fantasy, enjoining people to imagine a "nongendered transhuman existence"' where gender no longer matters (2006, pp. 312, 323). His accounts of trial data in the prosecution of transphobic hate crimes reveal intense gender and sexual anxieties on the part of defendants – anxieties specifically about manhood and masculinity ('I can't be fucking gay, I can't be fucking gay', shouted one of the defendants who murdered Gwen Araujo in California in 1992) (2006, p. 318). Thomas' thinking, like that of Butler, Cabral, and a number of recent feminist theorists, charts the violence intrinsic to gender itself. A more radical, *trans*formative move would be to go beyond a transgender to a transhumanist ethics and explore what that would embrace. Thomas claims to be doing this with his revaluation of the 'inhuman', but he does not begin to imagine what this would mean with regard to human relationships to other species, the planet, all living things, and some not living. In the twenty-first century, when the planet, its environment, and many plant and animal species are in grave peril from an arrogant humanism that has for 300 years anointed itself the decider of boundaries between the human and the inhuman, and for thousands of years proclaimed lordship over the inhuman, it is past time to find some new grounding for ethical responsibility.

The transphobic anxieties Thomas describes are disturbingly reminiscent of the trans-species anxieties that thread through the entire history of European racism – what Stephen Jay Gould called 'the search for signs of apish morphology in groups deemed undesirable' (1981, p. 113; see also Chapter 7). Humanism's racist legacy makes clear the historical, constructed nature of beasts and monsters, thus the affinity between scientific judgements about nonhuman species and about gender and sexual 'dysphoria'. Because discourses of human versus animal distinction are part of the deep hard wiring of racial, gender, and sexual hierarchies, deconstructing those discourses is a key step in the project of developing a transhumanist ethics. Toward this end, we can draw upon a long tradition of philosophical debate concerning the moral status of nonhuman animals, even as it may challenge the underlying assumptions and vocabulary of human rights. In a comprehensive synthesis and critique of this debate, Gary Steiner (2005) reviews a wide range of modern and postmodern philosophers who have questioned the strictly rationalist distinction between 'persons' and 'things' inherited from Kant, by reconsidering the moral ties between human beings and other animals.[25] Steiner faults most of these philosophers for remaining surreptitiously anthropocentric if not downright hierarchical (privileging the human over the nonhuman animal), whether through their emphasis on sentience and utility, cognitive awareness, self-reflection, or language. While exposing their inconsistencies and latent humanism,[26] Steiner none the less identifies certain elements, particularly in the ideas of Levinas and Derrida, that push beyond humanism.

Levinas' entire approach to ethics rests on a rejection of the autonomous individual in favour of the Other and the Other's freedom; 'Desire for others', 'the face' (*le visage*), challenges my autonomy and calls me to responsibility. Moreover, he tells us, 'the face is not exclusively a human face' and may express itself in non-linguistic ways (Levinas 2003, pp. 30–31). The story of the dog (Bobby) in the labour camp ('The Name of a Dog, or Natural Rights') shows 'the radical possibilities that can be opened up when the reach of the ethical question *who is my neighbour?* is widened to include nonhuman acquaintances'.[27] Dogs, or what Haraway (2004) calls 'companion species', not only remind us of our humanity; they help us transcend it. Steiner (2005) cites several key texts in which Derrida's rethinking of the subject and of intersubjectivity leads to a questioning of the boundary between human beings and other living beings. In 'Force of law: the "mystical foundation of authority"', Derrida wrote, 'we must reconsider in its totality the metaphysico-anthropocentric axiomatic that dominates, in the West, the thought of just and unjust' (1992, p. 19). In *Aporias*, he asserted (against Heidegger), 'any border between the animal and the *Dasein* of speaking man [is] unassignable' (quoted in Steiner 2005, p. 220). And in the essay 'Eating well', his fullest treatment of this subject, Derrida envisioned 'a radicalization of language' opening up possibilities (marks, iterations, deconstructions) that 'are themselves not only human' (quoted in Steiner 2005, pp. 218–222).[28] Likewise, Nussbaum argues that since justice requires us 'to secure a dignified life for many different kinds of beings "across the species barrier"' we need to treat (nonhuman) 'animals as subjects and agents, not just as objects of compassion' (2006, pp. 326, 350–351).

All this points to a very different kind of ethics from the contaminated humanism with which human rights discourse has up to now been burdened. It suggests, in Derrida's phrase, a 'responsibility toward the living in general', or what others call an ethics of 'biocentrism'. In such an ethics, human stewardship would replace human dominion over the biosphere, based on the principle – and the reality – of trans-species, transgender, transcultural, transnational interdependence. This biocentric approach:

> Recognizes that human beings are part of a shared community of life with other living beings; that living beings are part of a web of interdependence; that 'all organisms are teleological centers of life in the sense that each is a unique individual pursuing its own good in its own way'; and that 'humans are not inherently superior to other living things.'
>
> (Paul W. Taylor, quoted in Steiner 2005, p. 250)[29]

As Nussbaum (2006) argues that 'since [nonhuman] animals will not in fact be participating directly in the framing of political principles, and thus there is much danger of imposing on them a form of life that is not what they would choose', human beings have an even greater responsibility to treat them with care and respect (p. 352). (The same argument can be made, of course, regarding the responsibilities of mentally competent adult human beings toward children, the mentally infirm elderly, and those who are cognitively impaired.)[30] Indeed, *homo sapiens* has a singular and profound obligation to preserve 'the shared community of life' precisely because it is the species with the greatest capacity – and the longest and most devastating practice – of doing harm to itself and all other forms of life.

On individualism, autonomy, and relationality

An ethics grounded in what Levinas (2003) calls 'Desire for Others' and extended to the biosphere, has immediate implications for how we think about sexuality and sexual rights. The very focus on desire signals a departure from the disembodied, rational, autonomous, subject in favour of relationality and interconnection. Its implication is that the self has meaning only in and through others, that otherness and intentionality belong to other creatures beyond humans, and that the responsibility of humans in an ethical universe is one of caring for the 'web of interdependence' that makes life possible for all species and the planet. Both Levinas and Butler root such an ethics in human (and, in Levinas' case, other animal) embodiment. Because we are embodied – and paradoxically as a consequence of the vulnerability and solitude of that inescapable condition, we are, from before birth to death, inextricably bound up with others – our bodies depend on others to survive, form ideas and thoughts, speak, experience pleasure, heal, and make love. Moreover, we are continually disturbed by the deaths and suffering of others, of the Other's 'face', reminding us of our own culpability and the precariousness of our lives and life in general.[31] Butler stresses that the compelling pull of this ethical responsibility has nothing to do with the Other being like me, a face that mirrors mine; the deaths of the (unnamed) Iraqi family in Mahmudiyah, or Gwen Araujo, must be as painful to us as that of Daniel Pearl, the American Jewish journalist killed by Pakistani terrorists (Butler 2004a, pp. 37–38, 44). Such recognition carries not just a heavy burden but also a life-affirming promise: 'The face of the Other calls me out of narcissism towards something finally more important'; this call is the necessary condition for language, for discourse, for community (Butler 2004a, pp. 27, 138–139).

Just as a biocentric ethics seems to raise problems for a human-centred concept of rights, so would an ethics focused on community and relationality seem to disturb the inherent individualism of sexual and bodily rights. Sexual rights, both negative and affirmative, are not merely group rights but refer to the experiences and sensations of individual bodies and the agency of individual decision makers. Can a relational, biocentric ethics make space for individual self-actualization, desire of/for the self? That some concept of self-determination remains indispensable becomes evident when we consider the relentless barrage of violence, physical and verbal, that queer people and women and girls seeking sexual pleasure or abortion face, across the globe. They are accused, assaulted, and sometimes killed for having, in the words of the Vatican (1995), 'a hedonistic mentality unwilling to accept responsibility in matters of sexuality' and 'a self-centered concept of freedom', or for dishonouring the family for the sake of 'foreign' values and selfish lust.

Here is where we need to distinguish between a crude, libertarian individualism, based on a model of an autonomous self unfettered by social constraints or regulatory norms, and a *relational individualism* that assumes individual persons are always socially defined and connected. The dichotomy between individual autonomy and community is itself a discursive construct of modernity not confined to any particular region, religion, or culture (Euben 1999). The atrocities of the twentieth century remind us that both individualism and collectivism become toxic, even genocidal, when taken to extremes; together, they mediate one another and are the indispensable conditions of life. Butler (2004b) reminds us that we always need some notion of bodily integrity and autonomy in order to make claims on behalf of gays, lesbians, transsexuals, transgenders, and heterosexual women and girls to sexual freedom and self-determination, and of intersex people to be who they are, 'free of coerced medical, surgical, and psychiatric interventions' (p. 21). We would add that any coherent notion of pluralism is impossible without recognition of the individual differences and desires that constitute it.

Yet life itself warns that our bodies 'are not quite ever only our own'; they remain necessarily bound up in concentric circles of relationship. Indigenous feminist perspectives are especially helpful in emphasizing the 'reciprocal' relationship between 'collective and individual rights'. For indigenous women's organizations such as the Foro Internacional de Mujeres Indigenas, it is impossible to separate indigenous people's rights (to territories, cultural self-determination, natural resources) from indigenous women's rights (to sexual and reproductive health, political and economic participation, gender justice); 'my body' and 'my people' are mutually dependent (FIMI 2005). To admit that bodily autonomy or self-ownership is at best a strategic construct and at worst an illusion is not to deny the body's agency, but to recognize that we always express and seek our desires in highly mediated conditions not of our own choosing. This is an ontological and ethical premise, since 'the social conditions of my embodiment' include the relations with others that enable us to live well or to survive at all (Butler 2004b, pp. 20–21, Mahmood 2005). The relationality of the self also reminds us that bodily rights and integrity are inextricably linked with social justice. To say that 'the body has its invariably public dimensions' means that to fully realize such rights and to fulfil our responsibilities toward others requires new social arrangements and a more just distribution of resources and power. Social justice and economic justice are the enabling conditions of sexual rights.

Derrida is correct that human rights norms are both indispensable and insufficient; we need a human rights framework reconceived as relationally individual and social at the same time. What Eisenstein (2004) calls 'the polyversal status of individuality' requires that we '[hold] onto the notion of the social, communal self which has obligations to others but rights as well' (pp. 215–216). It must also be a form of human rights that explicitly calls for human responsibility in regard to other species and the biosphere. Sexuality is the space where we most directly encounter the paradox of simultaneous aloneness and togetherness; the body's vulnerability and its power; its passion to be free and its irrevocable connection to others.

Is relational individualism an answer to the core philosophical problem of human rights – how to define 'universal human values' without suppressing local differences and particularities? It is an immediately vexing problem in a world rife with resurgent and competing religious dogmatisms, and especially so for feminists who have pointed out time and again how invocations of local culture, tradition, and religious duty often mask systematic practices that abuse and subordinate women and girls. On the one hand, a relational and situational ethics is necessary for cross-cultural, cross-species understanding, environmental health, and global peace. It 'leaves open the possibility that we might also be remade in the process of engaging another's worldview, that we might come to learn things that we did not already know before we undertook the engagement' (Mahmood 2005, pp. 36–37). It presents us with 'an infinite task of translation, a constant reworking of [our] own particular position' (Žižek 2002, p. 66), and in this way holds out a shred of hope that human beings might not destroy one another and every single living thing. On the other hand, we cannot let go of a human rights perspective that defends individual bodies and their sexual pleasure and self-determination. This is so for two reasons. First, because human beings are the most destructive species on the planet and the most likely to suffer violence and deprivation from their own kind, they need special (remedial) attention. Second, it is only from our body's experience of pleasure and danger that we have the capacity to recognize the rights, needs, and desires of others.

Reaffirming pleasures in a world of dangers

> [T]he ability to say 'no' to what one does not desire is hugely conditioned on the capacity to recognize, delight in, and respond to one's desire to say 'yes' free of limiting stereotypes and with knowledge of the implications for one's safety and contentment.
>
> (Miller 2000, p. 93)

Reacting to decades of single-minded attention to abuses, victimization, and torture by feminist and human rights activists (see Chapters 8 and 9), writers on sexual rights since 2000 have shifted the balance toward the 'pleasure' side of the pleasure and danger equation. At issue here is the principle that 'positive' or affirmative rights – those that explicitly enhance capabilities, the range of freedoms, and the enabling conditions necessary to exercise them – are as important as 'negative' rights – those that prohibit abuses and violence (Garcia and Parker 2006, Petchesky 2000). With respect to sexuality, the Programme of Action (1994) adopted in Cairo defined 'sexual health' in terms of people being 'able to have a satisfying and safe sex life' aimed at 'the enhancement of life and personal relations, and not merely counselling and care related to reproduction and sexually transmitted diseases' (Para. 7.1). A decade later, Paul Hunt, the UN's Special Rapporteur on the Right to Health, likewise defined 'sexual health' as 'a state of physical, emotional, mental and social well-being related to sexuality, not merely the absence of disease, dysfunction, or infirmity'. In addition to his inclusion of sexual orientation in the 'fundamental human rights' related to sexuality (see Chapter 8), Hunt remarked that 'sexual health requires a positive and respectful approach to sexuality and sexual relationships, as well as the possibility of having pleasurable and safe sexual experiences, free of coercion, discrimination and violence' (Hunt 2004, pp. 14–15).

Implicit in these definitions is an awareness that positive and negative rights are inseparable:

> Not only does a person's right to fully develop and enjoy her body and her erotic and emotional capacities depend on freedom from abuse and violence, and on having the necessary enabling conditions and material resources [to make such enjoyment possible]; it may also be that awareness of affirmative sexual rights comes as a result of experiencing their violation.
>
> (Petchesky 2000, p. 97)

None the less, as religious and ideological conservatism have strengthened their hold on policy making in many national and international arenas (see Part 1), it remains far easier and more acceptable to oppose abuses, discrimination, and hate crimes than to assert 'pleasurable and safe sexual experiences' as a positive right – particularly for unmarried women, youth, and all varieties of sexual and gender outlaws. This is because of external threats (the political risks of being accused (from the left and the right) of 'hedonism', 'narcissism', and 'bourgeois' or 'Satanist' values) but also internal divisions including the confusions and disagreements among feminist and lesbian, gay, transgender, and intersex activists about what positive, collective values for sexual pleasure and well-being we actually share. At the same time, restricting advocacy to negative freedoms has unacceptable costs:

> The negative, exclusionary approach to rights, sometimes expressed as the right to 'privacy' or to be 'let alone' in one's choices and desires, can never in itself help construct an *alternative vision* or lead to fundamental structural, social, and cultural transformations. Even the feminist slogan 'my body is my own', while rhetorically powerful, may be perfectly compatible with the hegemonic global market, insofar as it demands freedom from abuse but not from the economic conditions that compel a woman to sell her body or its sexual or reproductive capacities.
>
> (Petchesky 2000, p. 91)

Freud's *Civilization and Its Discontents* (1962), often seen as a pessimistic resignation to the irresolvable conflict between Eros and Thanatos in modern societies, may seem an unlikely source to draw on here. However, this early twentieth-century text may also be read as a cautious critique of 'civilization's' inability to tolerate unfettered love, and an argument on behalf of 'sexuality as a source of pleasure in its own right'.[32] Later

Foucault (1978, p. 157), hardly a follower of Freud, famously called for a 'counterattack against the deployment of sexuality' as a domain of power and biopolitical regulation, a counterattack that could have as its motto 'bodies and pleasures'. Many researchers on sexuality and advocates of sexual rights across sexual and gender differences have taken up this call, beginning with Rubin's (1984) conceptualization of erotic justice and injustice, and her appeal for 'rich descriptions' that would abandon 'hierarchies of sexual value' and simply document 'bodies and pleasures' in all their enormous variety.[33] This literature reflects an attempt to escape the focus on normalization, 'sexual scripts', and the techniques of biopolitics – that is, the very view of sexuality as discourse and regulatory power that Foucault exposed – and to focus instead on what Gary Dowsett (2000) has called 'bodies in desire'; what people feel and do in everyday life. As Connell and Dowsett remark, 'social framing theory', more commonly known as social construction (see Chapter 5), has a 'tendency to lose the body' and intimate relationships in its preoccupation with discourses and techniques (1999, p. 191).

One example of this recent critical literature is Peter Jackson's detailed ethnographic exploration of the 'explosion of Thai identities' and the ways they 'are simultaneously gendered and sexualized'. Jackson elucidates the 'endless circuit of mutual referencing' between 'the categories of gender and sexuality' as they became manifest in the profusion of popular discourses for expressing different ways of being sexual, having sex, and doing gender in mid-twentieth-century Thailand. He challenges the frameworks of theorists like Foucault and Sedgwick who tend to separate 'sexuality' from gender. Instead, Jackson wants to 'talk of "eroticism" and "discourses of the erotic"' and to frame 'Thai identities as eroticized genders rather than sexualities' (Jackson 2007, pp. 352, 343). In doing so, he implicitly recasts Thai erotic subjectivities as active agents, self-naming and living their desire, rather than as objects of regulatory 'discipline'.

In a different way, Sylvia Tamale (2006) defies stereotypes of African women as always victimized by 'harmful traditional practices', and recovers local forms in which African women may redeploy such practices as vehicles of women's sexual empowerment. In a study of the Ssenga (female erotic teachers and counsellors) among the Baganda people of Uganda, Tamale finds a complex mix of aims and effects in sexual initiation rituals. Along with messages to young women and girls that convey strict heteronormativity and the need to fulfil wifely duties, she uncovers a strong sense of entitlement to sexual pleasure and well-being for women.[34] In addition to messages about the importance of economic independence from husbands and rights to be free from cruelty and abuse, Ssengas (whose practices have now become commercialized) convey information about aphrodisiacs, lubricants, 'sexual paraphernalia and aids', and a variety of sexually suggestive terms. Tamale even defends the traditional practice of elongating the labia of pre-menarchal girls, condemned by WHO as a form of female genital mutilation (FGM), as pleasure enhancing for both women and men. Among the younger generation of Ssenga trainees, many are rejecting the more traditional gender norms that privilege male sexuality, make motherhood women's ultimate identity, and fail to train men in how to please their women partners. These young Baganda women 'regard sex not primarily for procreation but for leisure and pleasure, relocating sex from the medicalized/reproduction plane to the erotic zone' (Tamale 2006, p. 93).

As we suggested earlier, it may be one of the strange ironies of the HIV/AIDS pandemic, particularly in Africa and South Asia, that it has created a space for more open talk about sexuality, sexual behaviour, and erotic pleasure. The Pleasure Project (2007) cites evidence that HIV prevention and safer sex programmes incorporating and promoting sexual pleasure can increase the consistent use of condoms and thus improve public health outcomes. The project has identified a wide range of such programmes in countries as diverse as Cambodia, India, Sri Lanka, Mozambique, Zambia, and Zimbabwe. Some, focusing on the familiar 'target groups' such as men who have sex with men, sex workers, and youth, involve interventions by peers and co-workers; others, focusing on married couples, involve such unlikely participants as 'local Catholic priests and nuns'. The project catalogues a surprising array of techniques for eroticizing both the male and female condom and using them to enhance stimulation. It introduces sexy language and tasty lubricants in training people how to use tongues, lips, hands, and eyes to make insertion a sensual experience, and it uses media campaigns to convey the general message that safer sex (with condoms) is exciting, 'natural', and fun (Knerr and Philpott 2006, Philpott *et al.* 2006). Reminiscent of decades of feminist campaigns for safe, effective, and female-friendly contraceptives, these programmes are committed to a 'power of pleasure' message as well as to the enabling conditions of availability, affordability, and good quality. All, they imply, are essential components of sexual rights as human rights.[35]

The 'sexy' marketing of safer sex products may seem like an instrumentalist co-optation of 'pleasure in its own right' – pleasure as a means toward prevention. Yet, to the extent that millions of people across the globe – disproportionately young African, South Asian, and African-American women – receive knowledge of sexuality filtered through the prism of HIV and AIDS, there is no better site in which to move pleasure to the foreground. This solemn coupling of health crisis and the erotic should remind us that 'the construction of sexual desirability' is 'already social', whatever the context (Connell and Dowsett 1999, pp. 191–192). HIV and programmes to address it are very prominent scenarios for producing gendered and sexual 'scripts' (Paiva 2000, Simon and Gagnon 1999), but they merely illustrate the reality that 'bodies and pleasures' are never unmediated. Alas, Foucault was right; they are always and every-where produced, shaped, and made intelligible through a field of discursive meanings (Butler 1993, Fausto-Sterling 2000). This in turn raises questions about the complex variety of whatever we may mean by 'pleasure', and the uneasy tension between pleasure as an infinitely variable lived experience and the more inflexible categories of 'rights':

> The idea of sexual pleasure, its definitions, its language, its expres-sion, all typically come from below, from the local context where people experience life. These interpretations emerge from cultural systems of meaning and significance that are a mélange of popular culture intersecting with elite culture, mechanically reproduced and ideologically mediated.... The tendency of *categorizing* rights does not easily lend itself to the multiple and fluid interpretations of pleasure and desire.
>
> (Garcia and Parker 2006, pp. 24–25)

Lewis and Gordon (2006) make a compelling case for why the call to bring 'pleasure' back into sexual rights may be rhetorically appealing but glosses over the enormous ambiguities and complexities the 'idea of sexual pleasure' involves. Enumerating dozens of hypothetical contexts in which sexual encounters occur, or reasons why people may engage in sexual acts – along a broad continuum from coercion to lust – they observe that 'the possibility and nature of "pleasure" is utterly different in all these situ-ations'.[36] Not only does 'context [shape] sexualities and sexual encoun-ters'; it also shapes what pleasure feels like (p. 110). A few of their examples illustrate this dramatically:

> If your children or grandparents are starving or ill, if you are unem-ployed or poor, if you are in a conflict zone far from home, then a paid sexual encounter could be joyful not because of actual physical or emotional satisfaction, but because you are accessing possibilities of affirmation.... If you are far from home in a risky conflict situation, far from the intimacies of family or community, living in discomfort, facing the unknowns of danger, injury or death, under pressure to keep up a 'front' in mostly male company, then the pleasure of sex with a local woman, enabled by financial exchange, may not be just about orgasm, but involve a whole range of reassurances and comfort. If you live in a civil war, with collapsed social infrastructure, wide-spread abject poverty and minimal family resources and violence in the home, your sexual experience with the older sugar daddy (who is enabling your only possible access to education as a girl) may also be the kindest, most pleasuring relation you have.
>
> (Lewis and Gordon 2006, p. 111)

Here we are reminded of the classic narrative by the nineteenth-century African-American former slave, Harriet Jacobs, when she begs her readers to stretch their moral compass to understand why she, as a 15-year-old enslaved girl, would willingly give herself to an older, unmarried man 'who is not her master': 'There is something akin to freedom in having a lover who has no control over you, except that which he gains by kindness and attachment' (Jacobs 1987 [orig. 1861], p. 385). Pleasure comes in many forms and may involve successful trades within conditions of racial-ized and gendered subordination, or warding off 'the fragile edges of pride, anxiety, humiliation and rejection that haunt traditional masculinities' (Lewis and Gordon 2006, p. 115).

But this kind of careful attention to the infinite nuances of pleasure and the 'contextual realities of real relations, real bodies in real life situations of survival' seems to require an entirely different vocabulary from that of human rights. Lewis and Gordon ask, 'is the language of "needs to be met" and "rights to be fulfilled" radically off key, dissociating sexual pleasure from social context and insulating it from the tides of ordinary daily lives?' (2006, p. 113). Once again we come up against the limitations of rights as an ethical framework and discourse; the ways in which its tendency to press 'sexuality' into discrete identity categories and to focus 'on violations' fails to capture either the range of erotic experience or 'the sexual diversity within each of us' (Sharma 2006, p. 55).

One way to address this problem is to broaden our understanding of eroticism itself and thus of what a human rights of sexuality might encompass. We need to return to something closer to Audre Lorde's (1984) conception of 'the uses of the erotic' and the ways in which eroti-cism is about empowering and energizing not only my body but also my community. This is similar to what Brazilian psychologist and AIDS activist Vera Paiva suggests in proposing a form of public education around HIV/AIDS that would merge a Freirian approach to politicization as self and community empowerment with a Brazilian cultural affirmation of the erotic potential in all of us. From this perspective, eroticism and public, communal engagement are entirely interdependent: '[E]ncouraging people to be the agents of their whole life – subjects who are capable of choosing and deciding' and 'to look beyond [their] own narcissistic reflec-tion [toward] psycho-social emancipation' is a means for creating political agency and stimulating desire at one and the same time (Paiva 2003, pp. 200–201).

When the National Network of Sex Worker Organizations in Kerala insists on both 'an enabling environment ... in which [sex workers] can live as free citizens' and 'the right to safe and pleasurable sex', its actions reflect a similar understanding (see Chapter 9). So does Outsiders, the UK-based organization for people with various forms of disability, when it holds sex parties for differently abled people of diverse sexual and gender orientations, making recognition of their sexual lives as important as access to physical, public spaces (Ilkkaracan and Jolly 2007). Erotic justice and social justice are not one and the same, but they are deeply tied to one another; and a human rights framework worth fighting for must embrace their deep interconnections.

Postscript
Dreaming and dancing – beyond sexual rights

The appeal to relink bodies with communities, and erotic justice with social justice, brings us back from the nebulae of ethics to the more solid but shifting ground where this book starts and ends: politics. But what sorts of politics will make these linkages possible in the world as it currently is? A quarter of a century ago, Derrida's dream of dancing beyond all the sexual binaries – 'feminine-masculine, ... bi-sexuality, ... homosexuality and heterosexuality' – was a vision of queerness that anticipated the eruption of 'incalculable choreographies' of sexual and gender variance across the globe (Derrida 1982, p. 76). Today, that vision seems like more than a dream, still much less than a liveable reality free from stigma and harassment, for the millions who attempt to live it. The issue we inevitably come back to is how to transform visions into practical possibilities: What obstacles still exist to bridging theory and practice? What concrete strategies, organizational forms, and ways of building viable coalitions are beginning to emerge for sexual rights activism? In addition, to what extent can that activism overcome some of the troubling limits of human rights as discussed earlier?

An inhospitable global landscape makes these questions all the more daunting. In scornful reaction to the choreographies of pleasure, the three forces that have cast their shadow over our discussions in the preceding chapters – rampant militarism, hegemonic capitalism, and dogmatic religiosity – continue to produce violent, commodified, covert, apologetic, or otherwise distorted forms of sexuality. The institutions of states and intergovernmental organizations, to which previous generations looked for social solidarity and the promise of equality, have become discredited by corruption, privatization, paralysis, and complicity with militarism, global capitalism, and radical religion. Meanwhile religious institutions are themselves caught in scandals of sexual predation (the Catholic Church) and agendas of military aggrandizement (imperial Christianity, radical Islam, Hindutva communalism, militant Zionism). In the interstices of these large-scale forces – at the level of the micropolitics of everyday life – biomedical authorities continue to pathologize, and police sanctions to criminalize and persecute, sexual deviants of many kinds. New local and transnational actors constantly emerge, but they face, on the one hand, scarce resources and marginalization within, or on the fringes of, left and feminist movements that have themselves become increasingly fragmented and marginalized; and on the other hand, the risks of co-option that come from reliance on international development agencies and donor agendas.

Yet, external forces and constraints are only part of the picture. A revitalized language and politics of sexual freedom need to overcome a number of binary traps – false double binds – that hobble our movements and keep political practice lagging behind recent theoretical advances regarding sexuality and gender that this book has attempted to bring into view. Among these traps, the following are most worrisome.

Culture versus political economy

A division between erotic justice and social justice (and consequently between movements for sexual rights, and those aimed at economic development and ending poverty and war) derives from an epistemological error that extracts intimate and bodily experience from its social matrix. Such a division makes no sense in the context of real people's lives. A sex worker's struggle against poverty, police brutality, HIV, and moral stigma is a multi-pronged struggle for a whole and dignified life. A transgender or intersex person's capacity to be who she/he is, in public without shame, or to access necessary health and prenatal care, is inseparable from her/his ability to find work in an environment free of discrimination and harassment. Iraqi women's exposure to daily threats of sectarian, sexual, and gender-based violence, and their exclusion from the political space, are part and parcel of their collective oppression due to the US-led military invasion and occupation.

Treating sexuality as something separate from political economy ignores the fact that health care access, affordable housing, adequate nutrition, safe environments, and secure livelihoods are indispensable for safe and pleasurable erotic experience to be real. This false dichotomy not only obscures the necessary enabling conditions for sexual rights across lines of gender, class, race, ethnicity, and geography. It also disregards the *materiality* of sexual expression and well-being, a materiality rooted, not in some essential biological drive or genetic predisposition, but rather in the ways that bodies 'matter' and become materialized through the same regulatory norms and power relations that produce gender, class, race, ethnicity, and geography to begin with (Butler 1993; see also Chapter 5). If bodies themselves – genes, hormones, sexual and reproductive organs – are always imbued with, and made intelligible through, norms and practices, the cultural and economic/political dimensions of those norms are also closely intertwined. And the *indeterminacy* of these relations (fluid, unpredictable, changing) makes it all the more urgent that advocacy for erotic justice and advocacy for economic justice be similarly bound together.

Secularity versus religion

As this writing comes to a close, the US presidential elections crowd the mainstream media with speeches by leading candidates professing 'faith' and belief in the divinity of Jesus Christ. At the same time, militant Islamists in Sudan call for the death of a British teacher who allowed her pupils to name a teddy bear Muhammed, and a religious court in Saudi Arabia sentences a female rape victim to 300 lashes for being seen in a car with men to whom she was not related. In such a climate, many advocates of both erotic justice and economic justice must feel pressed into a staunch defence of secularism – indeed, they must even feel nostalgia for what seemed to be a calmer, more rational era in which secularity governed public space, and religion was a matter of private conviction and ritual. But it is precisely because religion has become so intensely politicized in the post-Cold War world that secularity has taken on an aura of either a lost golden age, or the demonic and godless opposite of religious virtue. In other words, as this book has sought to emphasize (see Chapter 3), we again confront a false dichotomy, a highly rhetorical construction, that evades the complex ways in which 'faith' and 'reason', religion and politics, have always been interpenetrating, overlapping domains, though in different ways and in different historical and local contexts.

In the present geopolitical context – and possibly for the foreseeable future – feminist and sexual rights activists and intellectuals will need to re-engage with religion without 'returning' there. What this means, in terms of political analysis and strategy, is bringing a critical perspective to bear on religion as a continuous but changing aspect of political and social reality, not its 'opposite'. On the one hand, this kind of critical engagement means challenging – loudly and forthrightly – the injustices perpetrated in the name of religion, however and wherever they occur, while also disavowing Islamophobia, anti-Semitism, and other forms of religious bigotry sometimes proclaimed in the name of sexual rights. On the other hand, it could also mean opening doors that a dogmatic or defensive secularism leaves closed – for example, examining the spiritual, ecstatic, and mystical dimensions of sexuality, or forging alliances with religious identified groups where we share common goals and values. Sisters in Islam in Malaysia,[1] the Coalition for Sexual and Bodily Rights in Muslim Societies,[2] and Catholics for a Free Choice[3] provide examples of groups that have moved in this direction.

Individual versus community

Both the Marxist Left and the religious Right dismiss claims concerning sexual freedom and expression as 'individualist' by definition and therefore 'bad' – whether because such claims are subordinate to the presumably 'collective' aims of ending poverty, securing universal health care, empowering workers, and so on, or because they represent 'selfish' and 'hedonistic' moral values. Throughout the preceding chapters we have rejected this dichotomy and argued instead for a vision that encompasses *both* singularity and interdependence (of bodies, persons, desires). By insisting on the singularity of bodies we point to the indeterminacy and infinite variety of desire, even as bodies and pleasures are always lived within, and dependent on, multiple relationships and social ties. We also remind ourselves that economic and social rights accruing to communities (for safe water, health care, livelihoods) are ultimately about the individual bodies that need these resources to live. Rights are always individual and social at the same time, just as persons are. No one else can get inside 'my' body and experience its particular pain, terror, yearning, or ecstasy. But the pain, terror, yearning, and ecstasy are the effects of power relations and interdependencies that make us who or what we are, embed us within community and kin networks, and simultaneously produce community and kin as social constructs.

Identity versus humanity

The project of reconceptualizing individual claims within matrices of community and kin relationships – a holistic perspective that emphasizes the social and relational dimensions of sexual rights – is closely linked to that of rethinking identity politics. Here again we are faced with an array of imagined dichotomies that end up enervating social movements and weakening their capacity for radical transformation. In the realm of sexual and gender politics, at several points in this book we have alluded to the tensions between two unsatisfactory tendencies. First we have the totalizing and gratuitously additive character of acronyms (LGBT, LGBTQ, LGBTQI) that glibly cover over the specifically different situations of each subgroup, as well as the power differentials among them. Second, the prospect, and the reality, of 'splinterings', in which each of the subgroups breaks away into its own identity-based enclave, is also troubling. The contempt that some gay men, lesbians, and straight feminists have sometimes shown toward trans-men and -women who wish to join their gatherings, and the reaction of trans- and intersex groups who seek to establish clearly defined communities of their own, reinforce the fragmentation that critics of identity politics have bemoaned for some 15 years. Just as problematic is the reluctance of many HIV and AIDS groups to take on and defend issues of sexual diversity, equality, and pleasure, in addition to the safer discourses of public health. All this replays the tensions between commonality and difference (of race, ethnicity, class, region, sexual orientation) that have disturbed feminist politics for decades.

How therefore do we create meaningful and politically viable linkages across a wide range of identity-based groups without erasing the real social differences among them or returning to the empty and historically contaminated (and anthropocentric) abstraction of 'humanity as a whole'? The vision here is one of a politics of the body and its integrity, freedom, social connectedness, and pleasures that would prepare the ground for working coalitions and solidarity across many diverse activist groups – whether feminist, lesbian, gay, transgender, queer, intersex, and people living with HIV, or groups mobilized against torture, militarism, racism, and ethnic violence and those for health care, reproductive justice, comprehensive sex education, food security, and disability rights. Good models for such work across identity boundaries do exist, but they are still few and far between. At the national level, they include the campaigns in Turkey to reform the civil and penal codes (Ilkkaracan 2007); the human rights response to HIV and AIDS in Brazil (Vianna and Carrara 2007); and the fight to revoke Section 377 in India (Chapter 3; see also Ramasubban 2007). At the international level, they include the drafting and adoption of the Yogyakarta Principles (2006) and the coalitions working to bring awareness of sexual, reproductive, and health rights to the UN Human Rights Council.

Here there are lessons to be learned from another, related false dichotomy: that between the local and the global. All the examples of good models cited above are ones in which key actors have combined deep knowledge of local conditions, institutions, and cultures with awareness of, and experience in, shaping international human rights principles. They exemplify the observation made earlier that the global and the local are intersecting spaces rather than separate spheres, particularly in conditions of globalization and Internet communication. Yet tensions between these spaces persist, as illustrated by the *Zina* cases in Nigeria in which international activists attempted to intervene in complete disregard of the strategies of local sexual rights activists (see Chapter 3).

Imam's (2005, p. 66) caveat that we must privilege neither local nor global norms but retain a critical stance towards both reminds us once again that human rights/sexual rights discourse and practice constitute a terrain of political struggle that is constantly shifting. We cannot dispense with the language of human rights, but neither can we accept it as fully adequate or complete. Rather, the political project of human rights and sexual rights is to continually reinvent their meanings so that they are social and individual, global and local, theoretical and practical, inclusive and specific, visionary and operational, about the body and about the collective body, all at the same time. The 'beyond' beyond dichotomous thinking is political solidarity.

Glossary of terms

Acronyms

ACSF Analyse de Comportements Sexuels en France (National Survey on Sexual Behaviour, France)

ANRS Agence Nationale de Recherches sur le Sida (National AIDS Research Council, France)

CEDAW/Women's Convention Convention on the Elimination of All Forms of Discrimination Against Women

CPS Contraception Prevalence Surveys

DMZ Demilitarized zone

FTA Free Trade Agreement

FWCW Fourth World Conference on Women

GATT General Agreement on Tariffs and Trade

Health GAP Health Global Access Project

ICCPR International Covenant on Civil and Political Rights

ICESCR International Covenant on Economic, Social and Cultural Rights

ICPD International Conference on Population and Development

IDRF India Development Relief Fund

IIJG International Initiative for Justice in Gujarat

ITPA Immoral Traffic in Persons Prevention Act, 1986 (India)

MRC Medical Research Council

NACO National AIDS Control Organization (India)

NATSAL National Survey of Sexual Attitudes and Lifestyles (UK)

NGO Non-governmental organization

NHSLS National Health and Social Life Survey (USA)

NIH National Institutes of Health (USA)

PEPFAR President's Emergency Plan for AIDS Relief (USA)

PNAC Project for the New American Century

SAPs Structural adjustment programmes

SITA Suppression of Immoral Traffic in Women and Girls Act, 1956

TAC Treatment Action Campaign (South Africa)

TRIPS Trade-related intellectual property rights
TVPRA Trafficking Victims Protection Reauthorization Act (USA)
UDHR Universal Declaration of Human Rights
WFS World Fertility Survey

Global/regional institutions

APEC Asia Pacific Economic Community
AU African Union
CARICOM Caribbean Community
HRC United Nations Human Rights Council
ICC International Criminal Court
ICJ International Commission of Jurists
IMF International Monetary Fund
IUSSP International Union for the Scientific Study of Population
Mercosur Mercado Común del Sur (Southern Common Market)
NRC Norwegian Refugee Council
SADC Southern Africa Development Community
USAID United States Agency for International Development
WCC World Council of Churches
WHO World Health Organization
WTO World Trade Organization

Groups/organizations

ABIA Brazilian Interdisciplinary AIDS Association
ACLU American Civil Liberties Union
ACT-UP AIDS Coalition to Unleash Power
AI Amnesty International
AKP Islamist Party, Turkey
ARC ARC International, Canada
ARROW Asia-Pacific Resource and Research Organization for Women
BBC British Broadcasting Corporation
BD Bajrang Dal, youth arm of the Vishwa Hindu Parishad
BJP Bharatiya Janata Party
CARASA Committee for Abortion Rights and Against Sterilization Abuse
CAT Coalition Against Trafficking
CCR Center for Constitutional Rights
CHANGE Centre for Health and Gender Equity
CRR Center for Reproductive Rights
CWGL Centre for Women's Global Leadership
DAWN Development Alternatives with Women for a New Era
FIMI Foro Internacional de Mujeres Indigenas
GIRE Information Group for Reproductive Choice (Mexico)

HRW   Human Rights Watch
HSS   Hindu Swayamsevak Sangh
IGLHRC   International Gay and Lesbian Human Rights Commission
ILGA   International Lesbian and Gay Association
IRRRAG   International Reproductive Rights Research Action Group
MADRE   International women's human rights organization
MSF/DND   Médecins Sans Frontières, Drugs for Neglected Disease
    working group
OIC   Organization of Islamic Conference
OSI   Open Society Institute
PAN   Partido de Acción National (Mexico)
RSS   Rashtriya Swayamsevak Sangh: Hindu nationalist organization
    (India)
SAMOIS   Lesbian S/M organization (USA)
SCIRI   Supreme Council for the Islamic Revolution in Iraq
SexPol   German association for a proletarian sexual policy
SOS Corpo – Grupo de Saúde da Mulher   (formally SOS Corpo – Insti-
    tuto Feminista para a Democracies: Brazilian women's health NGO)
SPW   Sexuality Policy Watch
USCRI   United States Committee for Refugees and Immigrants
VHP   Vishwa Hindu Parishad: a Hindu organization that is an offshoot
    of RSS (India)
WEDO   Women's Environment and Development Organization
WLUML   Women Living Under Muslim Laws

Terminology

ABC   Abstinence, be faithful, condoms
ARV   Anti-retroviral medication
Big PHARMA   Global pharmaceutical corporations
FGM   Female genital mutilation
IDP   Internally displaced persons
LGBT   Lesbian, gay, bisexual, transgender
LGBTI   Lesbian, gay, bisexual, transgender, intersex
LGBTQ   Lesbian, gay, bisexual, transgender, queer
LGBTQI   Lesbian, gay, bisexual, transgender, queer, intersex
MSM   Men who have sex with men
SRHR   Sexual and reproductive health and rights
STI   Sexually transmitted infections

United Nations institutions and programmes

CESCR   Committee on Economic, Social, and Cultural Rights
CHR   Commission on Human Rights

CRC Committee on the Rights of the Child
CSW Commission on the Status of Women
ECOSOC Economic and Social Council
HRC Human Rights Council
UNAIDS Joint United Nations Programme on HIV/AIDs
UNCHR United Nations Commission on Human Rights
UNDP United Nations Development Programme
UNFPA United Nations Population Fund
UNGASS United Nations General Assembly Special Session
UNHCR United Nations Refugee Programme
UNICEF United Nations Children's Fund
UNIFEM United Nations Fund for Women

Notes

Introduction

1 We are increasingly uncomfortable with this acronym that strings together a number of distinct movements whose unity is far from clear; see below.

I Landscaping sexualities

1 The Ukrainian-born medical doctor and political activist, Wilhelm Reich, then living in Vienna, created SexPol, and the initiative expanded further when he moved to Berlin. In 1931, as Nazi forces were gaining power, Reich wrote 'The sexual struggle of youth', which was used in the mobilization of more than 50,000 young people against capitalism and for sexual liberation. In 1933, forced to leave Germany, Reich went to Norway before moving to the USA in 1939 where his theories and writings regained visibility in the 1960s (see Reich 1973a).

2 Since the late 1990s, developing countries have contested US and EU hegemony in trade negotiations (note also trade-related tensions between the USA and EU themselves). In Asia, economic tensions between Japan, China, and more recently India, have also been growing. The rise in oil prices after the Iraq war has given new leverage to oil-producing countries in the Middle East, Central Asia, and Latin America, particularly in the emergence of Russia, Venezuela, and Iran as regional and global players. Meanwhile China is expanding its role as a global power, investing heavily in Africa. Moreover, high- and low-intensity armed tensions and conflicts, often related to the control of natural resources, have spread (for example, in Angola, Sierra Leone, and Darfur).

3 These same premises were the basis for the 1945 creation of the Bretton Woods institutions – the International Monetary Fund (IMF) and World Bank – and the General Agreement on Tariffs and Trade (GATT). For an overview, see Cohen 2002.

4 In Europe the trailblazer of these policies was the UK's Margaret Thatcher, Prime Minister from 1979 to 1990. In the USA, the Reagan administration adopted neo-liberal economic frameworks, which were not entirely abandoned during the Clinton era and were fully revived under Bush (although the Bush administration is definitely Keynesian in regard to military investments).

5 The antecedent of the Group of 7, or G7, was the Group of 6, made up of the finance ministers of France, Germany, Italy, Japan, the UK, and the USA, which first met in 1974 to discuss the effects of the 1973 oil crisis. In 1976,

when Canada joined the group, the G7 was created and started to meet annually in various locations to discuss economic and other policies with global effects. By the 1990s, the G7 had become an icon of Northern-led globalization, and its composition was contested by new emerging economies and other developing countries. In 1994, at the annual meeting held in Naples, Russia was invited to become a member of the group, and the name was changed to the G8. In parallel, developing countries established their own platform to engage in dialogue with the G8 as a block. This led to the creation of the so-called Group of 20, or G20, which comprises the G8 plus Argentina, Australia, Brazil, China, India, Indonesia, Mexico, Saudi Arabia, South Africa, South Korea, and Turkey. Southern members of the G20 are invited to discuss specific issues with G8 members in their annual meetings.

6 Castells (1997) analyses the effects of the media and corruption in European countries. In 2004, UNDP examined perceptions of democracy in Latin America and concluded that because the promised democratization of the 1980s did not resolve social and economic inequalities, popular preferences were rapidly shifting toward authoritarianism. The political evolution in countries such as Venezuela, Bolivia, and Ecuador in the years that followed proved this assessment to be correct. Freedom House (2007) also concluded that freedom and civil rights were losing ground in many settings because democratic institutions remain fragile and disorganized.

7 With regard to human rights defenders working in the field of sexuality, the 2005 IGLHRC and CWGL report *Written Out: How Sexuality is Used to Attack Women's Organizing*, quotes Dr Hina Jilani, the UN special representative on human rights defenders, on the effects of the current climate on organizations working in the fields of HIV/AIDS and human rights:

> [I]nformation on HIV/AIDS, reports of alleged human rights abuses by members of a governing political party or statements critical of the human rights impacts of government security policies have all been claimed by states to be information whose publication is a threat to national security.
> (IGLHRC and CWGL 2005, p. 45)

8 Although not an exhaustive list, just a few examples of this trend in major cinematic works might include Louis Malle's *The Lovers* (1958), Fellini's *Satyricon* (1969), Bergman's *Cries and Whispers* (1971), Bertolucci's *Last Tango in Paris* (1972), Liliana Cavani's *The Night Porter* (1974), or Oshima's *The Realm of Senses* (1976).

9 Mention should be made of the subtle homoeroticism of such films as *From Here to Eternity* (Fred Zimmermann, 1953), *Suddenly Last Summer* (Joseph L. Mankievicz, 1959), *Handsome Antonio* (Mario Bolognini, with a Pasolini script, 1959), and *Death in Venice* (Visconti, 1971). Between 1961 and 1975, Pasolini directed 26 movies, the last one being *120 Days of Sodom*. Fassbinder has directed 43 movies since 1966, and Almodovar 29 since 1974.

10 One example is the Indian film *Fire* (Deepa Mehta, 1996), which tells the story of a love affair between two women. It sparked angry demonstrations by Hindu revivalists when it was first shown in India but attracted audiences worldwide. In the past three years we have witnessed the global successes of the Hollywood hits *Brokeback Mountain*, *Capote*, and *Transamerica*, as well as films produced in Southern countries, such as *Amarelo Manga* (Brazil, 2002), *Beautiful Boxer* (Thailand, 2003), *Dakan* (Guinea/France, 1997), *Madam Satā* (Brazil, 2002), *Mango Soufflé* (India, 2002), and *Plata Quemada* (Argentina, 2000).

11 A quick Internet search identifies 146 festivals worldwide, the large majority in the USA and Europe. But the list also includes four festivals in the global South: in Brazil, Hong Kong, India, and Mexico.

12 The Brazilian researcher and HIV activist Veriano Terto portrays these transformations as 'the "gayification" of heterosexual imagination and practices, particularly in the case of women' (personal communication, November 2006). Gregori (2004) calls attention to the increasing number of women, all over the world, who are using sex shop gadgets, exploring the conceptual and political dilemmas this poses for certain feminist streams of thinking.

13 The 'V' in V-Day stands for Valentine, Vagina, and Victory, linking love and respect for women to ending violence against women and girls.

14 This was the case in Uganda in 2004. In China, the production was staged with great success at a university in the south of the country but it was banned in Beijing where it would have had greater visibility.

15 Information on the project may be found online at www.empowerfoundation.org/kumjing.html (accessed 26 October 2007).

16 At the Round Tables Count Down 2015, sponsored by the International Planned Parenthood Federation in London in 2004 to commemorate the ten years of the International Conference on Population and Development, Sexuality Policy Watch and the International Women's Health Coalition organized the Sexuality Track. In the debates of the event, Victor Bernardtz, representing the Youth Coalition, talked about his personal experience as well as about the theatre group, of which he was a member. It is worth noting that Bernardtz is now the anchor of a highly popular talk show on Swedish TV.

17 In addition to the major long-standing parades of San Francisco, New York, and Rome, gay pride events are proliferating and growing everywhere. For instance, participation in the São Paulo parade increased from 2000 people in 1997 to three million in 2006. Efforts to hold World Gay Pride 2006 in Jerusalem in 2006 met tremendous resistance – from the Vatican, the Israeli Supreme Court, religious leaders of the three main faiths, and Palestinians who saw it as a move that would give Israel undeserved recognition as a human rights haven. Although the original plan for a march through the city's centre was cancelled, thousands of demonstrators none the less gathered in a sports stadium 'under a heavy police guard' (Myre 2006).

18 The Gay Games, originally called the Gay Olympics, started in San Francisco in 1982 when 1300 athletes participated. In the 2006 Chicago Gay Games, it is estimated that 12,000 people participated in the competition. When Montreal was defined as the location for the 2006 Games, a conflict emerged between the local committee and the Federation of Gay Games, which led to major dissidence and to the establishment of the Out Games, first held in 2006 in Montreal and scheduled for Copenhagen in 2009.

19 Evangelical churches own a number of radio and TV channels in the USA and many countries in the developing world. In Brazil, one main TV channel – with branches in Lusophone Africa, Latin America, and the USA itself – belongs to the Universal Church of the Kingdom of God, a Brazilian Pentecostal initiative. The investment and presence of the Catholic Church in the print media, radio, and television have also expanded enormously in the past ten to 20 years. Opus Dei, the extremely conservative Catholic organization, operates the Navarra Institute in Spain that provides training on new media technologies and re-engineering of press enterprises, particularly for Latin American journalists, editors, and managers. While the training is not openly ideological but rather technical (which explains its great appeal among media professionals), it

constitutes an opportunity for Opus Dei to identify potential allies and construct an Ibero-Latin American media-based network.

20 We acknowledge Bina Srinivasan's important analysis of the bombardment of
India with Western cultural products. Bina was an Indian feminist involved in
many global initiatives, including the Feminist Dialogues organized at the
World Social Forum in Mumbai in 2004. She died prematurely in August 2007
as this book was being finalized.

21 Historical studies have identified tragic examples in the persecution of homosexuals by the Inquisition in Europe, particularly in Portugal and Spain and in
their American colonies (see Crompton 2003). One of the best-known episodes
is the condemnation of Felipa de Souza to exile in Angola, when the Portuguese
Inquisition held hearings in Bahia, Brazil in 1591. Since 1994, the International
Gay and Lesbian Human Rights Commission has granted a Felipa de Souza
Award to individuals and groups for outstanding work in defence of the
human rights of 'LGBTQ' people. See also Chapter 5.

22 For more on Mead and Malinowski, see Chapter 4. For a discussion of more
current anthropological work, see Chapter 5.

23 The surge and development of social movements when politics at large was
being increasingly discredited is an evident paradox that cannot be examined
more fully here. While some authors view this surge of new voices and
agendas as the sign of a renewal of politics (e.g., Benhabib 2002, Castells
1997, 1998, Fraser 1997, Giddens 2000), others interpret it as a phenomenon directly correlated with the demise of states, the primacy of market
forces, and philanthropic responses to social needs. Some theorists go further
and affirm that the political disenchantment of late capitalism may also be
attributed to postmodern interrogations of foundational political principles,
unitary subjects, history, and consensus, placing emphasis on differences and
interrogations.

24 In 1957 in the UK, the Wolfenden Report on Homosexual Offences and Prostitution recommended that homosexual behaviour in private between consenting
adult men (i.e., over 21 years) should be decriminalized but that curbs on prostitution should be tightened. Then, in July 1967, the Sexual Offences Act
received Royal Assent, partially decriminalizing sex between men (two men
over 21 'in private') but excluding from the norm persons belonging to the
armed forces or the merchant navy and applying only to England and Wales. In
West Germany, full decriminalization took place in 1969. The UK process
would be completed with *Dudgeon* v. *UK*, which was presented to the European Court of Human Rights in 1981. The European Court also issued positive
decisions with respect to other cases, such as *Norris* v. *Ireland* in 1985. In the
USA, progressive lawyers started a campaign in the 1960s to get states to pass
model penal codes. Illinois was the first state to adopt a version and decrimi-
nalize sodomy in 1961 – a process that culminated most recently in the US
Supreme Court's relatively liberal decision in *Lawrence* v. *Texas* (2002) (see
Chapter 3). In most of the socialist world and in Japan abortion was legalized
in the 1950s, but in Western countries legal reforms started in the late 1960s
when abortion was legalized in Australia, Canada, and the UK. In 1970 abortion was also legalized in New York, and in 1973 the US Supreme Court, in
Roe v. *Wade,* declared all the individual state bans on abortion during the first
and second trimesters to be unconstitutional. Legal reforms ensued in Europe
and elsewhere: Sweden (in 1974 legislation adopted in the 1930s and 1940s
was adjusted), France (1975), West Germany (1976), Israel (1976), New
Zealand (1977), Italy (1978), and the Netherlands (in 1980 legal reform was

finalized, but even before that abortion was accessible). In India, China, and Vietnam abortion was legalized as part of population control policies.

25 A number of events may be listed as key early moments in the transnationalization of civil society actors engaged with sexual politics. In 1978 the International Lesbian and Gay Association (ILGA) was created. In 1984, feminists from all over the world who were engaged in struggles for abortion and contraception and against forced sterilization met in Amsterdam where they created the Women's Global Network for Reproductive Rights and crafted a first global consensus on reproductive rights. At the UN Third World Conference on Women in Nairobi, Kenya, 1985, 14,000 women participated in the parallel NGO Forum, where issues such as abortion, female genital mutilation, and women's health were debated. Regional formations such as the Latin American and Caribbean Women's Health Network, established in 1984, and the Asia-Pacific Resource and Research Organization for Women (ARROW), founded in 1994, have also blossomed, while global networks on HIV prevention and research have rapidly evolved through autonomous civil society initiatives as well as the involvement of major institutional actors such as the World Health Organization (WHO), the World Bank, and, more recently, UNAIDS.

26 Feminist organizations from diverse regions, including lesbian groups, started engaging more systematically within UN processes at the 1975 First World Conference on Women in Mexico City. By the 1990s, they had gained much more knowledge and expertise about international institutions. Gay groups, sex worker organizations, and HIV-positive people, in contrast, remained mainly focused on national politics. The global nature of HIV/AIDS, however, would gradually shift their attention to international processes. The international AIDS conferences that started in the late 1980s played a key role in this regard, and the projects and programmes developed by the WHO, World Bank, and, later on, UNAIDS also enhanced the participation of many other actors in global HIV policy debates. By the early 2000s these diverse voices were visible and active in some key UN negotiations (see Chapters 2 and 7).

27 The Norway statement reads in part:

> At its recent session, the Human Rights Council received extensive evidence of human rights violations based on sexual orientation and gender identity, including deprivation of the rights to life, freedom from violence, and torture. We commend the attention paid to these issues by the Special Procedures, treaty bodies, and civil society. We call upon all Special Procedures and treaty bodies to continue to integrate consideration of human rights violations based on sexual orientation and gender identity within their relevant mandates. We express deep concern at these ongoing human rights violations. The principles of universality and non-discrimination require that these issues be addressed. We therefore urge the Human Rights Council to pay due attention to human rights violations based on sexual orientation and gender identity, and request the President of the Council to provide an opportunity, at an appropriate future session of the Council, for a discussion of these important human rights issues.
>
> (Available online at www.ilga.org/news_results.asp?LanguageID=1&FileCategoryID=44&File ID=944&ZoneID=7 [accessed 13 October 2007])

28 The International Commission of Jurists and Human Rights International Services led the initiative with the support of a wide range of human rights specialists and sexual rights advocates. See www.yogyakartaprinciples.org.

29 One of Elredge's critiques, for instance, reads:

> Sex is so clearly separated from pure reproduction in humans – and there is so much interplay between sex and economics, and even between economics and reproduction in human life – that this 'human triangle' of sex, reproduction, and economics makes us the very last creatures on the planet to conform to such strictures of evolutionary determinism.
>
> (Elredge 2004, p. 27)

30 For further discussions on these issues, see, for example, HRW 2007d, Kissling 1999, 2003, Lamberts-Bendroth 1999, Ortiz-Ortega 2005, Saghal and Yuval-Davis 1992, UN 2007.

31 The same group also circulated highly homophobic literature that equated homosexuality and lesbianism with 'paedophilia', 'prostitution', 'incest', and 'adultery' as a single toxic brew and blamed 'homosexuals' for 'behaviours which everyone knows spread HIV/AIDS' (quoted in Petchesky 2000, p. 87).

32 In the case of the process leading up to the Fourth World Conference on Women in Beijing, following the difficult debates of the final preparatory meeting a working group was created to define how gender would be addressed in the final document. Its final recommendation was that there was no need for a definition of the term 'gender' because the concept had been extensively used in United Nations documents.

33 In an article originally published in the *Huffington Post*, Dawkins develops the following reasoning: 'The political tendency currently in ascent attributes more value to stem cells than to adult persons. It is obsessively worried with gay marriage, in detriment of genuinely important issues that, in fact, would make a difference in the world' (translated and republished in *Folha de São Paulo*, 25 August 2007. Available online at http://www1.folha. uol.com.br/folha/ilustrada/ult90u322666.shtml (accessed on 26 October 2007)). He has also launched a massive Internet campaign calling for atheists to make themselves visible, which is openly inspired by sexual politics, as it is titled the Out Campaign. Available online at http://outcampaign.org (accessed 26 October 2007). However, Dawkins may still be characterized as an ultra-Darwinist and it is very difficult to foresee in the near future a more open and productive interaction between his followers and theorization of the field of sexuality as it has developed in recent decades (see Chapters 4 and 5).

2 The real politics of 'sex'

1 By the end of the nineteenth century the following countries had abolished sodomy laws: France (1791), Monaco, (1793), Luxembourg (1795), Netherlands (1811), Brazil (1830), Turkey (1858), Guatemala (1871), Mexico (1871), San Marino (1865), Japan (1880), Italy (1890), and Argentina (1886). By the 1940s: Peru (1924), Poland (1932), Denmark (1934), Uruguay (1934), Iceland (1940), Switzerland (1942), and Sweden (1944). This list is probably incomplete as the Ottosson study does not provide the dates of the reform adopted in a number of countries that may eventually fall into these categories (see n. 3).

2 Countries in this second wave include: Greece (1951), Thailand (1957), Jordan (1960), Czech Republic and Slovakia (former Czechoslovakia, 1962), Hungary (1962), United Kingdom (1967/1969), the USA (a few states in the late 1960s, full abolition 2003), Germany (1968/1969), Bulgaria (1968), Canada (1969), Costa Rica (1971), Austria (1971), Finland (1971), Norway (1972), Malta (1973), Australia (1975), Tasmania (1997), Croatia (1977), Slovenia (1977),

Montenegro (1977), Cuba (1979), and Spain (1979). It should be noted, however, that in most socialist countries, including Cuba, the abolition of laws prohibiting homosexual acts did not automatically imply the end of discrimination and persecution. In most of Eastern Europe, discrimination and abuses would only diminish after 1989.

3 Albania (1995), Armenia (2003), Azerbaijan (2000), Bahamas (1991), Belarus (1994), Bosnia–Herzegovina (1998/2000), Cape Verde (2004), Central African Republic (n/a), Chad (n/a), Chile (1998), China (1993), Colombia (1981), Cyprus (1998), Democratic Republic of Congo (n/a), Dominican Republic (n/a), Ecuador (1997), Estonia (1992), Former Yugoslavia (n/a), Republic of Macedonia (1996), Gabon (n/a), Georgia (2000), Iraq (2003), Ireland (1993), Israel (1988), Kyrgyzstan (1998), Latvia (1992), Liechtenstein (1989), Lithuania (1993), Moldova (1995), Mongolia (early 1990s), New Zealand (1986), Puerto Rico (2005), Romania (1996), Russia (1993), Serbia (1994), South Africa (1998), Tajikistan (1998), Timor-Leste (n/a), Ukraine (1991), and USA (full abolition in 2003). Ottosson's study identified another 34 countries where same-sex relations are not criminalized but for which no dates of reforms are provided: Bolivia, Burkina Faso, Burundi, Cambodia, Central African Republic, Chad, Comoros, Congo, Democratic Republic of Congo, Dominican Republic, El Salvador, Equatorial Guinea, Gabon, Haiti, Honduras, Indonesia, Ivory Coast, Laos, Madagascar, Mali, Netherlands Antilles, New Caledonia, Niger, North Korea, Palestine West Bank, Paraguay, Philippines, Rwanda, South Korea, Syria, Vanuatu, Venezuela, and Vietnam. In a few of these cases reforms may have occurred far back in time. Bolivia, Honduras, Paraguay, Venezuela, and Haiti are examples, as their respective legislation may have followed the early French/Latin American strands. In other settings, such as Rwanda, Burundi, Cambodia, and Laos, which experienced dramatic conflict in the 1980s and 1990s, more liberal legislation seems to be an outcome of post-conflict transitions. The same applies to Timor-Leste, which became independent in 2002.

4 The first group of countries includes: Bahrain, Bangladesh, Brunei, Cook Islands, Fiji, Gambia, Ghana, Grenada, Guyana, India, Jamaica, Kenya, Kiribati, Kuwait, Malawi, Malaysia, Mauritius, Myanmar, Namibia, Nauru, Nigeria, Niue, Northern Cyprus, Palau, Palestine-Gaza, Papua New Guinea, Qatar, Saint Kitts and Nevis, Saint Lucia, Seychelles, Sierra Leone, Singapore, Sri Lanka, Swaziland, Tanzania, Tokelau, Tonga, Tuvalu, Turkmenistan, Uganda, Uzbekistan, Western Samoa, Zambia, Zimbabwe, and The Chechen Republic. The second group includes: Algeria, Angola, Antigua and Barbuda, Barbados, Belize, Benin, Bhutan, Botswana, Cameroon, and The Republic of Djibouti. Dominica, Eritrea, Ethiopia, Guinea, Guinea-Bissau, Iran, Lebanon, Liberia, Libya, Marshal Islands, Mauritania, Morocco, Mozambique, Nepal, Nigeria, Oman, Pakistan, Saint Vincent and the Grenadines, São Tomé and Principe, Saudi Arabia, Senegal, Solomon Islands, Somali, Sudan, Togo, Trinidad and Tobago, Tunisia, United Arab Emirates, Yemen, and Zanzibar (Tanzania).

5 Iran, Mauritania, Saudi Arabia, Sudan, United Arab Emirates, Yemen, and some Northern States in Nigeria.

6 While Egypt falls in the first category, Brazil falls in the second. Debate about same-sex relations in the armed forces – culminating in the dubious 'don't ask, don't tell' policy – was a main topic of sexual politics in the USA during the 1990s and beyond.

7 The Project for the New American Century (PNAC), founded in early 1997, is a US neo-conservative think-tank based in Washington, DC. The PNAC's

stated goal is 'to promote American global leadership' based on the assumption that 'American leadership is both good for America and good for the world'. It has exerted strong influence on high-level US government officials in the Bush administration, particularly in the development of military and foreign policies involving national security.

8 The 2001 Global Gag Rule revived the rules established by the so-called US/Mexico City policy adopted by the Reagan administration in 1984, which was formally suspended by Clinton in 1992, although limitations remained in place for specific funds. Abortion may appear to many as an unusual way to start exploring current 'sex wars', the main argument being that abortion might be a health and rights issue, or a moral concern, but not exactly a sexual matter. In our view, however, prescriptions aimed at disciplining bodies and moralities place abortion in the same 'damned' cluster as homosexuality, prostitution, and freedom of sexual expression. Furthermore, the logic behind the criminalizing of abortion cannot be fully comprehended without taking into account its meaning as a form of control over female sexuality. Thus, in a large number of countries, rape and risk to the woman's life are accepted legal exceptions to allow for abortion, the rationale being that women who have been raped or may die because of pregnancy do not deserve punishment because they did not behave badly. In contrast, the millions of women who resort to abortion in other circumstances are automatically subsumed in the category of those who are sexually irresponsible and must be punished, either because they had sex out of wedlock or, in a less moralistic perspective, simply because they have not practised birth control.

9 Public Law 108–125.

10 The language on prostitution is very similar in the PEPFAR Act and TVPRA, stating that funds cannot be used to 'promote or advocate the legalization or practice of prostitution or sex trafficking' (PEPFAR) or to support organizations that 'have not stated in either grant application, a grant agreement, or both, that it does not promote, support, or advocate the legalization or practice of prostitution' (TVPRA). See CHANGE 2005b, Ditmore 2007, Girard 2004, Sex Workers Project 2007.

11 Colorado's Marilyn Musgrove and 81 co-sponsors presented the amendment to the Republican-dominated House of Representatives. In November 2003, the Senate introduced a similar amendment, which would later be slightly revised to preserve the possibility of civil unions.

12 Among other related comments in the speech he declared:

> A strong America must also value the institution of marriage.... Activist judges, however, have begun redefining marriage by court order, without regard for the will of the people and their elected representatives. On an issue of such importance, the people's voices must be heard. If judges insist on forcing their arbitrary will upon the people, the only alternative left to the people will be the constitutional process. Our nation must defend the sanctity of marriage.
>
> (Cited in Girard 2004, p. 19)

13 It should be noted that the banned procedure is the one doctors consider safest for pregnant women and that abortions conducted later than 20 weeks comprise only 1.2 per cent of all abortions in the USA; 88 per cent, or nine out of ten of all abortions, occur in the first trimester of pregnancy. Available online at www.guttmacher.org/in-the-know/timing.html (accessed 21 October 2007).

14 In line with these backward trends, in February 2006 South Dakota state legislators approved a bill banning access to abortion except in cases of rape and

risk to the mother's life (the *New York Times*, 6 March 2006). Available online at www.nytimes.com/2006/03/06/politics/06cnd-abort.html (accessed 30 September 2007). The bill was contested in a referendum mobilized by local women's health groups, Planned Parenthood, and the American Civil Liberties Union (ACLU) in November 2006; voters rejected the bill by a vote of 55 per cent against 45 per cent.

15 In April 2004, the images of sexual abuse and torture committed by American soldiers in the Abu Ghraib prison in Iraq revealed that, beyond this screen of sexual morality, other factors such as oil interests, war, race, torture, gender, sexuality, and religion were, in fact, intersecting in complex and perverse ways. In Petchesky's words:

> Like a cruel mockery of the sexual rights and freedom movements that had surfaced in country after country during the previous decade, this horror show of military sadism and sexual coercion stands at once as a sign of imperial impunity and the truth of sexuality as a punitive weapon in the hands of the Christian Army of God.
>
> (Petchesky 2005, p. 475)

16 For the most comprehensive and useful overview see D'Emilio and Freedman (1988).

17 The Reagan administration suspended funding to UNFPA immediately after the UN Conference on Population (Mexico City, 1984) and initiated the USAID programme to promote 'natural' methods of contraception worldwide.

18 Globalization, while fuelling and sustaining US domestic growth after 2002, has also increased internal inequality, unemployment, and greater uncertainty for a wide range of social sectors. It has also deepened US dependence on other economies, particularly in the financing of its growing fiscal deficit. More importantly, it has effectively expanded the possibilities for other countries or entire regions – such as China or the European Union – to threaten US economic hegemony. These threats to US hegemony are one main motif of neo-conservative analyses and projections.

19 In fact, the neo-conservative architects of the Bush administration's geopolitical policies, including those on Iraq, are secularists or Jews who have little interest in the Christian Right's stands on abortion, stem cell research, gay marriage, and sexual nonconformity (Vice-President Dick Cheney's daughter is openly a lesbian). We would argue, however, that neo-conservatives have exploited the alliance with right-wing evangelicals in order to secure an electoral base and to claim an ideological advantage.

20 See PEPFAR Watch at www.pepfarwatch.org.

21 As described in a HRW briefing:

> The lead defendant, Sherif Farhat, was a businessman related by blood and marriage to eminent Egyptians. State security officers arrested him weeks before the others. A few of his co-workers and acquaintances were also taken in; the rest of the men were strangers to him, trawled in and framed to create the illusion of a homosexual 'organization'. Many of Farhat's family believe he was the victim of a political vendetta aimed at his relatives. One defendant jailed with him says Farhat, in prison, called the trial 'a revenge match between two big families in the country'.
>
> (HRW 2004c, p. 22)

22 The most popular version of this encounter says that Castro took Museveni aside and said: 'Brother you have a problem!'

23 Jacobson also reminds us that President Museveni's wife is a born-again Christian and that the Catholic Church is very strong in the country.

24 Sarah Mukasa of Akina Mama reported the episode in March 2005 at a panel discussion to launch *Written Out* (IGLHRC and CWGL 2005) at the 59th session of the CSW commemorating and reviewing progress of the Beijing Fourth World Conference on Women.

25 One of the conclusions of the report is that:

> Same-sex practicing people in Uganda are also disproportionately affected by the abuse of police powers, extortion, and arbitrary arrests in violation of Article 6 of the African Charter. In the uneven application of the so-called sodomy laws, Ugandan police and government officials are denying Ugandans their right to liberty.
>
> (IHRC and SMU 2006, p. 1)

26 A third woman, Afsatu Abukabar, was also condemned and successfully appealed with the support of Nigerian feminists and lawyers. But her case never attracted global attention (Imam 2005).

27 Harsh controversies have been evolving in relation to the 2008 Lambeth Conference, the ten-yearly gathering of the Church's 850 bishops. In May 2007, the Archbishop of Canterbury, Dr Rowan Williams, announced that Gene Robinson, the gay Bishop of New Hampshire, USA, would not be invited. But even so the Southern conservative leaders have said they will boycott the conference and once again Dr Akinola has been active in the debate (*Daily Telegraph* 2007).

28 As the legislative process gained momentum, tensions developed, since some international groups had taken action without giving due recognition to the critical role played by local NGOs or respecting the rhythm of internal advocacy. Their actions have clearly contributed to flare-ups that accelerated the processing of the bill in early 2007.

29 Among the many sources documenting the increasing visibility of these groups in India, see Csete 2002, Fernandez 2002, John and Nair 1998, Menon 1999, Narrain 2001, People's Union of Civil Liberties-Karnataka 2003, Ramasubban 1995, 2007, Sangini 2005.

30 For an overview of this debate, see Ramasubban 2007; see also Aggarwal 2002, Gupta 2002, Lawyers Collective 2001, Voices Against 377 2004.

31 These initiatives include the Sonagachi cooperative created in 1992 by a public health scientist in one main red-light district of Kolkata (West Bengal), which is now run by sex workers themselves, and the Sangram programme that supports sex workers in Sangli (Maharashtra). But other less well-known sex worker-led organizations have been active for many years, such as Bharatiya Patita Udhar Sabha, founded in Delhi in 1984; the Pune Devadasi Sanghatana, founded in Pune, Maharashtra, in 1981; and the Asahaya Nari Tiruskrit Sangh, a women's organization of sex workers that was formed in the red-light area of Mumbai. In all three cases brothel keepers are directly involved.

32 The legal framework consists mainly of the Immoral Traffic in Persons Prevention Act, 1986 (ITPA) but other laws, including the penal code as well as ordinances covering state-level police, railways, beggary, and health, are more often used to tackle prostitution. The ITPA resulted from the 1986 reform of the Suppression of Immoral Traffic in Women and Girls Act of 1956 (SITA), which tolerates prostitution as a necessary social evil. Prostitution by a person on her/his own, within her/his own premises, is not considered a criminal act and clients are not subject to punishment. However, anyone maintaining a brothel,

living off the earnings of a prostitute, or procuring or detaining a woman for the sake of prostitution is subject to punishment, as is any person who solicits or seduces for the purpose of prostitution or carries sex work into the vicinity of public places. The conflation of trafficking and prostitution in the law allows police to raid brothels without a warrant on the grounds that an offence is being committed under the ITPA (Kotiswaran 2001).

33 The first position is one historically adopted by the Coalition Against Trafficking (CAT) and more recently by the Bush administration. The second is in line with the law adopted in Sweden in 1998, which gained visibility under the spell of new US HIV/AIDS and trafficking policies and is often quoted by CAT members and US officials as a 'promising model'. The third, known as 'emancipationist', is supported by a wide range of sex workers' organizations and networks in all regions (Kempadoo 2005).

34 *The Times of India* (1 October 2005) reported:

> The government is planning to revise anti-prostitution laws drastically to provide for the imprisonment and fine for anyone caught with prostitutes and to drop provisions, which make soliciting a crime. The existing law provides for action only against prostitutes. The amendment, proposed by the department of women and child and awaiting cabinet clearance, provides for three-month imprisonment and a fine of R20,000 for the patrons. The department has also proposed to do away with sections 8 and 20 of the Immoral Trafficking Prevention Act (ITPA), which makes soliciting a punishable offence. The proposed change is being justified on the grounds that most sex workers are victims of circumstances.

35 In late October, the two American male directors of Restore International entered the area to take photographs without police support and without permission. A conflict ensued in which a mob reacted and attacked the two men. The collective of sex workers convinced the mob to leave the men alone and neither pressed charges against the community or Sangram. However, there followed a public protest by sex workers demanding that action be taken against the men for harassing and terrorizing the community (Sangram 2005).

36 It may yet be revived since in India, as elsewhere, one key trait of sex politics battles is that they never entirely end. Quite frequently regressive policy proposals remain dormant before suddenly resurging when the adversaries of sexual plurality consider that circumstances are once again favourable to push for their cause.

37 On 13 February 2007 the Associated Press reported that the 80-year-old AIDS activist, Gao Yaojie, was blocked from leaving her home in Shangai by plain-clothes police to prevent her from applying for a US visa, which she needed to travel to New York to accept an award from the Vital Voices Global Partnership, a non-profit group supported by US Senator Hillary Clinton.

38 The well-known exception is Romania, where during the Ceausescu regime abortion was prohibited as part of a pro-natalist policy. As maternal mortality rates skyrocketed in the years that followed, Romania became a prime case, used extensively by international organizations and abortion activists, to argue for abortion to be addressed as a major public health problem (Kligman 1998).

39 In October 2007, as this book was being finalized, the conservative Law and Justice Party led by the Kaczynski brothers collapsed over a corruption probe. The ensuing election had the highest turnout since 1989 (55 per cent) and the Centre–Right Civic Platform defeated the Kaczynskis' coalition by 44 to 31 per cent.

40 For articles on these sequential episodes, visit the LGBTQ section at the Human Rights Watch website, available at www.hrw.org/doc/?t=lgbt (accessed 16 October 2007).

41 For instance, the AKP government based its arguments against the penal code reforms on 'national values' rather than on religious concerns. 'Indeed, renowned secular jurists and academics supported the religious conservatives in their opposition to amendments of articles concerning honour and virginity, agreeing that these articles were in line with Turkish customs and traditions' (Ilkkaracan 2007, p. 260).

42 It should also be noted that the reform proposed by the feminist campaign was successful in relation to practically all the main demands. The matter of same-sex relations was one exception, a sign that homophobic ideologies remain entrenched in Turkish culture and politics.

43 We include a brief review of conservative state politics on abortion here, not only because the criminalization of abortion must be interpreted as a punishment for women's 'bad sexual behaviour', but also because, in the current abortion wars, the actors, factors, and forces at play are, by and large, the same ones that constitute obstacles to sexual plurality.

44 Paragraph 107k of the Beijing Platform for Action reaffirms and expands paragraph 8.25 of the ICPD Programme of Action and reads as follows: (k) Para. 8.25 of the Programme of Action of the International Conference on Population and Development states:

> In no case should abortion be promoted as a method of family planning. All Governments and relevant intergovernmental and non-governmental organizations are urged to strengthen their commitment to women's health, to deal with the health impact of unsafe abortion as a major public health concern and to reduce the recourse to abortion through expanded and improved family-planning services. Prevention of unwanted pregnancies must always be given the highest priority and every attempt should be made to eliminate the need for abortion. Women who have unwanted pregnancies should have ready access to reliable information and compassionate counselling. Any measures or changes related to abortion within the health system can only be determined at the national or local level according to the national legislative process. In circumstances where abortion is not against the law, such abortion should be safe. In all cases, women should have access to quality services for the management of complications arising from abortion. Post-abortion counselling, education and family-planning services should be offered promptly, which will also help to avoid repeat abortions. Consider reviewing laws containing punitive measures against women who have undergone illegal abortions.

45 The first group of countries includes: Benin (2003), Bhutan (2003), Burkina Faso (2003), Chad (2002), Colombia (2006), Ethiopia (2004), Guinea (2000), Mali (2000), Saint Lucia (2004), Swaziland (2005), and Togo (2007). In the majority of cases, extremely restrictive legislation was changed to include new circumstances for abortion, such as rape, incest, or grave foetal abnormalities, but also, in many cases, to ensure the protection of women's physical and mental health.

46 Argentina, Bolivia, Brazil, Ghana, Mozambique, Nigeria, Peru, the Philippines, Trinidad and Tobago, Uruguay, among others.

47 Bernstein and Politi (1996) describe how William Casey, then director of the

CIA and a practising conservative Catholic, visited Rome several times for religious retreats in the Vatican, where he helped to craft these geopolitical strategies.

48 In the two conferences, as well in the five-year reviews, Nicaragua systematically aligned itself with the Vatican and other conservative forces. Feminist organizations were not invited to be part of the country delegations and were constantly attacked by the conservative media and government officials. See Girard 2007, Petchesky 2003, and Chapter 8.

49 In the late 1990s Ortega was accused of sexual abuse by his stepdaughter, Zoila America, an episode that would not, however, affect his political career. He went on to expand his alliances with conservative religious institutions and they backed him in the 2006 elections. In 2007, after being re-elected, Ortega announced that Cardinal Miguel Obando – who in the 1980s led the internal struggle against liberation theology – was to join his cabinet as coordinator of the new council of national reconciliation (*La Prensa*, 2 February 2007). Available online at www.laprensa.com.ni/archivo/2007/febrero/ 02/noticias/portada/ (accessed 20 March 2007).

50 In this extremely difficult political environment the Rosita case reared up again; the girl was once again found to be pregnant after allegedly being raped by her stepfather. In investigating the case the police and the minister of family affairs found out that in 2005 she had already had a baby. Feminists who were following the case told the press that they knew about the latest pregnancy and had been told by Rosita and her family that the father was a young boy who studied with her. The government and other conservative forces are using the episode to accuse reproductive rights advocates engaged in the 2003 campaign of manipulation and irresponsibility. Activists, for their part, have told the press they trust the family and the care they have provided to Rosita. They have also underlined the similarities between Rosita's case and the episode of Zoila America, the stepdaughter of Daniel Ortega, who in the 1990s accused him of sexual abuse.

51 According to Nicaraguan abortion rights activists, in personal exchanges, in 2006, when the therapeutic abortion clause was abolished, Ortega promised Sandinista women leaders and other progressive actors that the abolition would be temporary, as he would do his best to reinstate the clause when the full reform of the penal code was discussed. However, this has not happened.

52 The 'Act on Family Planning, Human Embryo Protection and Conditions of Permissibility of Abortion'.

53 In recent years, Poland has systematically played a conservative role in European Union debates on health, human rights, and other relevant matters. Poland did not ratify Protocol XIII to the European Convention on Human Rights and Biomedicine concerning biomedical research. In September 2007, it was the only state to present a veto against the European Commission's initiative to establish the European Day against the Death Penalty and to issue a joint resolution condemning capital punishment.

54 Gretkowska also stated:

> This poster is intended to shatter stereotypes in the anachronistic world of politics, which is more often dominated by uncommunicative men with their black tie outfits.... We are beautiful, nude, proud. We are true and sincere, body and soul. This is not pornography, there is nothing to see in terms of sex, our faces are intelligent, concerned, proud.
>
> (Available online at
> www.telegraph.co.uk/news/main.jhtml?xml=/news/2007/09/25/wpoland1
> 25.xml [accessed 10 October 2007])

3 The sad 'return of the religious'

1 This title is inspired by Derrida's (1998) elaboration on the 'sad return of the religious' to describe contemporary fundamentalism that implies, among other things, a deep interrogation on the inexorable secularization of societies projected by modern political thinkers.

2 Both secularity and *laïcité* denote the principle of separation between political and religious power. In the Western historical experience, secularity and *laïcité* have usually been combined with the correlate principle of freedom of religion. But in the course of the twentieth century, particularly in a socialist world, secularity was compulsory and freedom of religion was curtailed (these rules remain to a large extent in place in China, for instance). *Laïcité* rules of separation between politics and religion, however, are deeper and more strict than those observed in political systems guided by the principle of secularity. For instance, they explicitly prohibit religious teaching (as a matter of faith) in the public educational system, as well as the use of religious symbols in or by public institutions.

3 Their leaders included Alexander Campbell (1788–1866), an early leader of the Christian Restoration Movement, and Joseph Smith (1805–1844), the founder of the Mormon Church.

4 For example, the liberal Presbyterian Charles Briggs was charged with heresy and prosecuted in 1891, in New York. The case attracted front-page headlines and stimulated much public debate (Armstrong 2000).

5 The feminists Victoria Woodhull, Tennessee Claflin, Ida Craddock (who subsequently committed suicide), and Emma Goldman were also prosecuted under the Act, as were Reverend Henry Beecher (who was accused of adultery) and the writer D.M. Bennet (condemned for publishing a liberal piece titled 'Letter to Jesus'). The second case raised against Sanger led to the 1932 Supreme Court decision suspending the ban on contraception. However, the other portions of the law remained in place even when a series of judicial controversies occurred in respect of the interpretation of 'obscenity'. See Chesler (2007); see also 'Hearing on obscenity prosecution and the constitution held by a committee of the US Senate'. Available online at www.ksg.harvard.edu/presspol/news_events/news_archive/PDFs/Schauer_Testimony_031605.pdf (accessed 9 September 2007).

6 Between 1914 and 1918 three major conferences on The Bible and Prophecy were organized when the participants revised the Scofield Reference Bible, published in 1909, in search of the signs of the evil times approaching.

7 The newly created American Civil Liberties Union (ACLU) and the lawyer, Clarence Darrow, defended Scopes, and gained international visibility with the case.

8 The WLUML states:

> The use of the term 'fundamentalism' has been debated in WLUML over the years (some of us do not use it; others find it is widely understood and consider it the least shocking for describing the phenomenon). However we agree on the broad nature of the phenomenon as... 'the use of religion (and often ethnicity and culture) to gain and to mobilize power'.
>
> (WLUML 1997, p. 5)

9 Among this group of Republicans, Richard Vignerie, Howard Phillips, and Paul Weyrich were particularly disappointed when Ronald Reagan indicated he would choose Richard Schweiker, a moderate, as his running mate if nominated by the party to contest the presidential election. They thus decided to break

ranks with the Republican Party to mobilize against liberal hegemony in American society (Armstrong 2000).

10 This battle included the judgement and silencing of the theologians Hans Kung, Leonardo Boff, and Yvonne Gebara, among others, as well as the steady erosion of liberation theology in Latin America and the substitution of progressives in the hierarchy by conservative bishops and cardinals all over the world. The purge was personally conducted by Cardinal Ratzinger, the present Pope Benedict XVI, who for many years headed the Congregation for the Doctrine of Faith, described by many as a remnant of the Inquisition.

11 For instance, in Peru following the demise of Fujimori, a member of the controversial Catholic organization, Opus Dei, became minister of health and later prime minister (Cáceres *et al.* 2007). In Uruguay, in 2004, in the weeks preceding a Senate vote on a reproductive health law that included a provision to allow abortion on demand up to the twelfth week of pregnancy, senators were flooded with protest messages from Brazilian Catholic organizations. The law was defeated by a narrow margin of four votes. Later that year, the Left coalition, Frente Amplio, won the presidential election, but, even before his inauguration, Tabare Vasquez, the new president – a doctor whose son is a priest – announced he would veto the bill if it was retabled and approved. Even though Uruguay is known in Latin America as strongly attached to secular values, at the time of writing this deadlock had not yet been resolved (Corrêa 2006). In Brazil, in 2003, the supposedly left-wing Lula administration appointed a known conservative Catholic as federal attorney, and in 2007 pushed for the early retirement of a Supreme Court judge in order to nominate a member of the extremely conservative Catholic Association of Jurists.

12 One case in point is Afghanistan, where secular ideas gained acceptance among the elites in the late nineteenth century.

13 In the words of the then supreme leader of the RSS, M.S. Golwalkar,

> The foreign races in Hindusthan [India] must adopt the Hindu culture and language, must learn to respect and hold in reverence Hindu religion, must entertain no idea but those of the glorification of the Hindu race and culture, i.e., of the Hindu Nation and must loose [*sic*] their separate existence to merge in the Hindu race, or may stay in the country, wholly subordinated to the Hindu Nation, claiming nothing, deserving no privileges, far less any preferential treatment – not even citizen's rights. There is, at least, should be, no other course for them to adopt. We are an old nation; let us deal, as old nations ought to and do deal, with the foreign races who have chosen to live in our country.
> (Quoted in Sabrang and The South Asian Citizens Web 2003, pp. 25–26)

14 Chakravarti (2000) analyses how *Hindutva* ideologues reject rulers such as Ashoka, a pacifist influenced by Buddhism, or the Mughal sultans, who were acknowledged for their administrative abilities and tolerance. They glorify leaders like Chandragupta, a ruler of the Mauryia dynasty, who minimized alien cultures or religions and whose army defeated the Greek invaders led by Alexander. Significantly, *Chanakya*, a popular 1980s television series about Chandragupta, projected the Hindu male as a self-controlled ascetic hero who saves the nation from both external and internal enemies.

15 In 1988, the BJP leader, Advani, dressed as Rama, toured the country in a car altered to resemble an ancient chariot (Swamy 2003). Since the mosque was destroyed the site has remained controversial, and in 2005 was bombed by Islamic extremists.

16 In September 2007, the first hit in a web search using the word 'Ratzinger' (Cardinal Ratzinger, now Pope Benedict XVI) was the Ratzinger Fan Club.

17 Augustine dramatically portrayed desire of the flesh as the *libido* painfully trailing across the *cloaca mundi* (the dirtiness of the world). This conception would be repeatedly re-elaborated, as in the writings of Saint Hildegard about a man and a woman lying together, side by side, gently perspiring, and then

> the woman would become pregnant with the man's perspiration and, while they laid thus sweetly asleep, she would give birth painlessly from her side ... in the same way God brought Eve forth from Adam and that the Church was born from the side of Christ.
>
> (Quoted in Jantzen 2000, p. 229)

18 As Foucault (1985) points out, the rules adopted to guide self-examination and confession in the case of the 'sins of flesh' immediately preceded and connected with modern techniques of sex disciplining that have prevailed since the eighteenth century.

19 The following excerpt illustrates the tone and tropes utilized in this argument:

> The Greeks – not unlike other cultures – considered *Eros* principally as a kind of intoxication, the overpowering of reason by a 'divine madness' which tears man away from his finite existence and enables him, in the very process of being overwhelmed by divine power, to experience supreme happiness.... The Old Testament firmly opposed this form of religion, which represents a powerful temptation against monotheistic faith, combating it as a perversion of religiosity. But it in no way rejected *Eros* as such; rather, it declared war on a warped and destructive form of it, because this counterfeit divinization of *Eros* actually strips it of its dignity and dehumanizes it. Indeed, the prostitutes in the temple, who had to bestow this divine intoxication, were not treated as human beings and persons, but simply used as a means of arousing 'divine madness': far from being goddesses, they were human persons being exploited.
>
> (Vatican 2005b, p. 2)

20 The text distorts pre-Christian discourses on love to strengthen its heterosexual argument, affirming that the Greeks conceptualized *Eros* as the love between men and women, a clear attempt to obscure realities of Greek male homoeroticism. Later the text equates the extraction of Eve from Adam to the famous myth of divided beings debated in Plato's *Symposium*. Once again the objective is to deny and evict same-sex love, as Plato's divided beings were of three natures: the ones split into a male half and a female half, those divided between two male halves, and those divided into two female halves.

21 This is illustrated in the writings of the medieval philosopher Imam Ghazali (1050–1111), which provide a glaring contrast to Christian sexual doctrines of the same period. Mernissi notes that Ghazali's ideas are much closer to Freud than to the fathers of the Church, as in:

> God the almighty created the spouses; he created man with his penis, his testicles and his kidney (believed to be the semen producing gland). He gave woman a uterus, the receptacle and repository of the seed. He burdened men and women with the weight of sexual desire.
>
> (Mernissi 2000, p. 20)

22 The groups involved in the cases and related activities aimed at demystifying Sharia are Baobab for Women's Rights, Constitutional Rights Project, Women's

Action Collective, Women's Action Research and Documentation, and the Nigerian Office of the International Human Rights Law Group, and individuals included Snusi Lamiso Sanusi and Ayesha Imam.

23 Note that there have been many other cases of *Zina* involving men accused of homosexuality or cross-dressing (see Chapter 2).

24 This assertion is not only substantive in conceptual and political terms. It is also directed at international actors involved in the *Zina* cases, who did not acknowledge local groups or engage with them on which global strategies to adopt.

25 Sabrang and the South Asia Citizen Web (2003) provide detailed information on these US-based organizations, including: The Hindu Swayamsevak Sangh (HSS), which, according to one of its flyers, '[Was] started in the USA and other parts of the world to continue what RSS is doing in India'; Overseas Friends of BJP, the BJP support group in the USA; VHP-America, the US counterpart of Vishwa Hindu Parishad, which was the main force behind the violent takeover and destruction of a sixteenth-century Babri mosque in Ayodhya; HinduUnity.org, a website run from the USA that claims to be the official website of the Bajrang Dal (the paramilitary wing of the VHP); India Development and Relief Fund (IDRF), which primarily funds the Sangh through its Sewa Vibhag operations (Sewa Vibhag being the service branch of the RSS). Given the connections between these groups and the timing, the Gujarat episode must also be examined in light of the escalation of anti-Islamic discourses in the USA during the period, even though the *Hindutva* ideology of Islamophobia long preceded the 11 September 2001 attacks on the USA. If nothing else, the US climate in early 2002 may have led the leaders of the riots to imagine that the incident would not attract much international attention. They were not entirely wrong, as the mainstream media did not report fully on what happened in Gujarat.

26 The images and temples of Ardhanarishvara are clear remnants of early Hinduism, as in the case of the beautiful sculpture preserved in the Elephant Island temple. But the Hindu–Right discourses often conflate *hijras* with 'emasculated Hindu men', and some of its more radical versions go so far as to say that the *hijra* tradition is a 'corruption' of Hindu tradition brought about by the Mughal invasion.

27 The emphasis on ecumenism necessarily implied the dissolution of boundaries between religions and the priority of social justice among progressive Catholic sectors and political groups – such as the socialists and communists – who had historically promoted the tenets of secularization.

28 Gadamer (1998) recalls the debates following the Second World War on the tragic effects of dogmatic atheism adopted by fascist regimes, but that it was only after 1989 that this critique extended to the anti-democratic, or even coercive, nature of compulsory secularization implemented under communism (and still in place in China, Vietnam, and North Korea).

29 The Religious Consultation on Population, Reproductive Health, and Ethics is led by the progressive Catholic theologian, Daniel McGuire. See the materials it produces online. Available at www.religiousconsultation.org/. See also ICPC 2004.

30 Information about these various initiatives may be found at:
www.rimaweb.com.ar/aborto/28_septiembre/campana2001.html
www.mujeresdelsur.org.uy/
www.convencion.org.uy/
www.libertadeslaicas.org.mx/paginas/Enciclopedia/EncicloLegisla.htm.

31 In critiquing Kant's Christian-European chauvinism, Derrida makes more or less the same point when he suggests that 'tolerance' was a concept adopted by Europeans to signify their own moral superiority: 'The lesson of tolerance was first of all an exemplary lesson that the Christian deemed himself alone capable of giving to the world.... In this respect, the French Enlightenment ... was ... essentially Christian' (1998, p. 11).

32 These linguistic roots are the Latin *relegere*, 'bringing together in order to return and begin again; whence *religio*, scrupulous attention, respect, patience, even modesty, shame or piety – and, on the other hand ... *religare* ... obligation, ligament ... debt, etc., between men or between man and God' (Derrida 1998, pp. 36–37).

33 Slavoj Žižek makes a similar argument when he says that 'the fundamental divide' in today's world is not that between Islamic fundamentalism and secular rationalism but rather 'the one between those included into the sphere of (relative) economic prosperity and those excluded from it' (Kordela 2005, p. 124; Žižek 2002).

34 Kordela (2005) concludes that insofar as both the Left and the Right see no alternative to hegemonic global capitalism, secular (liberal) rationalism has completely exhausted itself; the only remaining site of oppositional movement is faith (p. 225).

35 Tully and Masani (1988) argue that Nehru's approach to democracy, drawing a sharp division between public and private, saw religious ritual of any sort as out of place in public life, but that this distinction may have little meaning in 'the popular mind' in modern India (pp. 22–23).

36 The fact that prominent Islamic feminists, including the Egyptian Nawal Al-Saadawi and leading members of Women Living Under Muslim Laws, have spoken in full support of the French government's position does not lessen the paternalistic, protectionist aspect of the French state's ban on veiling and headscarves in public schools.

37 Their focus is primarily on right-wing evangelical Protestantism, but this focus ignores the extent to which a conservative evangelical movement has progressed within the Catholic Church and a strong and historically unprecedented alliance between right-wing Catholics and Protestants in the USA formed around anti-abortion politics in the 1980s and further developed in the movement against gay and lesbian rights, including marriage. See www.theocracywatch.org and Petchesky 1990, ch. 7.

38 Jakobsen and Pellegrini (2003, p. 36) make exactly this criticism of Kennedy's 1996 decision in *Romer* v. *Evans*, where, again in a 6–3 decision, the court denied the constitutionality of a Colorado statute intended to repeal state ordinances prohibiting discrimination on the basis of sexual orientation.

4 The modernization of 'sex' and the birth of sexual science

1 The Freudian notion of pre-Oedipal bisexuality is attached to the evolutionary frame analysed above. As Gayle Rubin pointed out, it conceives of sexual development as though the child would travel through a series of organic stages until reaching a kind of anatomic destiny that is necessarily heterosexual – unless development has been arrested at some preliminary point along the way (Rubin 1975). But Rubin also recognized that Freud's insights on pre-Oedipal bisexuality potentially offered a critical conceptual tool for understanding how gender systems are constituted, and for destabilizing the rigid binary logic that they imply. In her view the revolutionary potentiality of the notion of bisexual-

ity was never fully explored by psychoanalysis itself due to the conservatism prevailing in the field at large. For further discussion of these issues see Chapter 5.

2 Bullough (1985) reports that during this period the Council made 470 grants to more than 100 investigators, supporting the work of as many as 585 scientists. Much of this support went to biologists and physicians working on biomedical aspects of sexuality, but some also went to a wide range of social science research, like the cross-cultural comparisons of anthropologists such as Ford and Beach, described above, and, in particular, after 1941, to the work of the Kinsey group.

3 Kinsey rejected this criticism throughout his career, arguing that in a random sample not all those included would answer the questions that were put to them and that the sample would therefore be biased (Bullough 1998, p. 130).

4 One of the most striking things about the negative reactions to Kinsey's work, beyond the heated nature of the criticisms, is the ongoing attention it has received over time, even decades after the research was carried out. High-profile critiques include books published by Judith Reisman, which charge Kinsey with fraud and criminal behaviour, including child sexual abuse, albeit without providing any convincing evidence (see, e.g., Reisman 1998). The conservative Family Research Council made similar claims of sexual interaction with children in its video, *The Children of Table 34*, but has focused even more strongly on Kinsey's work on homosexuality and sexual orientation. Similarly charged interpretations have been made by a number of Kinsey's biographers, in particular by James H. Jones in his book, *Alfred C. Kinsey: A Public/Private Life* (Jones 1997), which describes Kinsey as bisexual and suggests that he also practised masochism. Leading progressive thinkers such as Martin Duberman (1997) have refuted such charges. What is remarkable is the extent to which Kinsey, long after his death in 1956, continues to serve as a polarizing figure in the battles over sexuality that have been such a major part of the so-called 'culture wars' in the USA (see Radosh (2004) on the 'culture wars' and sexuality more broadly; see also Chapter 5).

5 Rusk announced the end of funding for the Kinsey Institute at the same time that he announced funding for a major project by the Union Theological Seminary, whose president had publicly criticized Kinsey's finding on the frequency of homosexual behaviours. In announcing the grant, Rusk is quoted as stating that 'some of the projects formerly supported [by the Foundation], including that of Dr. Kinsey, are now in a position to obtain support from other sources' (Pomeroy 1972, p. 285). In fact, Kinsey received no other foundation support up until his death a few years later and much of the data he collected have never been written up or published.

6 See, for example, the Institute of Medicine/National Academy of Sciences (1986) report, *Confronting AIDS: Directions for Public Health, Health Care, and Research*, and the National Research Council's influential volume, *AIDS: Sexual Behavior and Intravenous Drug Use* (Turner et al. 1989, pp. 73–185).

7 The funders of the NHSLS included, in addition to the Robert Wood Johnson Foundation, the Henry J. Kaiser Family Foundation, Rockefeller Foundation, Andrew Mellon Foundation, The John D. and Catherine T. MacArthur Foundation, New York Community Trust, and American Foundation for AIDS Research. Later, the Ford Foundation provided additional support for data analysis.

8 For an overview of this field and the principal donors involved in it, see Hartmann 1995, chs 6 and 7; see also Corrêa 1994 and Petchesky 1990, ch. 2.

9 For a more detailed and compelling history of Galton's contributions to scientific racism and the origins and rise of the eugenics movement in Europe and the USA, see Ewen and Ewen 2006, chs 17–20.

10 For overviews of the role of eugenics in relation to the birth control/contraceptive movement, see Ellen Chesler (2007) on Sanger's life and work. See also Gordon 1976, chs 6 and 7, and Petchesky 1990, ch. 2. Chesler makes clear that, although Sanger tried to distance herself from some of the worst racist excesses of the eugenicists, she none the less sought the backing of eugenic-minded professionals and scientists and supported compulsory sterilization laws (especially for the 'feebleminded' and 'handicapped'). Ironically, however, the eugenicists mostly denounced birth control and kept their distance from Sanger, whom they regarded as a sex radical.

11 For a detailed discussion of the relationship between eugenics and social demography in the interwar period, see, in particular, Ramsden 2003. More broadly, see also Gordon 1976, Petchesky 1990, Ross 1998, Weeks 1981.

12 For early overviews of survey findings, see, e.g., Cleland and Hobcraft 1985, Cleland et al. 1987.

13 For more on the debates around fertility decline see, e.g., UNFPA 2006.

5 The social construction of sexual life

1 On interactionist theory, in addition to Gagnon and Simon 1973, see Brake 1982, Plummer 1975, 1982. On psychoanalysis and its appropriation in post-structuralist and feminist analysis, in addition to Lacan 1968, 1977, see Benjamin 1988, Chodorow 1978, 1991, Deleuze and Guatarri 1977, Hocquenghem 1978, Mitchell 1974. On Foucault and early work on the history of sexuality, in addition to Foucault 1978, see D'Emilio and Freedman 1988, Padgug 1979, Trumbach 1977, Weeks 1979, 1981, 1985. On key anthropological work during this period, see Blackwood 1986, Fry 1982, Herdt 1981, Newton 1972, Ortner and Whitehead 1981, Rubin 1975, 1984, Vance 1984.

2 While many of their key ideas were already laid out in their first major book, Sexual Conduct, published in 1973, both Gagnon and Simon continued to pursue active research careers over the next three decades, exerting significant influence on the field of sexuality research, particularly after the increase in research activity that followed the emergence of the AIDS epidemic (see below). Although Simon died in 2000, readers interested in his later work should see his book, Postmodern Sexualities (Simon 1996). For a collection of Gagnon's essays that provides a useful overview of the development of his thinking, see his collection, An Interpretation of Desire (Gagnon 2004). As important as their long-term contributions have been, however, it is worth emphasizing how groundbreaking their early work was, in many ways pre-dating and anticipating the slightly later notion of the 'productive discourses' of sexuality that would come to be most closely associated with Foucault, as well as the later notions of the 'performative' nature of gender and sexuality that have come to be associated with writers such as Judith Butler (see the discussion below).

3 While Mitchell was among the first wave of feminist thinkers to engage with psychoanalysis, primarily through the opening created by Lacan's work, many others have explored a similar set of issues (see, e.g., Gallop 1982, 1987, Grosz 1990).

4 The work carried out by Deleuze and Guattari has had widespread impact, particularly in literary studies and the humanities. For detailed introductions to

their work, see Goodchild 1996, Holland 1999. For an important extension of their critique focusing specifically on homosexual desire, see Hocquenghem 1978. For an extremely helpful reading of their work and its impact on the analysis of sexuality, see Weeks 1985, 1986, 2000; see also Chapter 4.

5 For a sense of their influence on Foucault's work, see Foucault's Preface to *Anti-Oedipus: Capitalism and Schizophrenia* (Foucault 1977b), originally published in French in 1972, just four years before the publication of *The History of Sexuality* (Foucault 1978).

6 While the first volume of Foucault's *The History of Sexuality* (1978) has been by far the single most influential text, a range of other studies have followed similar lines of analysis (see, e.g., Halperin 1990, Katz 1995, Padgug 1979, Weeks 1981, 1985.

7 Foucault's work, as well as the secondary literature on Foucault's thinking and its impact, is extensive. The first volume of *The History of Sexuality*, originally positioned as the introduction to a multi-volume project, was originally published in French in 1976 and then in English in 1978. While the nature of this project would change quite dramatically after the publication of the first volume, it is still worth consulting the second and third volumes of this project, published shortly before Foucault's death in 1984 and later translated into English as *The Uses of Pleasure* (Foucault 1985) and *Care of the Self* (Foucault 1988). In addition to these main works, many of Foucault's ideas on sexuality and the politics of sexuality may be accessed in his published Collège de France lectures – see, in particular, *Society Must Be Defended* (Foucault 2003) – and in his interviews and miscellaneous political writings – see, for example, *Power/Knowledge: Selected Interviews and Other Writings, 1972–1977* (Foucault 1980) and *Foucault Live: Interviews, 1961–1984* (Lotringer 1996). The secondary literature on Foucault is massive, and not always interesting. Particularly worthwhile is the biography of Foucault by Didier Eribon (1991). For recent analysis of Foucault's continued importance in shaping our thinking about sexuality, as well as the need to remember his transgressive qualities rather than sanctifying him, as some streams of cultural studies seem to do, see Halperin 2002b, Weeks 2005.

8 For a discussion of the rise of demography, the study of population, and their relationship to biopower as well as to racism, see lecture 11, 17 March 1976, in Foucault 2003, pp. 239–264.

9 For key references on ancient Greece or Rome, see, for example, Boswell 1980, Halperin 1990, Padgug 1979. For pre-industrial societies, see Brown 1986, Ng 1990, Trumbach 1977. For the nineteenth and early twentieth centuries, see Chauncey 1994, Smith-Rosenberg 1985, Vicinus 1985, Weeks 1981. For the post-Second World War era, see Berube 1990, D'Emilio 1983, D'Emilio and Freedman 1988, Kennedy and Davis 1993, Weeks 1977.

10 For pioneering and contemporary work on sub-Saharan Africa, see Baylies and Bujra 2000, Heald 1995, Moodie *et al.* 1988, Preston-Whyte 1995, Preston-Whyte *et al.* 2000, Shepherd 1987. On Asia, see Boellstorf 2005, Jackson 1989, Manderson 1992, Najmabadi 2005, Stoler 1997, Tan 1996. On Latin America, see Cáceres 1996, Carrier 1976, 1995, Carrillo 2002, Fry 1982, Kulick 1998, Lancaster 1992, Parker 1987, 1991, 1999, Taylor 1985.

11 For pioneering early work carried out in the 1970s and particularly in the 1980s, see, for example, Blackwood 1986, Brandes 1980, Carrier 1976, Fry 1982, Gregor 1985, Lancaster 1992, Nanda 1990, Parker 1987, 1991, Strathern 1972, Vance 1984, Williams 1986.

12 Rubin's theoretical and empirical work has also been linked to her own

activism not only as a key combatant in the lesbian and feminist 'sex wars' during the 1980s (see Duggan and Hunter 2006), but also as a founding member of SAMOIS, a lesbian S/M organization which flourished in San Francisco in the late 1970s and early 1980s (see Califia 1981, Rubin 2003), followed by The Outcasts, which was founded in 1984 and active into the 1990s (see Rubin 1996). Rubin's ethnographic research on the gay male leather subculture in San Francisco has provided important empirical documentation of sexual resistance and dissidence in the USA during the 1970s and 1980s (see Rubin 1982, 1991, 1997, 2000, 2002).

13 The term 'queer theory' was originally coined at an academic conference in the USA by the feminist film and cultural studies scholar, Teresa de Lauretis (1991). It was quickly appropriated by a wide range of voices, including the mainstream media, in ways that led de Lauretis herself to question and even reject the term not long after she had introduced it (see de Lauretis 1994a, 1994b).

14 The literature that is typically labelled queer theory is now immense, and far too extensive to summarize here. For readers who wish to explore this work further, in addition to the work of Sedgwick (1990, 1993) and Warner (1991, 1993, 2000), see also Abelove et al. 1993, Edelman 1994, 1995, Fuss 1991, Halperin 1996, 2002. For an overview of this emerging body of work in the mid-1990s, see Jagose 1996. For a discussion of the impact of queer theory in the social sciences (as opposed to literary criticism and the humanities), see Seidman 1996, Stein and Plummer 1994.

15 The term 'heteronormativity' is closely associated with queer theory and has come to be widely used in much academic writing. Michael Warner initiated the use of the term in his introduction to a special issue of Social Text published in 1991 (Warner 1991).

16 It is important to also note that even if queer theory originated and flourished most extensively in Western academic settings, in the age of the Internet and global information flows these ideas have circulated widely in the South as well as the North, and have helped to shape the analysis of gender and sexuality across a wide range of diverse societies outside the Anglo-European world.

6 After AIDS

1 It is worth remembering in this regard that public health emerged over the course of the twentieth century mainly from medicine and social medicine and that most schools of public health were originally departments in schools of medicine (see Fee 1997). Public health has come, over time, to provide an important emphasis on the broader population base of health and illness – and through this emphasis, at times, an important critique of much biomedical thinking – despite its traditionally dependent status within the social organization of biomedical knowledge and research.

2 A similar interaction between political climate, or context, and the conduct of research may be seen in relation to biomedical investigation. For a detailed and nuanced account of the relations between social and political context and biomedical AIDS research, see, in particular, Epstein 1996.

3 For further discussion of this approach, and its roots in what has been described as 'interpretive anthropology', see Parker 1991; also Geertz 1973, 1983.

4 The literature that could be cited here is now extensive. See, for example, Aggleton 1996a, Carrier 1995, Carrillo 2002, González Block and Liguori

1992, Jackson 1997, 2007, Kahn 1996, Kulick 1998, Lancaster 1992, Padilla 2007, Parker 1991, 1999, Prieur 1998, Tan 1999, Terto Jr. 2000. One of the key outcomes of this research was to problematize the uncritical use of biomedical categories such as 'homosexuality' and 'heterosexuality' cross-culturally, as well as to classify those who may not self-identify using such terms. Yet even this critique would create its own problems, as the use of the term 'MSM' (men who have sex with men) makes clear. While originally developed by community-based organizations as part of a critique of biomedical categories (see Deverell and Prout 1999), the term 'MSM' was quickly adopted by biomedical and epidemiological researchers and public health officials as a way of describing populations with no reference to self-identity or reflexivity. This practice, in turn, would quickly erase meaningful social and cultural differences (see Muñoz-Laboy 2004).

5 Perhaps not surprisingly, since sexual interactions between women have been thought to be relatively unproblematic in terms of HIV transmission, work focusing on same-sex relations between men has received far more attention than work focusing on lesbians. This situation began to change in the past decade, stimulated less by HIV and AIDS than by developments in queer theory and lesbian and gay studies (see, e.g., Blackwood and Wieringa 1999; also Kennedy and Davis 1993, Morgan and Wieringa 2005, Wieringa et al. 2007).

6 See, for example, Aggleton 1999, Brennan 2004, Hunter 2002, Kempadoo 1999, Kempadoo and Doezema 1998, Meekers and Calves 1997, Padilla 2007, Truong 1990, Preston-Whyte et al. 2000, Wojcicki 2002.

7 See, for example, Currah et al. 2006, Halberstam 1998, Narrain 2004, Reddy 2005.

8 Again, the literature here is extensive. For an overview of such arguments, see, for example, Farmer 1999, Farmer et al. 1996, Parker et al. 2000b.

9 In many of the inner cities in the USA, for example, processes of social disintegration and environmental devastation similar to those found in poorer countries have been identified as playing a key role in the spread and impact of the epidemic (see, e.g., Fullilove 2005, Wallace et al., 1994). Recent analyses of social and economic change during the 1980s and 1990s have also emphasized how growing disparities between rich and poor in virtually all countries of the world – what Manuel Castells has described as 'the rise of the Fourth World', as much in the fully industrialized or post-industrial West as in the industrializing countries – have been associated with a range of social and environmental ills, including HIV and AIDS (see Castells 1998).

10 On migration and HIV, see, for example, Decosas et al. 1995, Farmer 1992, 1995, Herdt 1997, Webb 1997.

11 For a critical overview of the ways in which World Bank policies have impacted upon the HIV epidemic, see Simms 2004.

12 However, more recent studies show a more mixed pattern regarding the relation between armed conflict, displacement, and HIV risk. A major difference seems to be between protracted conflict zones where populations are relatively isolated, as in Sierra Leone and Sudan, and those (especially post-conflict) where there is more mobility in and out of the affected zone, as in Uganda and the Democratic Republic of the Congo. See Part III, as well as Bartlett et al. 2004, Petchesky and Laurie 2007, Spiegel 2004, UNFPA 2006.

13 The literature on women's vulnerability to HIV infection is now extensive. In addition to the examples cited here, see also Gupta and Weiss 1993, Parker et al. 2000a, Sobo 1995.

7 On the indispensability and insufficiency of human rights

1 On the 'capabilities' approach to social justice, see Nussbaum 1999, 2006, Nussbaum and Glover 1995, Sen 1999. For cogent critiques of this approach, see Asad 2003, Benhabib 1995, Phillips 2002. On global public goods, see Kaul *et al.* 1999, the critique in Petchesky 2003, and the discussion in Chapter 9.

2 The following discussion was adapted in part from Petchesky 2003, ch. 1.

3 See statement, 'International Civil Society Denounce UN Meeting on AIDS as a Failure'. Available online at www.pepfarwatch.org/pubs/release_june%202_UNGASS_AIDS.doc (accessed 7 October 2007).

4 Contrary to some interpretations, we do not read Foucault's analysis as rejecting rights of the body or human rights but rather as situating those ideas within historically particular contexts and political constraints.

5 For a sample of these frequent critiques, see Grewal 1998, Kapur 2005, Kothari and Sethi 1991, Tushnet 1984.

8 Inventing and contesting sexual rights within the UN

1 Some of these principles are contained in legally binding multilateral instruments: the International Covenant on Economic, Social, and Cultural Rights (1976); the Convention on the Elimination of All Forms of Discrimination against Women (1981); and the Rome Statute of the International Criminal Court (1998). Others are in documents with mainly moral and political authority; for example, the Programme of Action of the International Conference on Population and Development (Cairo, 1994); the Platform for Action of the Fourth World Conference on Women (Beijing, 1995); the Commission on Human Rights Resolution 33, 'Access to Medication in the Context of Pandemics such as HIV/AIDS' (2001); and the UN General Assembly Special Session on HIV/AIDS Final Declaration (2001).

2 See Amartya Sen 1999, pp. 227–231 for an example of this critique.

3 For earlier accounts of feminist campaigns and strategies to secure recognition of reproductive and sexual rights as human rights, especially for women and girls, see Petchesky 2000, 2003.

4 On the naivety of women's groups at the UN about the Vatican's attack on 'gender' discourse, see Girard 2007, pp. 334–336, and Chapter 9. Girard gives a striking quote from her interview with a member of the Swedish delegation to the Beijing Women's Conference: 'I regret that we did not photograph the mullahs and the Vatican priests in the UN corridors and the hotels, sitting and preparing their joint texts together' (2007, p. 337).

5 See Bunch and Reilly 1994, Copelon 1994, 2000, Fried and Landsberg-Lewis 2000, Miller 2004, Spees 2003 for illuminating documentation of these feminist global campaigns.

6 Girard notes that 'several Islamic and African countries could not follow the Holy See all the way on "various forms" because of their support for polygamous families' (2007, p. 326). However, the prevalence of female-headed households in the Americas and especially the Caribbean also played a crucial role in opening up governments' receptivity to seeing families as multiple.

7 It is noteworthy that the US delegation, comprised mainly of women from the Democratic Party allied with the Clinton administration, not only backed off from this effort but played a significant role in crafting the strongly heterosexist compromise text. Nervous about the power of right-wing conservatives at home, the US delegates submitted an interpretive statement during the delibera-

tions on paragraph 96 that emphasized, at three different times, the phrases 'relationships *between women and men*' and 'freedom from coercion, discrimination and violence', thus deflecting any possible interpretation that would highlight lesbian identity or women's right to sexual pleasure (US Government Delegation, Statement to the Main Committee of the Fourth World Women's Conference [*sic*], 14 September 1995). This kind of equivocation – too often accommodating rather than challenging right-wing politics – is what we have come to expect of Bill and Hillary Clinton and the mainstream of the Democratic Party in the USA.

8   See especially quotes from Barbara Klugman in Girard 2007, pp. 338, 340.

9   The first and one of the most important of these opinions was that rendered by the UN's Human Rights Committee (different from the Commission) in *Toonen* v. *Australia* in March 1994 (see Saiz 2004, p. 49; see also Chapter 2).

10 Since such affirmation directly contradicts current US government policy (under the Bush administration and PEPFAR), it is noteworthy that the USA was not a member of the CRC at the time this progressive language was adopted.

11 Girard's account of the ill-fated 'Brazil resolution' is, again, the most thorough documentation of this episode currently available (see Girard 2007, pp. 341–353). The text of the resolution expressed 'deep concern at the occurrence of violations of human rights in the world against persons on the grounds of their sexual orientation' and stressed 'that human rights and fundamental freedoms are the birthright of all human beings, that the universal nature of these rights and freedoms is beyond question, and that the enjoyment of such rights and freedoms should not be hindered in any way on the grounds of sexual orientation'. It called 'upon all States to promote and protect the human rights of all persons regardless of their sexual orientation' and requested 'the UN High Commissioner for Human Rights to pay due attention to the violation of human rights on the grounds of sexual orientation' (Girard 2007, p. 343).

12 Quotes from Girard (2007, pp. 342, 353) are from her oral interviews with Brigid Inder, Susanna Fried, John Fisher, and Frederico Meyer. See also ARC 2006.

13 The ARC document contains detailed statements relating to specific country violators by the UN High Commissioner for Human Rights, Louise Arbour; the Special Representative of the Secretary General on Human Rights Defenders, Hina Jilani; the Working Group on Arbitrary Detention; the Special Rapporteur on extra-judicial, summary or arbitrary executions, Philip Alston; the Special Rapporteur on contemporary forms of racism, racial discrimination, xenophobia, and related intolerance, Doudou Diène; the Independent Expert on Minority Issues, Gay McDougall; the Special Rapporteur on violence against women, Yakin Ertürk; the Special Rapporteur on the promotion and protection of the right to freedom of opinion and expression, Ambeyi Ligabo; the Special Rapporteur on torture and other cruel, inhuman, or degrading treatment or punishment, Manfred Nowak; and the Special Rapporteur on freedom of religion, Asma Jahangir.

14 The Yogyakarta Principles (2007) comprise a comprehensive document analysing the specific ways in which every major international human rights principle embodied in the UDHR, the covenants, and the conventions applies to 'persons of diverse sexual orientations and gender identities'. See also ARC 2007b, and Chapter 1.

9 Transnational debates: sexuality, power, and new subjectivities

1 The folding of sexual rights into reproductive rights in the context of the ICPD had political and pragmatic as well as problematic conceptual roots; see the discussion in Chapter 8.

2 Sexual and reproductive health and rights were originally defined in the 1994 ICPD Programme of Action, paras 7.2 and 7.3, and again in the 1995 Fourth World Conference on Women Platform for Action, paras 94–96. According to these documents, signed by most countries in the world, reproductive health means 'a state of complete physical, mental and social well-being, and not merely the absence of disease or infirmity, in all matters relating to the reproductive system and to its functions and processes'. It 'implies that people are able to have a satisfying and safe sex life and that they have the capability to reproduce and the freedom to decide if, when and how often to do so'. Reproductive rights include 'the basic right of all couples and individuals to decide freely and responsibly the number, spacing and timing of their children and to have the information and means to do so' as well as 'the right to make decisions concerning reproduction free of discrimination, coercion and violence'. For full discussion of the definitions and debates surrounding 'sexual rights' in the UN, see Chapter 8.

3 We feel obliged to note that Corrêa and Petchesky used this simplified linking of reproductive and sexual in relation to rights in the 1994 article 'Reproductive and sexual rights: A feminist perspective' (republished in Parker and Aggleton 2007), but just a few years later both authors substantially revised this too easy conceptual solution (see Corrêa 1997, Petchesky 2000), which, we also note, still requires further examination and reframing.

4 On these complexities, see, among others, Butler 2005, Cabral and Viturro 2006, Currah 2003, Fausto-Sterling 2000, Feinberg 1996, Halberstam 1998, Halperin 2002a; see also Chapter 10.

5 It is important to note that interestingly, at least in Latin America, developments have been registered in regard to this critical intersection. Vianna and Carrara (2007) analyse how, in Brazil, productive dialogues around abortion have been evolving between feminists and LGBTQ activists. In 2007, in Uruguay, the demonstration organized on 28 September, the Latin American Day for the Decriminalization of Abortion, coincided with the Montevideo Gay Pride Parade.

6 Thanks to Róisín Ryan-Flood and Dean Spade (in presentations at the workshop on Sexing Reproductive Regulation: Gendering Health and Human Rights, Keele University, UK, June 2007) for making us aware of the struggle of some transpeople (who may be masculine in appearance and self-presentation but have female reproductive systems) and lesbians in same-sex couples to be treated respectfully and gain access to services in obstetric settings.

7 International law differs from this approach. The Protocol to Prevent, Suppress and Punish Trafficking in Persons, Especially Women and Children – informally known as the Palermo Protocol – which supplements the United Nations Convention against Transnational Organized Crime (G.A. Res. 55/25, UN GAOR, 55th Sess., Supp. No. 49 (2000)), does not require that prostitution be criminalized but rather leaves it to ratifying states to determine how to respond. Moreover, the Protocol requires proof of coercion or abuse in determining the matter of consent (thanks to Alice Miller for this clarification).

8 For a compilation of responses to, and materials on, PEPFAR and the 'prostitution pledge', see OSI 2007 and CHANGE 2005b.

9 These USAID funds were not applied in the national HIV programme, but transferred through the government to NGOs doing HIV/AIDS prevention work in keeping with Brazil's strict regulations about bilateral and multilateral funds. The amount lost with the suspension of the USAID–Brazil agreement in relation to HIV is not substantial when compared with the total Brazilian public health budget (approximately US$20 billion annually). However, it was quite significant for NGO work because the suspension coincided with the end of the third World Bank loan to the Brazilian National AIDS Programme, which, since 1993, has included an important component for prevention work by NGOs. Although not yet fully evaluated, the end of USAID funding for Brazilian HIV/AIDS NGOs can certainly be counted as one example of the long-term detrimental effects of US government policies on sexuality.

10 In Zambia, young women have rates of infection three times higher than those of young men, while in Kenya – where the epidemic is actually declining – the rates are seven times higher (UNAIDS 2006).

11 Zuma had been head of the South Africa National AIDS Council and has often been portrayed as the potential next president of the country. During his trial, Zuma stated that it was his duty as a Zulu man to have sex with the young woman because of the way she sat and dressed, and that he didn't bother to use a condom, thinking there wasn't much risk because he took a shower after having sex.

12 See Petchesky (2003) for a more detailed account.

13 TRIPS (Trade-Related Intellectual Property Rights) is the multilateral system set up in the 1990s under the WTO to balance trade interests, particularly patent rights, and public interests such as health.

14 This reprieve may be temporary, depending on the outcome of the ongoing political struggle in Thailand. In September 2006, a military coup deposed the increasingly troubled but democratically elected government of Prime Minister Thaksin Shinawatra. This crisis was met with considerable alarm in the Western press, yet it is interesting that, in the midst of a major constitutional struggle and 'period of turmoil' (in the words of the *New York Times*), the military rulers chose to move forward with the compulsory licence against Merck and to defy the US trade regime. As of this writing, the USA had suspended negotiations on the FTA with Thailand pending the restoration of 'democracy' (Gerhardsen 2007, Mydans 2007). Situations such as this raise serious questions once again about the contradictions of 'democracy' and its meanings in the era of globalization.

15 Developing countries comprise 72 per cent of the world's population but only 13 per cent of the world's drug market; all of Africa accounts for only 1 per cent of world drug sales. See MSF/DND 2002, Petchesky 2003, Rosenberg 2001.

16 See Camargo and Mattos (2007) for a critique of this tendency within the World Bank.

17 On the debates concerning circumcision, see, for example, Cohen 2005, USAID 2003, World Bank 2006, WCC 2006, as well as the more cautious analyses of social researchers such as Aggleton (2007) and Dowsett and Couch (2007).

18 The concept of 'global public goods' originated in the late 1990s, coinciding with the anti-globalization movement and appealing to the pragmatists in the treatment access movement. It seeks to create a macroeconomic framework for valuing and financing 'goods whose benefits reach across borders, generations and population groups' and are thus 'under-provided by local and national governments'. Unlike ordinary commodities, the market handles such goods

poorly or has no interest in them because they are, in economists' terms, 'non-excludable' and 'non-rivalrous in consumption', meaning their ownership and use cannot be packaged, transferred, and privately appropriated (Kaul *et al.* 1999, pp. ix–xxi). Not only are there few market incentives to provide them, but the mechanisms of international cooperation to make sure they are provided are weak. Universal access to essential medicines and supplies (e.g., condoms) and vaccines to free the world of infectious diseases are perfect examples. See Kaul *et al.* (1999) and Stiglitz (2002) for other examples.

19 See Petchesky (2003) and Standing (1999) for further critiques of this model.

20 A jarring example was the refusal of the committee to allow the display of a powerful series of posters, sponsored by Catholics for a Free Choice, showing couples of various races, ethnicities, and genders using condoms. This was in contrast to the ubiquitous display of commercial ads of drug companies and others.

21

> Freedom from discrimination is a fundamental human right founded on universal and perpetual principles of natural justice. The core international human rights instruments – the Universal Declaration on Human Rights, Convention Against Torture, Inhuman and Degrading Treatment, International Covenant on Civil and Political Rights, International Covenant on Economic, Social and Cultural Rights, International Convention on the Elimination of All Forms of Discrimination Against Women, and the Convention on the Rights of the Child – prohibit discrimination based on race; colour; sex; language; religion; political or other opinion, national, ethnic, or social origin; property; disability; fortune; birth; or other status. The right to non-discrimination is also detailed in such regional instruments as the African Charter on Human and People's Rights, the American Convention on Human Rights, and the European Convention on Human Rights.
>
> (Maluwa *et al.* 2002, p. 8)

22 The Committee apparently backtracked on some of the more far-reaching implications of its *Toonen* decision in a more recent ruling concerning the extension of pension rights accorded to unmarried different-sex couples to unmarried same-sex couples. In *X* v. *Colombia* (2007), it held that countries which are party to the International Covenant on Civil and Political Rights may not discriminate against same-sex couples in the awarding of such benefits. But it also seemed to overrule the interpretation that discrimination on grounds of 'sex' also included 'sexual orientation', implying that the two are distinct (Wintemute 2007).

23 See the discussion in Chapter 8.

24 Compare Garcia and Parker, who note, with regard to the complexity of human sexuality, 'the tension between recognizing its fluidity, social construction and historical contingency, on one hand, and the need to create categories and identities to "operationalize" sexual rights, on the other hand' (2006, p. 20). See also Sharma 2006.

25 See articles by Currah and Minter, in Currah *et al.* 2006. Minter defines transgender 'as an umbrella term including transsexuals, transvestites, cross-dressers, drag queens and drag kings, butch and femme lesbians, feminine gay men, intersex people, bigendered people, and others who, in Feinberg's words, "challenge the boundaries of sex and gender"'. He distinguishes this from the terms 'gay' and 'lesbian', referring distinctly to an identity or status based on 'sexual object choice' alone, and 'queer', which includes 'lesbian, gay, bisexual

and transgender people' (Minter 2006, p. 159, n. 1). The term 'gender outlaw' comes from Feinberg 1996.

10 At the outer limits of human rights: voids in the liberal paradigm

1 These figures include those fleeing from economic emergencies, natural disasters, and political threats as well as armed conflict. Numbers vary depending on the method of counting and who is doing the counting (see Weiss and Korn 2006). In its 2007 report (on 2006), UNHCR notes that 'the number of stateless persons had more than doubled in 2006 compared with ... 2005' but that this figure understates the magnitude of the problem due to the unavailability of statistical data on statelessness (2007b, p. 5).

2 See www.globalsecurity.org (2007) for this data.

3 See www.globalsecurity.org.

4 Deaths attributed to 'coalition forces' have declined as a total proportion of deaths in Iraq since 2004 but have continued to increase in number. See Burnham *et al.* 2006, p. 10.

5 Mixed reports on level of HIV risk and access to reproductive and maternal health services reflect differing conditions in refugee camps. For those who are relatively isolated, away from constant inflows of combatant or migrant men (e.g., Sierra Leone and Sudan), women's and girls' HIV prevalence rates may actually be lower than in their communities of origin. Likewise, women and girls may have better access to reproductive and maternal health services in refugee camps than they would within either the host or origin countries, unless levels of armed conflict and insecurity make it too dangerous for service providers to remain in the camps – as in Darfur or many places in Iraq. See Hynes *et al.* (2002), McGinn and Purdin (2004), UNFPA (2006) for interesting examples.

6 On Abu Ghraib, see Danner 2004, Eisenstein 2007, Enloe 2007, Hersh 2004, Petchesky 2005. On Guantánamo and the CIA's 'secret interrogation program', where the same sexual humiliation tactics have been systematically deployed, see Mayer 2005, 2007.

7 On Rwanda, see HRW 1996, Landesman 2002; on Gujarat, see IIJG 2003.

8 An Iraqi tortured in Abu Ghraib was quoted in the *China Daily* in May 2004 as saying, 'It's OK if they beat me. Beatings don't hurt us.... But no one would want their manhood to be shattered. They wanted us to feel as though we were women, the way women feel, and *this is the worst insult, to feel like a woman*' (quoted in Susskind 2007, p. 20, emphasis added).

9 Puar (2004) also stresses this point. On Israeli checkpoints, see Peteet 2002; on Palestinian interrogation techniques, see Erlanger 2007.

10 For revealing historical accounts of this policy of co-optation, 'blowback', and renewed support of Islamist groups by US governments, see, e.g., Ali 2002, Johnson 2004, Khalidi 2004, Rashid 2000. The USA ostensibly went to war in Afghanistan in 2001 to defeat the extremist Taliban, rout Al Qaeda, and capture Osama bin Laden, but at this writing most of Afghanistan had reverted to chaos and warlord rule, the Taliban was back in control of significant areas, and Osama bin Laden remained at large somewhere in the mountains of Pakistan (Rhode and Sanger 2007).

11 By the summer and autumn of 2007, the strategy of US-led occupation forces had shifted to include conciliation of Sunni tribal leaders and parties as well.

12

> By summer 2003, Islamist 'misery gangs' were patrolling the streets in many areas, beating and harassing women who were not 'properly' dressed or behaved.... Across Iraq, cities were soon plastered with leaflets and graffiti warning women against going out unveiled, driving, wearing make-up, or shaking hands and socializing with men. Islamist 'punishment committees' sprang up, manned by the Badr Brigade of the US-backed SCIRI Party and its rival, the Mahdi Army.... [They] roamed the streets attacking people accused of flouting Islamic law.... Wearing pants or appearing in public without a headscarf became punishable by death.
>
> (Susskind 2007, p. 7)

13 Under the Baathist regime, despite its harshness toward all political opponents and rival groups, it is undisputed that women's status – in terms of educational levels, health, and access to professions and government jobs (though not the higher rungs of political leadership) – was higher than anywhere else in the Arab world. Most women in Saddam Hussein's secular state, moreover, did not feel compelled to wear the hijab (Lasky 2006).

14 Army and FBI documents secured by the American Civil Liberties Union through the Freedom of Information Act reveal numerous reports of rapes and other abuses of Iraqi women detainees by US military guards and interrogators, including the sodomization of a 73-year-old woman (see ACLU 2007), none of which appeared in the mainstream US press before 2006. See also Danner 2004, Eisenstein 2007, Harding 2004, Hersh 2004, Susskind 2007.

15 For extensive commentary on this evidence concerning complicity of the US Secretary of Defense, Attorney General, Vice-President, and President in matters related to Abu Ghraib and Guantánamo, see Danner 2004, Hersh 2004, Mayer 2007, Shane and Mazzetti 2007.

16 On 28 September 2006 the US Congress approved a bill on the handling of detainees, terrorist trials, and interrogation procedures that, in the words of the *New York Times*, 'gave Mr. Bush most of what he wanted'. The US Military Commissions Act follows a broad definition of 'illegal enemy combatants' that would include legal residents of the USA as well as foreign citizens living in their own countries, and effectively denies the right of habeas corpus for such detainees. Furthermore, it abrogates much of the Geneva Conventions' meaning concerning torture and degrading treatment, leaving it up to the president to decide what methods of interrogation are permissible; sets up a system of military tribunals for trying so-called enemy combatants, denying the power of judicial review to civilian courts; and, not least, defines sexual offences so narrowly that the wide array of sexual violence, abuse, and intimidation now defined as war crimes and crimes against humanity under international law (the ICC Statute particularly) – such as those committed famously in Abu Ghraib – would not count as torture (*New York Times* 2006a, 2006b, Zernike 2006).

17 Public reactions to these events led President Bush to intimate that he might consider closing Guantánamo, which was still open and running, with some prisoner releases, at the time of writing. But closing Guantánamo would not end the Guantánamo syndrome; its prisoners would simply be reshuffled through the grid of what Chalmers Johnson (2004) calls the US Empire's 'globe-girdling Baseworld'.

18 Emily Grabham (2007) makes a similar point in critiquing what she calls 'the hyper-embodiment of intersexual [*sic*] people by the medical profession': 'Their

"abnormal" corporeality renders [intersex infants, youth, and adults] somehow more "mappable" and, crucially, less autonomous than people who appear to be more clearly sexed', she observes. Similar to drug addicts, disabled people, or pregnant teenagers, they are read as 'being controlled by their bodies' and thus as prime candidates for biopolitical interventions (pp. 42–43).

19 All of Zillah Eisenstein's work, from *The Female Body and the Law* (1988) to *Sexual Decoys* (2007), continues to raise this critical question.

20 Sharma (2006) defines 'a queer perspective' as 'one which recognizes the dangers of narrowly defined identity politics, challenges heteronormativity, and locates itself in a framework of intersectionality, which takes account of the connections between different types of struggles and the interplay of multiple identities' (p. 57, n. 2).

21 In Turkey, where honour crimes have persisted, pressures from the EU and changes in the national criminal law have meant more prosecutions and long jail sentences for such crimes. Rather than diminishing the crimes, however, the result has been a rise in forced suicides of girls, to prevent the conviction of men. 'Women's groups [in Turkey] say the evidence suggests that a growing number of girls considered to be dishonored are being locked in a room for days with rat poison, a pistol, or a rope, and told by their families that the only thing resting between their disgrace and redemption is death.' Derya, a 17-year-old girl who had secretly met a boy from school, was ordered by her uncle to kill herself for the shame. After jumping into the Tigris and surviving, then trying to hang herself, then slashing her wrists with a kitchen knife, she finally took refuge in a local women's shelter (Bilefsky 2006). See also Ilkkaracan 2007.

22 Most of the murders have taken place in Kwa Zulu Natal province, which, perhaps not coincidentally, has one of the highest HIV/AIDS rates in South Africa (and thus worldwide). During July 2007 Sizakele Sigasa, age 34, and Salome Masooa, age 24, were shot to death execution-style, and Thokozane Qwabe, age 23, was stoned to death. One source described this as a 'state of emergency' for women, and particularly lesbians, in South Africa.

23 This is what Butler (2004b) appears to mean by 'the inherently conservative function of the norm' and its paradoxical status as being both socially integrative and 'exclusionary or violent' (pp. 2, 221).

24 For example, in defining David Reimer's 'precarious life', Butler (2004b) insists 'that it is precisely the ways in which he is not fully recognizable, fully disposable, fully categorizable, that his humanness emerges' (p. 73).

25 As Nussbaum puts it, 'For Kant, only humanity and rationality are worthy of respect and wonder; the rest of nature is just a set of tools' (2006, p. 347). In this sense, Kant typifies most of European Enlightenment thinking.

26 For example, the animal rights philosopher Tom Regan presents a thought experiment involving five survivors on a lifeboat, where four are human and the fifth is a dog, and one must be sacrificed or all will drown. He doesn't hesitate to throw the dog overboard (Steiner 2005, p. 11). Levinas, despite his story of a friendly dog he encountered in a Nazi labour camp whom he called 'the last Kantian in Nazi Germany', none the less reviled Heidegger for equating the concentration camps with commercialized food production, thus, he felt, trivializing the Holocaust (2005, pp. 214–215). And Derrida, after accusing Heidegger of 'carno-phallogocentrism' – i.e., '[asserting] the primacy of meat-eating, male, linguistic beings' – quickly dissociates himself from 'vegetarianism, ecologism, or ... societies for the protection of animals' (2005, pp. 218, 220).

27 Quoted from David Clark, 'On being "the last Kantian in Nazi Germany":
dwelling with animals after Levinas' (1997), in Steiner 2005, p. 215.

28 Derrida here echoes the words of Virginia Woolf, imagining the relationship
between Elizabeth Barrett and her dog Flush: 'After all, she may have thought,
do words say everything? Can words say anything? Do not words destroy the
symbol that lies beyond the reach of words?' (Woolf 1983 [orig. 1933], p. 37).

29 Cf. Nussbaum (2006), who makes much the same arguments.

30 Some would argue that relations between pregnant women and their foetuses –
not yet full human persons but distinctly part of the web of human and bios-
pheric life – also belong in this argument for care and stewardship. Our position, like that of many feminists, is, yes, but under very different conditions
from those that now exist. A feminism grounded in principles of social justice
does not require dogmatic adherence to life on any terms, but rather attention
to the conditions of a decent, 'liveable life' (Butler 2004b, p. 8). As long as
women's bodies are the vehicles of pregnancies and women remain mainly
responsible for the care of children after they are born, safe, legal abortion
must remain a clear option for all women. In the meantime, we must continue
to struggle for a world and societies in which all children born have the full
possibility of realizing their capacities in health, dignity, and freedom. Pregnancy is an ontological situation unlike any other relationship, uniquely one
where the 'other' is also, inextricably, a part of one's self. For societies to regulate and dictate the outcome of pregnancies, while providing little or nothing to
protect women from unnecessary maternal deaths and their children from
hunger and brutality, is little short of obscene (Petchesky 1990).

31 See Butler 2004a, pp. xiv, 20–28, 30–31, 46, 134, and Levinas 2003, pp. xxxiii
(Introduction by Richard A. Cohen) and 29–33. Cohen's Introduction is
particularly helpful in clarifying Levinas' thought.

32

> The requirement ... that there shall be a single kind of sexual life for
> everyone disregards the dissimilarities, whether innate or acquired, in the
> sexual constitution of human beings; it cuts off a fair number of them from
> sexual enjoyment, and so becomes the source of serious injustice.... [Even]
> heterosexual genital love, which has remained exempt from outlawry, is
> itself restricted by further limitations, in the shape of insistence upon
> legitimacy and monogamy. Present-day civilization makes it plain that it
> will only permit sexual relationships on the basis of a solitary, indissoluble
> bond between one man and one woman, and that it does not like sexuality
> as a source of pleasure in its own right and is only prepared to tolerate it
> because there is so far no substitute for it as a means of propagating the
> human race.
>
> (Freud 1962, pp. 51–52)

33 For a sample of this literature, reflecting diverse geographical sites, see
Amuchastegui and Aggleton 2007, Dowsett 2000, Feinberg 1996, Halberstam
1998, Ilkkaracan 2000, Jackson 2007, Manderson and Jolly 1997, Misra and
Chandiramani 2005, Nanda 2007, Parker 1991, 1999, Parker and Gagnon
1995, Parker et al. 2000.

34 On women's sense of entitlement in matters of sexuality and reproduction, see
Petchesky and Judd 1998. On this sense of entitlement among African women
specifically, and their attempts to shape their own erotic lives, see Mama et al.
2005, McFadden 2003, and Osakue and Martin-Hilber 1998.

35 The project publicizes the slogan 'because sex education is rarely sexy/and
erotica is rarely safe/putting the sexy into safer sex'.

36 The list includes:

> marital duty or fear of abandonment; ... the need to perform and prove yourself; because you have no choice; business; education funding; fear of violence; self-esteem boosting; boredom; kindness and generosity; pity; fear that the man's balls will burst or he will go mad; worn down by constant demand; to be allowed to sleep; to have children; to feel powerful; for exercise; self-affirmation; love; ... for revenge; because there are electricity cuts at night; ... to lose weight;... because you cannot sleep; to reduce tension in the home; to share intimacy ... to forward your career; to get good grades.
>
> (Lewis and Gordon 2006, p. 111)

Postscript: dreaming and dancing – the 'beyond' beyond sexual rights

1 www.sistersinislam.pd.jaring.my.
2 www.wwhr.org.
3 www.catholicsforchoice.org.

Bibliography

Abelove, H., Barale, M.A., and Halperin, D.M. (eds) (1993) *The Lesbian and Gay Studies Reader*, New York and London: Routledge.

Aberle, S.D. and Corner, G.W. (1953) *Twenty-five Years of Sex Research: History of the National Research Council Committee for Research in Problems of Sex*, Philadelphia: W.B. Saunders.

Abu-Lughod, L. (2005) Comments on Panel, 'Rethinking the Intersections of Gender, Religion, and Human Rights', Conference on Women and Power, National Council for Research on Women, City University of New York, 7 June. Available online at www.ncrw.org/interest/2005annconf/rtiograhr.htm (accessed 25 November 2007).

Accad, E. (2000) 'Sexuality and sexual politics: conflicts and contradictions for contemporary women in the Middle East', in P. Ilkkaracan (ed.) *Women and Sexuality in Muslim Societies*, Istanbul: Women for Women's Human Rights.

ACLU (American Civil Liberties Union) (2007) 'Torture documents released under FOIA'. Available online at www.aclu.org/safefree/torture/torturefoia.html (accessed 26 September 2007).

Action Aid (2004) 'Blocking progress: how the fight against HIV/AIDS is being undermined by the World Bank and the International Monetary Fund', Washington, DC. Available online at www.actionaidusa.org/pdf/blockingprogress.pdf (accessed 4 September 2007).

Adam, B., Duyvendak, J., and Krouwel, A. (eds) (1998) *The Global Emergence of Gay and Lesbian Politics: National Imprints of a Worldwide Movement*, Philadelphia: Temple University Press.

Agamben, G. (1998) *Homo Sacer, Sovereign Power and Bare Life*, trans. D. Heller-Roazen, Stanford: Stanford University Press.

—— (2005) *State of Exception*, trans. K. Attell, Chicago: The University of Chicago Press.

Aggarwal, S. (2002) 'ABVA writ petition for repeal of Section 377', in B. Fernandez (ed.) *Humjinsi: A Resource Book on Lesbian, Gay and Bisexual Rights in India*, Mumbai: India Center for Human Rights and Law.

Aggleton, P. (ed.) (1996a) *Bisexualities and AIDS: International Perspectives*, London: Taylor & Francis.

—— (1996b) 'Global priorities for HIV/AIDS intervention research', *International Journal of STD & AIDS*, 7(Suppl. 2): 13–16.

—— (ed.) (1999) *Men Who Sell Sex: International Perspectives on Male Prostitution and HIV/AIDS*, London: University College London Press.

—— (2007) 'Just a snip? A social history of male circumcision', *Reproductive Health Matters*, 15(29): 15–21.

Aggleton, P., Ball, A., and Mane, P. (eds) (2006) *Sex, Drugs and Young People: International Perspectives*, London and New York: Routledge.

AI (Amnesty International) (2003) 'Uganda'. Available online at http://web.amnesty.org/report2003/uga-summary-eng (accessed 4 September 2007).

—— (2006) 'Uganda: fear for safety/harassment'. Available online at http://web.amnesty.org/library/Index/ENGAFR590072006?open&of=ENG-370 (accessed 6 January 2007).

—— (2007) 'Report 2007 – state of the world human rights'. Available online at http://thereport.amnesty.org/eng/A-year-in-campaigning/War-on-terror (accessed 23 August 2007).

Ajzen, I. and Fishbein, M. (1980) *Understanding Attitudes and Predicting Social Behavior*, Englewood Cliffs, NJ: Prentice-Hall.

Ali, T. (2002) *The Clash of Fundamentalisms: Crusades, Jihads and Modernity*, London and New York: Verso.

Almond, G.A., Appleby, R.S., and Sivan, E. (2003) *Strong Religion: The Rise of Fundamentalisms around the World*, Chicago: University of Chicago Press.

Alonso, A.M. and Koreck, M.T. (1989) 'Silences: "Hispanics", AIDS and sexual practices', *Differences*, 1: 101–124.

Altman, D. (1986) *AIDS and the New Puritanism*, London: Pluto Press.

—— (1994) *Power and Community: Organizational and Cultural Responses to AIDS*, London: Taylor & Francis.

—— (1995) 'Political sexualities: meanings and identities in the time of AIDS', in R. Parker and J.H. Gagnon (eds) *Conceiving Sexuality: Approaches to Sex Research in a Postmodern World*, New York and London: Routledge.

—— (2001) *Global Sex*, Chicago: The University of Chicago Press.

Amuchastegui, A. and Aggleton, P. (2007) ' "I don't know if she got pregnant": gender, responsibility and autonomy among young Mexican men', *Sexualities*, 10: 61–81.

APDC (Action Population and Development Canada) (2004) Sexual Orientation Resolution at the upcoming Commission on Human Rights, *Friday Facts* Vol. 5 Issue 2 – March 19. Available online at acdp.ca/fridayfacts.cfm/en/section/fridayfacts/ff120 (accessed 23 August 2007).

Appadurai, A. (1996) *Modernity at Large: Cultural Dimensions of Globalization*, Minneapolis: University of Minnesota Press.

Araloff, S. (2006) '100 days of Kazimierz Marcinkiewicz: euro-pragmatism victory', Axis Information and Analysis: Global Challenges Research. Available online at www.axisglobe.com (accessed 4 September 2007).

ARC (ARC International) (2006) 'Norwegian statement on sexual orientation and gender identity – 3rd Session of the United Nations Human Rights Council', Geneva, 1 December. Available online at www.arc-international.net/norwaystatement.html (accessed 9 September 2007).

—— (2007a) 'Annual report 2006'. Available online at http://arc-international.net/report2006.html (accessed 9 September 2007).

—— (2007b) 'References to sexual orientation, gender identity and related issues in reports submitted to the council'. Available online at www.arc-international.net (accessed 26 September 2007).

Armstrong, K. (2000) *The Battle for God: Fundamentalism in Judaism, Christianity and Islam*, New York: Ballantine.

Asad, T. (2003) *Formation of the Secular: Christianity, Islam, Modernity*, Stanford: Stanford University Press.

—— (2005) 'Reflections on läicité & the public sphere', *Social Science Research Council, Items and Issues*, 5(3). Available online at http://publications.ssrc.org/items/v5n3/index.html (accessed 22 November 2007).

Bahgat, B. (2001) 'Explaining Egypt's targeting of gays'. Available online at www.merip.org/mero/mero072301.html (accessed 29 October 2007).

Bahgat, H. and Afifi, W. (2007) 'Sexual politics in Egypt', in R. Parker, R. Petchesky, and R. Sember (eds) *SexPolitics: Reports From the Frontlines*, Sexuality Policy Watch. Available online at www.sxpolitics.org/frontlines/home/index.php (accessed 22 November 2007).

Bandarage, A. (1997) *Women, Population, and Global Crisis: A Political-economic Analysis*, London: Zed Books.

Bandura, A. (1977) *Social Learning Theory*, Englewood Cliffs, NJ: Prentice-Hall.

Bartlett, L., McGinn, T., and Purdin, S. (2004) 'Forced migrants – turning rights into reproductive health', *The Lancet*, 363: 76–77.

Bassett, M. (1993) 'Social and economic determinants of vulnerability to HIV infection: the Zimbabwe experience', *AIDS Analysis Africa*, July/August: 9–11.

Bateson, G. (1947) 'Sex and culture', *Annals New York Academy of Sciences*, 47: 647–660.

Baylies, C., Bujra, J. with the Gender and AIDS Group (2000) *AIDS, Sexuality and Gender in Africa*, London and New York: Routledge.

BBC World (2006) 'Pope's speech stirs Muslim anger'. Available online at http://news.bbc.co.uk/2/hi/europe/5346480.stm (accessed 28 November 2007).

Becker, M. and Joseph, J. (1988) 'AIDS and behavioral change to avoid risk: a review', *American Journal of Public Health*, 78: 384–410.

Bedford, K. (forthcoming) 'Governing intimacy in the World Bank', in S. Rai and G. Waylen (eds) *Analysing and Transforming Global Governance: Feminist Perspectives*, Cambridge: Cambridge University Press.

Beisel, N. (1997) *Imperiled Innocents: Anthony Comstock and Family Reproduction in Victorian America*, Princeton: Princeton University Press.

Bell, D. and Binnie, J. (2000) *The Sexual Citizen: Queer Politics and Beyond*, Cambridge: Polity Press.

Benhabib, S. (1995) 'Cultural complexity, moral interdependence, and the global dialogical community', in M. Nussbaum and J. Glover (eds) *Women, Development and Culture*, Oxford: Oxford University Press.

—— (2002) *The Claims of Culture. Equality and Diversity in the Global Era*, Princeton: Princeton University Press.

Benjamin, J. (1988) *The Bonds of Love: Psychoanalysis, Feminism, and the Problem of Domination*, New York: Pantheon.

Bernstein, C. and Politi, M. (1996) *His Holiness*, New York: Penguin.

Berquó, E. (ed.) (2000) *Comportamento Sexual da População Brasileira e Percepções do HIV/Aids*, Brasil: Ministério da Saúde.

—— (2006) 'Arranjos familiares no Brasil: uma visão demográfica – Elza Berquó', in Lílian Moritz Shwarzc (ed.) *História da Vida Privada no Brazil*, Companhi das Letras, São Paulo.

Berube, A. (1990) *Coming Out Under Fire: The History of Gay Men and Women in World War Two*, New York: The Free Press.

Bilefsky, D. (2006) 'How to avoid jail for honor killing? Honor suicide', *New York Times*, 16 July.

Birdsal, N., Kelly, A.C., and Sinding, S.W. (2001) *Population Matters*, Oxford: Oxford University Press.

Blackwood, E. (ed.) (1986) *Anthropology and Homosexual Behavior*, New York: Haworth Press.

Blackwood, E. and Wieringa, S. (eds) (1999) *Female Desires: Same-sex Relations and Transgender Practices Across Cultures*, New York: Columbia University Press.

Bloom, D.E., Canning, D., and Sevilla, J. (2003) *The Demographic Divided: A New Perspective on the Economic Consequences of Population Change*, Population Matters Monograph MR-1274, Santa Monica: Rand.

Bloomberg.com (2006) 'Pope condemns same-sex unions, calls gay love "weak"'. Available online at www.netscape.com/viewstory/2006/05/11/pope-gay-marriage -is-weak/?url=http%3A%2F%2Fwww.bloomberg.com%2Fapps%2Fnews %3Fpid%3D10000087%26sid%3Dawia81URdshw%26refer%3Dtop_world_n ews&frame=true (accessed 23 November 2007).

Boellstorff, T. (2005) *The Gay Archipelago: Sexuality and Nation in Indonesia*, Princeton: Princeton University Press.

Bond, G.C. and Vincent, J. (1997) 'AIDS in Uganda: the first decade', in G.C. Bond, J. Kreniske, I. Susser, and J. Vincent (eds) *AIDS in Africa and the Caribbean*, Boulder: Westview Press.

Bongaarts, J. (2005) 'The causes of stalling fertility transitions', paper presented at International Union for the Scientific Study of Population Conference, Tours, France, July.

Bornstein, K. (1994) *Gender Outlaw: On Men, Women and The Rest of Us*, New York and London: Routledge.

Borradori, G. (2003) *Philosophy in a Time of Terror: Dialogues with Jürgen Habermas and Jacques Derrida*, Chicago: University of Chicago Press.

Boseley, S. and Goldenberg, S. (2005) 'Brazil spurns US terms for AIDS help', *Guardian*, 4 May. Available online at www.guardian.co.uk/brazil/story/ 0,12462,1475966,00.html (accessed 9 September 2007).

Boswell, J. (1980) *Christianity, Social Tolerance, and Homosexuality*, Chicago: University of Chicago Press.

Bourdieu, P. (ed.) (1993) *La misère du monde*, Paris: Seuil.

—— (1998) *Practical Reason: On the Theory of Action*, Cambridge: Polity Press.

—— (1999) *Weight of the World: Social Suffering in Contemporary Society*, Cambridge: Polity Press.

—— (2002) *Masculine Domination*, Stanford: Stanford University Press.

Bozon, M. and Leridon, H. (1996) *Sexuality and the Social Sciences: A French Survey on Sexual Behaviour*, Aldershot: Dartmouth Publishing Group.

Brake, M. (1982) *Human Sexual Relations: Towards a Redefinition of Sexual Politics*, New York: Pantheon Books.

Brandes, S. (1980) *Metaphors of Masculinity: Sex and Status in Andalusian Folklore*, Philadelphia: University of Pennsylvania Press.

Brandt, A. (1987) *No Magic Bullet: A Social History of Venereal Disease in the United States Since 1880*, Oxford and New York: Oxford University Press.

Brennan, D. (2004) *What's Love Got to Do with It?: Transnational Desires and Sex Tourism in the Dominican Republic*, Durham, NC: Duke University Press.

Brown, J. (1986) 'Lesbian sexuality in medieval and early modern Europe', in M. Duberman, M. Vicinus, and G. Chauncey, Jr. (eds) *Hidden From History: Reclaiming the Gay and Lesbian Past*, New York: Meridian.

Brown, W. (1988) *Manhood and Politics: A Feminist Reading in Political Theory*, Totowa, NJ: Rowman & Littlefield.

Buckley, C. (2007) 'Gays living in shadows of new Iraq', *New York Times* (December), p. A8.

Bullough, V.L. (1985) 'The Rockefellers and sex research', *Journal of Sex Research*, 21(2): 113–125.

—— (1994) *Science in the Bedroom: A History of Sex Research*, New York: Basic Books.

—— (1998) 'Alfred Kinsey and the Kinsey Report: historical overview and lasting contributions', *Journal of Sex Research*, 35(2): 127–131.

Bunch, C. and Reilly, N. (1994) *Demanding Accountability: The Global Campaign and Vienna Tribunal for Women's Human Rights*, New Brunswick, NJ: Center for Women's Global Leadership.

Burke, K. (1945) *A Grammar of Motives*, Berkeley: University of California Press.

Burnham, G., Doocy, S., Dzeng, E., Lafta, R., and Roberts, L. (2006) *The Human Cost of the War in Iraq: A Mortality Study, 2002–2006*, Baltimore, and Baghdad, Iraq: Bloomberg School of Public Health, Johns Hopkins University and School of Medicine, and Al Mustansiriya University.

Butalia, U. and Sarkar, T. (1995) *Women and the Hindu Right*, New Delhi: Kali For Women.

Butler, J. (1990a) *Gender Trouble: Feminism and the Subversion of Identity*, New York and London: Routledge.

—— (1990b) 'Performative acts and gender constitution: an essay in phenomenology and feminist theory', in S.E. Case (ed.) *Performing Feminisms: Feminist Critical Theory and Theatre*, Baltimore: Johns Hopkins University Press.

—— (1991) 'Imitation and gender insubordination', in D. Fuss (ed.) *Inside/Out: Lesbian Theories, Gay Theories*, New York and London: Routledge.

—— (1993) *Bodies that Matter: On the Discursive Limits of 'Sex'*, New York and London: Routledge.

—— (2004a) *Precarious Life: The Powers of Mourning and Violence*, New York: Verso.

—— (2004b) *Undoing Gender*, New York and London: Routledge.

—— (2005) *Giving an Account of Oneself*, New York: Fordham University Press.

—— (2007) 'Interview with Judith Butler, gender trouble: still revolutionary or obsolete?' Available online at www.ilga.org/news_results.asp?LanguageID=1&FileID=1097&ZoneID=7&FileCategory=6 (accessed 22 August 2007).

Cabral, M. (2005) 'En estado de excepción: intersexualidad e intervenciones sociomédicas', paper presented at Seminario Regional Salud, Sexualidad y Diversidad en América Latina, Lima, Peru, 22–24 February, trans. A. Sarda.

Cabral, M. and Viturro, P. (2006) '(Trans)sexual citizenship in contemporary Argentina', in P. Currah, R.M. Juang, and S.P. Minter (eds) *Transgender Rights*, Minneapolis: University of Minnesota Press.

Cáceres, C. (1996) 'Male bisexuality in Peru and the prevention of AIDS', in P. Aggleton (ed.) *Bisexualities and AIDS: International Perspectives*, London: Taylor & Francis.

Cáceres, C., Palomino, N., and Cueto, M. (2007) 'Sexual and reproductive rights in Peru: unveiling false paradoxes', in R. Parker, R. Petchesky, and R. Sember (eds) *SexPolitics: Reports from the Frontlines*, Sexuality Policy Watch. Available online at www.sxpolitics.org/frontlines/home/index (accessed 28 November 2007).

Califia, P. (1981) 'A personal view of the history of the lesbian S/M community and movement in San Francisco', in SAMOIS (ed.) *Coming to Power: Writings and Graphics on Lesbian S/M*, Boston: Alyson Publications.

Camargo, K. and Mattos, R. (2007) 'Looking for sex in all the wrong places: the silencing of sexuality in the World Bank's public discourse', in R. Parker, R. Petchesky and R. Sember (eds) *SexPolitics: Reports from the Frontlines*, Sexuality Policy Watch. Available online at www.sxpolitics.org/frontlines/home/index.php (accessed 22 November 2007).

Cameron, E. (2002) 'Constitutional protection of sexual orientation and African conceptions of humanity', *South African Law Journal*, 118: 642–650.

Carballo, M., Albrecht, G., Caraël, M., and Cleland, J. (1989) 'A cross-national study of patterns of sexual behavior', *Journal of Sex Research*, 26: 287–299.

Carrier, J. (1976) 'Cultural factors affecting urban Mexican homosexual behavior', *Archives of Sexual Behavior*, 5: 103–124.

—— (1995) *De Los Outros: Intimacy and Homosexuality among Mexican Men*, New York: Columbia University Press.

Carrier, J. and Magaña, R. (1991) 'Use of ethnosexual data on men of Mexican origin for HIV/AIDS prevention programs', *Journal of Sex Research*, 28(2): 189–202.

Carrier, J., Ngyen, B., and Su, S. (1997) 'Sexual relations between migrating populations (Vietnamese with Mexican and Anglo) and HIV/STD infections in Southern California', in G. Herdt (ed.) *Sexual Cultures and Migration in the Era of AIDS: Anthropological and Demographic Perspectives*, Oxford: Clarendon Press.

Carrillo, H. (2002) *The Night is Young: Sexuality in Mexico in the Time of AIDS*, Chicago: University of Chicago Press.

Castelli, E. (2005) 'Comments on Panel, Rethinking the Intersections of Gender, Religion, and Human Rights', Conference on Women and Power, National Council for Research on Women, City University of New York, 7 June. Available online at www.ncrw.org/interest/2005annconf/rtiograhr.htm (accessed 27 November 2007).

Castells, M. (1996) *The Rise of Network Society*, Malden, MA: Blackwell.

—— (1997) *The Power of Identity*, Malden, MA: Blackwell.

—— (1998) *End of Millennium*, Malden, MA: Blackwell.

Castilhos, W. (2007) ' "Unshakable" position'. Available online at www.sxpolitics.org/mambo452/index.php?option=com_content&task=view&id=95&Itemid=119 (accessed 24 November 2007).

Césaire, A. (1972/2000) *Discourse on Colonialism*, New York: Monthly Review Press.

Chakravarti, U. (2000) 'A chaste hero rescues an emasculated nation', in M.E. John and J. Nair (eds) *A Question of Silence? The Sexual Economies of Modern India*, New Delhi: Kali for Women Delhi.

CHANGE (Centre for Health and Gender Equity) (2005a) 'Ugandan condom crisis'. Available online at www.genderhealth.org/uganda.php (accessed 4 September 2007).

—— (2005b) 'Implications of US policy restrictions on programs aimed at commercial sex workers and victims of trafficking worldwide'. Available online at www.pepfar.org (accessed 5 January 2007).

—— (2007) 'Centre for Health and Gender Equity (CHANGE) Applauds Senate Vote to Repeal the Global Gag Rule'. Available online at www.genderhealth.org/ (accessed 15 October 2007).

Chauncey, G. (1994) *Gay New York: Gender, Urban Culture, and the Making of the Gay Male World, 1890–1940*, New York: Basic Books.

Cheah, P. (1997) 'Positioning human rights in the current global conjuncture', *Public Culture*, 9(2): 233–266.

Chesler, E. (2007) *Woman of Valor: Margaret Sanger and the Birth Control Movement in America*, New York: Simon & Schuster.

Chodorow, N. (1978) *The Reproduction of Mothering*, Berkeley and Los Angeles: University of California Press.

—— (1991) *Feminism and Psychoanalytic Theory*, New Haven: Yale University Press.

Chouinard, A. and Albert, J. (eds) (1990) *Human Sexuality: Research Perspectives in a World Facing AIDS*, Ottawa: International Development Research Centre.

Ciezadlo, A. (2004) 'For Iraqi women, Abu Ghraib's taint', 24 May, *Christian Science Monitor*. Available online at www.csmonitor.com/2004/0528/p01s02-woiq.html (accessed 28 November 2007).

—— (2005) 'In Iraq, giving birth is complicated by war', 30 June, *Christian Science Monitor*. Available online at www.csmonitor.com/2005/0630/007s02-woiq.html (accessed 26 September 2007).

Citizen's Initiative (2002) 'How the Gujarat Massacre affected minority women? The survivors speak: a fact finding report by a women's panel'. Ahmedabad, 16 April. Available online at http://cac.ektaonline.org/resources/reports/womensreport.htm (accessed 23 November 2007).

Clark, D (1997) 'On being "the last kantian in Nazi Germany": dwelling with animals after Levinas', in J. Ham and M. Senior (eds) *Becoming Animality from the Middle Ages to the Present*, New York: Routledge.

Cleland, J. and Ferry, B. (eds) (1995) *Sexual Behavior and AIDS in the Developing World*, London: Taylor & Francis.

Cleland, J. and Hobcraft, J. (eds) (1985) *Reproductive Change in Developing Countries: Insights from the World Fertility Survey*, Oxford: Oxford University Press.

Cleland, J., Scott, C., and Whitelegge, D. (1987) *The World Fertility Survey: An Assessment*, Oxford: Oxford University Press.

Cochran, W., Mosteller, F., and Tukey, J. (1953) 'Statistical problems of the Kinsey Report', *Journal of the American Statistical Association*, 48: 673–716.

Cohen, B.J. (2002) 'Bretton Woods system', in R.J.B. Jones (ed.) *Routledge Encyclopedia of International Political Economy*, New York: Routledge.

Cohen, C.J. (1999) *The Boundaries of Blackness: AIDS and the Breakdown of Black Politics*, Chicago and London: The University of Chicago Press.

Cohen, J. (2005) 'Male circumcision thwarts HIV infection', *Science*, 309: 860.

Collet, A. (2006) 'Interrogating sexualities at Beijing Plus Ten', SPW Working Paper No. 3. Available online at www.sxpolitics.org/mambo452/index. php?option=com_docman&task=cat_view&gid=7&Itemid=2 (accessed 20 May 2007).

Connell, R.W. and Dowsett, G.W. (1999) ' "The unclean motion of the generative parts": frameworks in western thought on sexuality', in R. Parker and P. Aggleton (eds) (2007) *Culture, Society and Sexuality: A Reader*, London: University College London Press.

Cook, R.J. (1995) 'Human rights and reproductive self-determination', *The American University Law Review*, 44: 979–982.

Cooper, D. (1995) *Power in Struggle: Feminism, Sexuality and the State*, Buckingham: Open University Press.

Copelon, R. (1994) 'Intimate terror: understanding domestic violence as torture', in R. Cook (ed.) *Human Rights of Women: National and International Perspectives*, Philadelphia: University of Pennsylvania Press.

—— (2000) 'Gender crimes as war crimes: integrating crimes against women into International Criminal Law', *McGill Law Journal*, 46(3): 217–240.

Corrêa, S. (with Reichmann, R.) (1994) *Population and Reproductive Rights: Feminist Perspectives from the South*, London: Zed Books.

—— (1997) 'Empowerment in the feminist perspective: theoretical itineraries, challenges ahead', paper presented at the International Union for the Scientific Study of Population, Seminar on Female Empowerment and Demographic Processes: Moving Beyond Cairo, Lund, Sweden, 21–24 April.

—— (2006) 'Interlinking policy, politics and women's reproductive rights: a study of health sector reform, maternal mortality and abortion in selected countries of the South', DAWN. Available online at www.repem.org.uy/node/216 (accessed 29 August 2006).

Corrêa, S. and Jolly, S. (2006) *Sexuality, Development and Human Rights*. Available online at www.ids.ac.uk/ids/Part/proj/sexrights.html (accessed 18 August 2007).

Corrêa, S. and Parker, R. (2004) 'Sexuality, human rights and demographic thinking: connections and disjunctions in a changing world', *Sexuality Research and Social Policy*, 1(1): 15–38.

Corrêa, S. and Petchesky, R. (1994) 'Reproductive and sexual rights: a feminist perspective', in R. Parker and P. Aggleton (eds) *Culture, Society and Sexuality: A Reader*, London and New York: Routledge.

CREA, SANGAMA, and TARSHI (2005) *A Conversation on Sexual Rights in India*, New Delhi: Talking about Reproductive and Sexual Health Issues (TARSHI).

Crenshaw, K. (1991) 'Mapping the margins: intersectionality, identity politics, and violence against women of colour', *Stanford Law Review*, 43:1241–1299.

Crimp, D. (ed.) (1988) *AIDS: Cultural Analysis/Cultural Activism*, Cambridge, MA: MIT Press.

Crompton, L. (2003) *Homosexuality and Civilization*, Cambridge, MA: The Belknap Press/Harvard University Press.

CRR (Center for Reproductive Rights) (2002) *Bringing Rights to Bear: An Analysis of UN Treaty Monitoring Bodies on Reproductive and Sexual Rights*, New York: Center for Reproductive Rights.

—— (2003) 'Unconstitutional assault on the right to choose – federal abortion ban is an affront to women and the Supreme Court'. Available online at www.reproductiverights.org/pdf/pub_bp_uncon_assault.pdf (accessed 15 May 2007).

—— (2007) 'Abortion worldwide: twelve years of reforms'. Available online at www.reproductiverights.org/pr_05_0304abortion.html (accessed 29 August 2007).

Csete, J. (2002) 'HIV/AIDS in India: an epidemic of abuse', Human Rights Watch. Available online at http://hrw.org/english/docs/2002/07/10/india12865.htm (accessed 6 September 2007).

Currah, P. (2001) 'Queer theory, lesbian and gay rights, and transsexual marriages', in M. Blasius (ed.) *Identity/Space/Power*, Princeton: Princeton University Press.

—— (2003) 'The Transgender Rights Imaginary', *Georgetown Journal of Gender and the Law*, 4: 705–720.

Currah, P., Juang, R.M., and Minter, S.P. (eds) (2006) *Transgender Rights*, Minneapolis: University of Minnesota Press.

Daily Telegraph (2007) 'Anglican Church in a "mess" over gay bishop row', May 29. Available online at www.telegraph.co.uk/news/main.jhtml?xml=/news/2007/05/29/nchurch29.xml (accessed 4 September 2007).

Daniel, H. and Parker, R. (1993) *Sexuality, Politics and AIDS in Brazil*, London: Falmer Press.

Danner, M. (2004) *Torture and Truth: America, Abu Ghraib, and the War on Terror*, New York: New York Review of Books.

Darwin, C. (1859) *The Origin of Species*, London: John Murray.

—— (1871) *The Descent of Man and Selection in Relation to Sex*, London: John Murray.

Dawkins, R. (1976) *The Selfish Gene*, Oxford: Oxford University Press.

—— (2007) 'EUA são vítimas da política religiosa', *Folha de São Paulo*, Folha Ilustrada: E11.

de Alwis, M. (2004) 'The "purity" of displacement and the reterritorialization of longing: Muslim IDPs in northwestern Sri Lanka', in W. Giles and J. Hyndman (eds) *Sites of Violence: Gender and Conflict Zones*, Berkeley: University of California.

de Beauvoir, S. (1953 [orig. 1949]) *The Second Sex*, New York: Knopf.

de Boni, L.A. (1995) *Fundamentalismo*, Porto Alegre: EDIPUCRS.

D'Emilio, J. (1983) 'Capitalism and gay identity', in A. Snitow, C. Stansell, and S. Thompson (eds) *Powers of Desire*, New York: Monthly Review Press.

—— (1992) *Making Trouble: Essays on Gay History, Politics, and the University*, New York: Routledge.

D'Emilio, J. and Freedman, E.B. (1988) *Intimate Matters: A Social History of Sexuality in America*, New York: Harper & Row.

de la Dehesa, R. (2007) *Sexual Modernities: Queering the Public Sphere in Latin America*, Durham, NC: Duke University Press.

de Lauretis, T. (1991) 'Queer theory: lesbian and gay sexualities', *Differences: A Journal of Feminist Cultural Studies*, 3(2): iii–xviii.

—— (1994a) 'Habit changes', *Differences: A Journal of Feminist Cultural Studies*, 6(2–3): 296–313.

—— (1994b) *The Practice of Love: Lesbian Sexuality and Perverse Desire*, Bloomington: Indiana University Press.

de Zalduondo, B.O. (1999) 'Prostitution viewed cross-culturally: toward recontextualizing sex work in AIDS intervention research', in R. Parker and P. Aggleton (eds) *Culture, Society and Sexuality: A Reader*, London: University College London Press.

Decosas, J. (1996) 'HIV and development', *AIDS*, 10 (Suppl. 3): S69–S94.

Decosas, J., Anarfi, J., Kane, F., Sodii, K., and Wager, H.U. (1995) 'Migration and AIDS', *The Lancet*, 346: 826–828.

Delaney, C. (1995) 'Father, motherland and the birth of modern Turkey', in S. Yanagisano and C. Delaney (eds), *Naturalizing Power*, New York: Routledge.

Deleuze, G. and Guattari, F. (1977 [orig. 1972]) *Anti-Oedipus: Capitalism and Schizophrenia*, New York: Viking Press.

Derrida, J. (1982) 'Choreographies', *Diacritics*, 12(12): 66–76.

—— (1992) 'Force of law: "the mystical foundation of authority"', in D. Cornell, M. Rosenfeld, and D.G. Carlson (eds) *Deconstruction and the Possibility of Justice*, New York and London: Routledge.

—— (1998) 'Faith and reason: the two sources of "religion" at the limits of reason alone', in J. Derrida and G. Vattimo (eds) *Religion*, Stanford: Stanford University Press.

Derrida, J. and Vattimo, G. (1998) *Religion*, Stanford: Stanford University Press.

Deverell, K. and Prout, A. (1999) 'Sexuality, identity and community: the experience of MESMAC', in R. Parker and P. Aggleton (eds) *Culture, Society and Sexuality: A Reader*, London: University College London Press.

di Mauro, D. (1995) *Sexuality Research in the United States*, New York: Social Science Resource Council.

di Mauro, D. and Joffe, C. (2007) 'The religious right and the reshaping of sexual policy: an examination of reproductive rights and sexuality education', *Sexuality Research and Social Policy*, 4(1): 67–92.

Díaz, R.M. (2000) 'Cultural regulation, self-regulation, and sexuality: a psycho-cultural model of HIV risk in Latino gay men', in R. Parker, R.M. Barbosa, and P. Aggleton (eds) *Framing the Sexual Subject: The Politics of Gender, Sexuality, and Power*, Berkeley, Los Angeles, and London: University of California Press.

Ditmore, M.H. (2007) 'Sex work, trafficking, and HIV: how development is compromising sex workers' human rights', in A. Cornwall, S. Corrêa, and S. Jolly (eds) *Development with a Body*, London: Zed Books.

Djordjevic, J. (2006) 'Vagina sisters, crying men, soap opera stars and sushi: the story of the *Vagina Monologues* in Belgrade', in A. Cornwall and S. Jolly (eds) *Sexuality Matters, IDS Bulletin*, 37(5): 127–133.

Donzelot, J. (1978) *The Policing of Families*, New York: Pantheon.

Doward, J. (2007) 'Alarm at US right to highly personal data: religion and sex life among passenger details to be passed on to officials', *Observer*, 22 July Available online at www.guardian.co.uk/print/03302387-105744,00.html (accessed 21 September 2007).

Dowsett, G. (1996) *Practicing Desire: Homosexual Sex in the Era of AIDS*, Stanford: Stanford University Press.

—— (2000) 'Body play: corporeality in a discursive silence', in R. Parker, R.M. Barbosa, and P. Aggleton (eds) *Framing The Sexual Subject: The Politics of Gender Sexuality and Power*, Berkeley: University of California Press.

—— (2003) 'Some considerations on sexuality and gender in the context of AIDS', *Reproductive Health Matters*, 11(22): 21–29.

Dowsett, G. and Couch, M. (2007) 'Male circumcision and HIV prevention: is there really enough of the right kind of evidence?', *Reproductive Health Matters*, 15(29): 33–44.

Duberman, M. (1997) 'Kinsey's urethra: review of *Alfred C. Kinsey: A Public/Private Life* by James H. Jones', *The Nation*, 3 November: 40–43.

Duggan, L. (1995). 'Queering the state', in L. Duggan and N.D. Hunter (eds) *Sex Wars: Sexual Dissent and Political Culture*, New York: Routledge.

—— (2004) 'Holy matrimony!', *The Nation*, 15 March.

Duggan, L. and Hunter, N. (2006) *Sex Wars: Sexual Dissent and Political Culture*, 10th Anniversary Edition, New York and London: Routledge.

Durkheim, E. (2001) *The Elementary Forms of Religious Life*, New York: Oxford University Press.

Eck, D.L. (2000) 'Religion and the global moment', *Macalester International*, 8(spring): 3–26.

Edelman, L. (1994) *Homographesis: Essays in Gay Literary and Cultural Theory*, New York and London: Routledge.

—— (1995) 'Queer theory: unstating desire', *GLQ: A Journal of Lesbian and Gay Studies* 2(4): 343–346.

Eisenstein, Z. (1988) *The Female Body and the Law*, Berkeley: University of California Press.

—— (1996) *Hatreds: Racialized and Sexualized Conflicts in the 21st Century*, New York: Routledge.

—— (2004) *Against Empire: Feminisms, Racism and the West*, London: Zed Books/Melbourne: Spinifex Press.

—— (2007) *Sexual Decoys: Gender, Race and War in Imperial Democracy*, London and New York: Zed Books.

Ellis, H. (1932) *Views and Reviews*, Boston and New York: Houghton Mifflin.

—— (1936) *Studies in the Psychology of Sex*, New York: Random House.

Elredge, N. (2004) *Rethinking Sex and the Selfish Gene*, New York: W.W. Norton.

Engels, F. (1884) *The Origin of the Family, Private Property and the State*. Available online at www.marxists.org/archive/marx/works/1884/origin-family/index.htm (accessed 19 August 2007).

Enloe, C. (2000) *Maneuvers: The International Politics of Militarizing Women's Lives*, Berkeley: University of California Press.

—— (2007) *Globalization and Militarism: Feminists Make the Link*, Lanham, MD, and Plymouth, UK: Rowman & Littlefield.

Epstein, H. (2007) *The Invisible Cure: Africa, the West, and the Fight Against AIDS*, New York: Farrar, Strauss & Giroux.

Epstein, S. (1996) *Impure Science: AIDS, Activism, and the Politics of Knowledge*, Berkeley: University of California Press.

Eribon, D. (1991) *Michel Foucault*, Cambridge, MA: Harvard University Press.

Erickson, J.A. and Steffen, S.A. (1999) *Kiss and Tell: Surveying Sex in the Twentieth Century*, Cambridge, MA, and London: Harvard University Press.

Erlanger, S. (2007) 'A life of unrest (profile of Khaled Abu Hilal)', *New York Times Magazine*, 15 July.

Esiet, N. (forthcoming) 'Sexuality education as a human right: lessons from Nigeria', in A. Cornwall, S. Corrêa, and S. Jolly (eds) *Development with a Body*, London: Zed Books.

Euben, R. (1999) *Enemy in the Mirror*, Princeton: Princeton University Press.

Ewen, S. and Ewen, E. (2006) *Typecasting: On The Arts and Sciences of Human Inequality*, New York: Seven Stories Press.

Ewing, K.P. (2002) 'Legislating religious freedom: Muslim challenges to the relationship between church and state in Germany and France', in R.A. Shweder, M. Minow, and H.R. Markus (eds) *Engaging Cultural Differences: The Multicultural Challenge in Liberal Democracies*, New York: Russel Sage Foundation.

Ezzat, H.R. (2002) *Rethinking Secularism ... Rethinking Feminism*. Available online at www.islamonline.net/english/Contemporary/2002/07/Article01.shtml (accessed 19 January 2007).

Faria, V. and Potter, J. (2002) 'Televisão, novela e queda da fecundidade no Nordeste', *Novos Estudos CEBRAP*, 62 (March): 21–39.

Farmer, P. (1992) *AIDS and Accusation: Haiti and the Geography of Blame*, Berkeley and Los Angeles: University of California Press.

—— (1995) 'Culture, poverty, and the dynamics of HIV transmission in rural Haiti', in H. ten Brummelhuis and G. Herdt (eds) *Culture and Sexual Risk: Anthropological Perspectives on AIDS*, Amsterdam: Gordon & Breach.

—— (1999) *Infections and Inequalities: The Modern Plagues*, Berkeley and Los Angeles: University of California Press.

Farmer, P., Connors, M., and Simmons, J. (eds) (1996) *Women, Poverty and AIDS: Sex, Drugs and Structural Violence*, Monroe, ME: Common Courage Press.

Fausto-Sterling, A. (1992) 'Why do we know so little about human sex?', *Discover*, June: 28–30.

—— (1993) 'The five sexes: why male and female are not enough', *The Sciences*, 43: 20–24.

—— (2000) *Sexing the Body: Gender Politics and the Construction of Sexuality*, New York: Basic Books.

Fee, E. (1997) 'The history and development of public health', in F.D. Scutchfield and C.W. Keck (eds) *Principles of Public Health Practice*, New York: Delmar.

Feinberg, L. (1996) *Transgender Warriors: Making History from Joan of Arc to RuPaul*, Boston: Beacon Press.

Feldman, J. (1975) 'Les rapports nationaux sur les comportements sexuels: un exemple de deux types d'interaction science-societé', *Archives Européenes de Sociologie*, 26: 95–110.

Fernandez, H. (2002) *A Resource Book on Lesbian, Gay and Bisexual Rights in India*, Mumbai: India Center for Human Rights and Law.

FIMI (Foro Internacional de Mujeres Indigenas) (2005) 'Feminism with an indigenous perspective or an indigenous feminist vision?', *MADRE*. Available online at www.madre.org (accessed 26 September 2007).

Firestone, S. (1970) *The Dialectic of Sex: A Case for Feminist Revolution*, New York: Farrar, Straus & Giroux.

Fisher, J. (2006) 'Transforming the table – global advocacy on sexual orientation and gender identity – and the international response', paper presented at the International Commission of Jurists and International Services on Human Rights Expert Meeting on Human Rights, Sexual Orientation and Gender Identity organized, Yogyakarta, Indonesia, November.

Ford, C.S. and Beach, F.A. (1951) *Patterns of Sexual Behavior*, New York: Harper & Brothers.

Foucault, M. (1977a) 'Power and sex: an interview with Michel Foucault', *Telos*, 32 (summer): 152–161.

—— (1977b) 'Preface', in G. Deleuze and F. Guattari, *Anti-Oedipus: Capitalism and Schizophrenia*, New York: Viking Press.

—— (1978 [orig. 1976]) *The History of Sexuality, Volume 1: An Introduction*, New York: Pantheon.

—— (1980) *Power/Knowledge: Selected Interviews and Other Writings, 1972–1977*, New York: Pantheon.

—— (1985) *The History of Sexuality, Volume 2: The Uses of Pleasure*, New York: Vintage Books.

—— (1988) *The History of Sexuality, Volume 3: The Care of the Self*, New York: Vintage Books.

—— (2003) *Society Must Be Defended: Lectures at the College De France 1975–1976*, New York: Picador.

Fraser, N. (1997) *Justice Interruptus: Critical Reflections on the 'Postsocialist' Condition*, New York and London: Routledge.

Freedman, D. (2005). '¿Estado laico o estado liberal?', in La Trampa de la Moral Única: argumentos para una democracia laica. Campaña 28 de Septiembre por la Despenalización del Aborto, Campaña Tu Boca Contra los Funadmentalismos, Campaña por la Convención de los Derechos Sexuales y Reproductivos, Lima, Peru. Available online at www.isis.cl/MujerySalud/Sexual/Documentos/doc/latrampa.pdf (accessed 20 December 2007).

Freedom House (2007) *Freedom in the World 2006*, New York and Lanham, MD: Freedom House/Rowman & Littlefield Publishers.

Freitas, A. (2001) 'Linking through closed doors', in *Trade, AIDS, Public Health and Human Rights, DAWN Informs*, Special Supplement(August): 9–11.

Freud, S. (1905; standard edn 1953) 'Three essays on the theory of sexuality', in *Complete Psychological Works*, Vol. 7, London: Hogarth Press.

—— (1962) *Civilization and Its Discontents*, New York: Norton.

Fried, S.T. and Landsberg-Lewis, I. (2000) 'Sexual rights: from concept to strategy', in K. Askin and D. Koenig (eds) *Women's Human Rights Reference Guide*, New York: Transnational Press.

Fry, P. (1982) *Para Inglês Ver: Identidade e Política na Cultura Brasileira*, Rio de Janeiro: Zahar.

Fullilove, M.T. (2005) *Root Shock: How Tearing Up City Neighborhoods Hurt America and What We Can Do About It*, New York: Ballantine Books.

Fuss, D. (ed.) (1991) *Inside/Out: Lesbian Theories, Gay Theories*, New York and London: Routledge.

Gadamer, H.F. (1998) 'Dialogues in Capri', in J. Derrida and G. Vattimo (eds) *Religion*, Stanford: Stanford University Press.

Gagnon, J.H. (2004) *An Interpretation of Desire: Essays in the Study of Sexuality*, Chicago: University of Chicago Press.

Gagnon, J.H. and Parker, R. (1995) 'Conceiving sexuality', in R. Parker and J.H. Gagnon (eds) *Conceiving Sexuality: Approaches to Sex Research in a Postmodern World*, New York and London: Routledge.

Gagnon, J.H. and Simon, W.S. (1973) *Sexual Conduct: The Social Sources of Human Sexuality*, Chicago: Aldine.

Gago, V. (2006) 'Feminismo y izquierda en América Latina: relaciones peligrosas', *Página 12* (December). Available online at www.mulheresdeolho.org.br/?p=157 (accessed 27 December 2006).

Gallop, J. (1982) *The Daughter's Seduction: Feminism and Psychoanalysis*, Ithaca: Cornell University Press.

—— (1987) *Reading Lacan*, Ithaca: Cornell University Press.

Garcia, J. and Parker, R. (2006) 'From global discourse to local actions: the makings of a sexual rights movement', *Horizontes Antropológicos*, 12(26): 13–42.

Gaspari, E. (2007) 'O papa e o padre polonês anti-semita' *Folha de São Paulo*, 12 September. Available online at http://www1.folha.uol.com.br/fsp/brasil/fc1209200719.htm (accessed 28 November 2007).

Gebhard, P.H. and Johnson, A.B. (1979) *The Kinsey Data: Marginal Tabulations of 1938–1963, Interviews conducted by the Institute for Sex Research*, Philadelphia: W.B. Saunders.

Geertz, C. (1973) *The Interpretation of Cultures*, New York: Basic Books.

—— (1983) *Local Knowledge*, New York: Basic Books.

Gender Health (2007a) 'Policy brief: implications of U.S. policy restrictions for programs aimed at commercial sex workers and victims of trafficking worldwide'. Available online at www.genderhealth.org/pubs/ProstitutionOathImplications.pdf (accessed 10 September 2007).

—— (2007b) 'Timeline: application of the "Prostitution Loyalty Oath" in U.S. global AIDS policy'. Available online at www.genderhealth.org/loyaltyoath.php (accessed 10 September 2007).

General Assembly's Declaration on the Elimination of Violence against Women (1993) United Nations General Assembly Resolution 48/104 of 20. Available online at www.unhchr.ch/huridocda/huridoca.nsf/(Symbol)/A.RES.48.104.En (accessed 18 November 2007).

Gentleman, A. (2007) 'Setback for Novartis in India over drug patent protection', *New York Times*, 7 August.

Gerhardsen, T.I.S. (2007) 'Quiet TRIPS meeting expected'. Available online at www.ip-watch.org/weblog/index.php?p=499&res=1024_ff&print=0 (accessed 26 September 2007).

Gettleman, J. (2007) 'Chaos in Darfur rises as Arabs fight with Arabs', *New York Times*, 3 September.

Ghosh, H.A. (2002) 'Feminist perspective: September 11th and Afghan women'. Available online at http://www/ncmonline.como/content/ncn/2002/jan (accessed 21 January 2002).

Giami, A. (1991) 'De Kinsey au sida: l'evolution de la construccion du comportement sexuel dans les enquetes quantitatives', *Sciences Sociales et Santé*, 4: 23–56.

—— (1996) 'The ACSF survey questionnaire: the influence of an epidemiological representation of sexuality', in M. Bozon and H. Leridon (eds) *Sexuality and the Social Sciences: A French Survey on Sexual Behaviour*, Aldershot: Dartmouth Publishing.

Giddens, A. (1990) *The Consequences of Modernity*, Cambridge: Polity Press.

—— (1992) *The Transformation of Intimacy: Sexuality, Love and Eroticism in Modern Societies*, Cambridge: Polity Press.

—— (2000) *Runaway World*, London and New York: Routledge.

Girard, F. (2004) *Global Implications of U.S. Domestic and International Policies on Sexuality*, Sexuality Policy Watch. Available online at www.sxpolitics.org/mambo452/index.php?option=com_docman&task=cat_view&gid=7&Itemid=2 (accessed 18 August 2007).

—— (2007) 'Negotiating sexual rights and sexual orientation at the UN', in R. Parker, R. Petchesky, and R. Sember (eds) *SexPolitics: Reports from the Frontlines*, Sexuality Policy Watch. Available online at www.sxpolitics.org/frontlines/home/index.php (accessed 22 November 2007).

Girard, F. and Waldman, W. (2000) 'Ensuring the reproductive rights of refugees and internally displaced persons: legal and policy issues', *International Family Planning Perspectives*, 26(4): 167–173.

Glanz, J. (2007) 'Inspectors find rebuilt projects crumbling in Iraq', *New York Times*, 29 April. Available online at www.nytimes.com/2007/04/29/world/middleeast/29reconstruct.html?hp (accessed 28 November 2007).

Glanz, J. and Farrell, S. (2007) 'More Iraqis said to flee since troop rise', *New York Times*, 24 August. Available online at www.nytimes.com/2007/08/24/world/middleeast/24displaced.html?pagewanted=print (accessed 28 November 2007).

Glanz, J. and Grady, D. (2007) 'Cholera epidemic infects 7,000 people in Northern Iraq', *New York Times*, 12 September.

Global Rights (2006) 'Letter to President Obasanjo'. Available online at www.globalrights.org/site/DocServer/Letter_-_Obasanjo_-_3.pdf?docID=4803 (accessed 15 May 2007).

Goffman, E. (1959) *The Presentation of Self in Everyday Life*, New York: Doubleday.

—— (1963) *Stigma: Notes on the Management of Spoiled Identity*, New York: Simon & Schuster.

Golden, T. (2006) 'U.S. should close prison in Cuba U.N. panel says', *New York Times*, 20 May.

Goldenweiser, A. (1929) 'Sex and primitive society', in V.F. Calverton and S.D. Schmalhausen (eds) *Sex in Civilization*, New York: Macaulay.

González Block, M.A. and Liguori, A.L. (1992) *El SIDA en los Estratos Socioeconómicos de México*, Cuernavaca: Instituto Nacional de Salud Pública.

Goodchild, P. (1996) *Deleuze and Guattari: An Introduction to the Politics of Desire*, Newbury Park, CA: Sage.

Gordon, L. (1976) *Woman's Body, Woman's Right: A Social History of Birth Control in America*, New York: Grossman.

Gould, S.J. (1981) *The Mismeasure of Man*, New York: Norton.

Grabham, E. (2007) 'Citizen bodies, intersex citizenship', *Sexualities*, 10(1): 29–48.

Greenhalgh, S. (1996) 'The social construction of population science: an intellectual, institutional, and political history of 20th century demography', *Comparative Studies in Society and History*, 38(1): 26–66.

Greenhouse, L. (2006) 'Guantanamo case: military panels found to lack authority – new law possible', *New York Times*, 30 June.

Greer, G. (1970) *The Female Eunuch*, New York: Bantam Books.

Gregg, J. (2003) *Virtually Virgins: Sexual Strategies and Cervical Cancer in Recife, Brazil*, Stanford: Stanford University Press.

Gregor, T. (1985) *Anxious Pleasures: The Sexual Lives of an Amazonian People*, Chicago: University of Chicago Press.

Gregori, M.F. (2004) 'Prazer e perigo: notas sobre feminismo, sex-shops e S/M', in A. Piscitelli, S. Carrara, and M.F. Gregori (eds) *Sexualidades, Saberes, Convenções e Fronteiras*, Rio de Janeiro: Garamond.

Grewal, I. (1998) 'On the new global feminism and the family of nations: dilemmas of transnational feminist practice', in E. Shohat (ed.) *Talking Visions: Multicultural Feminism in a Transnational Age*, Cambridge, MA: MIT Press.

Grosz, E. (1990) *Jacques Lacan: A Feminist Introduction*, London and New York: Routledge.

Guimarães, R. (ed.) (2005) *The Inequality Predicament: Report on the World Social Situation*, New York: United Nations.

Gupta, A. (2002) 'Trends in the application of Section 377', in B. Fernandez (ed.) *Humjinsi: A Resource Book on Lesbian, Gay and Bisexual Rights in India*, Mumbai: India Center for Human Rights and Law.

—— (2005) 'Narratives of corruption', *Ethnography*, 6(1): 5–34.

Gupta, G.R. and Weiss, E. (1993) 'Women's lives and sex: implications for AIDS prevention', *Culture, Medicine and Psychiatry*, 17(4): 399–412.

Halberstam, J. (1998) *Female Masculinity*, Durham, NC, and London: Duke University Press.

Halper, S. and Clarke, J. (2004) *America Alone: The Neo-conservatives and the Global Order*, Cambridge: Cambridge University Press.

Halperin, D.M. (1990) *One Hundred Years of Homosexuality*, New York and London: Routledge.

—— (1996) *Saint Foucault: Towards a Gay Hagiography*, Oxford: Oxford University Press.

—— (2002) *How to Do the History of Homosexuality*, Chicago: University of Chicago Press.

Hamburger, E. and Buarque de Holanda, H. (2004) 'Sociologia, pesquisa de mercado e sexualidade na mídia: aundências vs. Imagens', in A. Piscitelli, S. Carrara, and M.F. Gregori (eds) *Sexualidades, Saberes, Convenções e Fronteiras*, Rio de Janeiro: Garamond.

Haraway, D. (2004) *The Haraway Reader*, New York and London: Routledge.

Harding, L. (2004) 'The other prisoners', *Guardian*, 20 May.

Harrell-Bond, B.E. (2002) 'Can humanitarian work with refugees be humane?', *Human Rights Quarterly*, 24(1): 51–85.

Hartmann, B. (1995) *Reproductive Rights and Wrongs: The Global Politics of Population Control*, Boston: South End Press.

Harvey, D. (2005) *A Brief History of Neoliberalism*, Oxford and New York: Oxford University Press.

Heald, S. (1995) 'The power of sex: some reflections on the Caldwells' "African Sexuality" thesis', *Africa: Journal of the International African Institute*, 65(4): 489–505.

Heilborn, M.L., Aquino, E., Bozon, M., and Knauth, D.R. (eds) (2006) *O Aprendizado da Sexualidade: Reprodução e Trajetórias Sociais de Jovens Brasileiros*, Rio de Janeiro: Editora Fiocruz and Editora Garamond.

Held, D., Goldblatt, D., McGrew, A., and Perraton, J. (1999) *Global Transformations: Politics, Economics and Culture*, Cambridge: Polity Press.

Henriksson, B. (1995) *Risk Factor Love: Homosexuality, Sexual Interaction and HIV Prevention*, Göteborg, Sweden: Göteborgs Universitet.

Herdt, G. (1981) *Guardians of the Flutes: Idioms of Masculinity*, New York: McGraw-Hill.

—— (ed.) (1992) *Gay Culture in America: Essays from the Field*, Boston: Beacon Press.

—— (ed.) (1997) *Sexual Cultures and Migration in the Era of AIDS: Anthropological and Demographic Perspectives*, Oxford: Clarendon Press.

Herdt, G. and Lindenbaum, S. (eds) (1992) *The Time of AIDS: Social Analysis, Theory, and Method*, Newbury Park, CA: Sage.

Hersh, S.M. (2004) *Chain of Command: The Road from 9/11 to Abu Ghraib*, New York: HarperCollins.

Hirsch, J. (2003) *A Courtship After Marriage: Sexuality and Love in Mexican Transnational Families*, Berkeley, Los Angeles and London: University of California Press.

Hocquenghem, G. (1978) *Homosexual Desire*, London: Allison & Busby.

Holland, E. (1999) *Deleuze and Guattari's Anti Oedipus: Introduction to Schizoanalysis*, New York and London: Routledge.

Holland, J., Ramazanoglu, C., Sharp, S., and Thompson, R. (1998) *The Male in the Head*, London: Tufnell Press.

Honigman, J.J. (1954) 'An anthropological approach to sex', *Social Problems*, 2(1): 7–16.

HRW (Human Rights Watch) (1996) *Shattered Lives: Sexual Violence During the Rwandan Genocide and its Aftermath*, Index No. 2084, New York: Human Rights Watch.

—— (1999) '*Annual Report* – section IV'. Available online at www.hrw.org/reports/1999/indiachr/christians8–04.htm (accessed 12 September 12 2007).

—— (2002) 'Epidemic of abuse: police harassment of HIV/AIDS outreach workers in India', 14(5): C. Available online at hrw.org/english/docs/2002/07/10/india12865.htm (accessed 22 November 2007).

—— (2004a) 'Hated to death: homophobia, violence, and Jamaica's HIV/AIDS epidemic', *Human Rights Watch*, 16(6).

—— (2004b) 'Scandal and stigma: the queen boat trials'. Available online at http://hrw.org/reports/2004/egypt0304/3.htm (accessed 5 May 2007).

—— (2004c) 'In a time of torture: the assault on justice in Egypt's crackdown on homosexual conduct'. Available online at http://hrw.org/reports/2004/egypt 0304/index.htm (accessed 29 October 2007).

—— (2005) 'China shuts down gay and lesbian event'. Available online at http://hrw.org/english/docs/2005/12/20/china12328_txt.htm (accessed 28 August 2007).

—— (2006a) 'Nigeria: Obasanjo must withdraw bill to criminalize gay rights'. Available online at http://hrw.org/english/docs/2006/03/23/nigeri13066_txt.htm (accessed 15 May 2007).

—— (2006b) 'Nigeria: anti-gay bill threatens democratic reforms'. Available online at http://hrw.org/english/docs/2007/02/28/nigeri15431.htm (accessed 29 August 2007).

—— (2007a) 'Christian leaders in US condemn Nigeria's anti-gay bill – persecution and hatred not Christian values'. Available online at http://hrw.org/english/docs/2007/02/27/nigeri15424.htm (accessed 15 May 2007).

—— (2007b) 'Poland: school censorship proposal threatens basic rights'. Available online at http://hrw.org/english/docs/2007/03/16/poland15512.htm (accessed 28 August 2007).

—— (2007c) 'Russia: gay rights under attack'. Available online at http://hrw.org/english/docs/2007/06/13/russia16174.htm (accessed 28 August 2007).

—— (2007d) 'Movements and moral panics'. Available online at http://hrw.org/wr2k5/anatomy/2.htm (accessed 23 August 2007).

—— (2007e) *Israel/Lebanon: Israeli Indiscriminate Attacks Killed Most Civilians.* Available online at http://hrw.org/english/docs/2007/09/06/isrlpa16781.htm (accessed 17 November 2007).

—— (2007f) *South Africa: Lesbians Targeted for Murder.* Available online at http://hrw.org/english/docs/2007/08/08/safric16617.htm (accessed 17 November 2007).

HRW (Human Rights Watch) and ILGA (International Lesbian and Gay Association), European Region (2007) ' "We have the upper hand" – freedom of assembly in Russia and the human rights of lesbian, gay, bisexual, and transgender people'. Available online at http://hrw.org/backgrounder/lgbt/moscow0607/ (accessed 4 September 2007).

Hubbard, R. (1990) *The Politics of Women's Biology,* New Brunswick: Rutgers University Press.

Hubert, M., Bajos, N., and Sandfort, T. (eds) (1998) *Sexual Behaviour and HIV/AIDS in Europe,* London: University College London Press.

Hunt, P. (2004) 'Economic, social and cultural rights: the right of everyone to the enjoyment of the highest attainable standard of physical and mental health', Report of the Special Rapporteur, UN Commission on Human Rights, 60th Session, 16 February.

Hunter, J.D. (1992) *Culture Wars: The Struggle to Define America,* New York: Basic Books.

Hunter, M. (2002) 'The materiality of everyday sex: thinking beyond "prostitution" ', *African Studies,* 61: 99–120.

—— (2005) 'Cultural politics and masculinities: multiple-partners in historical perspective in KwaZulu-Natal', *Culture, Health and Sexuality,* 7: 209–223.

Hynes, M., Sheik, M., Wilson, H.G., and Spiegel, P. (2002) 'Reproductive health indicators and outcomes among refugee and internally displaced persons in post-emergency phase camps', *Journal of the American Medical Association,* 288(5): 595–603.

ICJ (International Commission of Jurists) (2004) International Human Rights References to Non-discrimination on the Grounds of Sexual Orientation, Geneva. Available online at www.icj.org (accessed 28 September 2007).

ICPC (International Committee for Peace Council) (2004) 'Religion and women: an agenda for change', Declaration approved at meeting on Women and Religions in a Globalized World, Chiang Mai, Thailand, 29 February to 29 March.

Available online at www.peacecouncil.org/ChiangMai.html (accessed 25 November 2007).

IGLHRC (International Gay and Lesbian Human Rights Commission) (2007a) 'LGBT Nigerians' responses to the same-sex Prohibition Act'. Available online at www.iglhrc.org/site/iglhrc/section.php?id=5&detail=714 (accessed 15 May 2007).

—— (2007b) 'Voices from Nigeria'. Available online at www.iglhrc.org/site/iglhrc/ section.php?id=5&detail=695 (accessed 15 May 2007).

IGLHRC (International Gay and Lesbian Human Rights Commission) and CWGL (Center for Women's Global Leadership) (2005) *Written Out: How Sexuality is Used to Attack Women's Organizing*, New York: IGLHRC and CWGL.

IHRC (International Human Rights Commission) and SMU (Sexual Minorities Uganda) (2006) *Report on the Rights of Lesbian, Gay, Bisexual, and Transgender People in the Republic of Uganda under the African Charter of Human and People's Rights*. Available online at www.iglhrc.org/files/iglhrc/reports/ Uganda%20Shadow%20Report%20.pdf (accessed 15 May 2007).

IIJG (International Initiative for Justice in Gujarat) (2003) *Threatened Existence: A Feminist Analysis of the Genocide in Gujarat*, Bombay: Forum Against Oppression of Women.

ILGA (International Gay and Lesbian Association) (2007) *World Legal Survey*. Available online at www.ilga.info/Information/Legal_survey/ilga_world_legal_ survey%20introduction.htm (accessed 23 August 2007).

Ilkkaracan, P. (2000) *Women and Sexuality in Muslim Societies*, Istanbul: Women for Women's Human Rights – New Ways.

—— (2007) 'How adultery almost derailed Turkey's aspiration to join the European Union', in R. Parker, R. Petchesky, and R. Sember (eds) *SexPolitics: Reports from the Frontlines*. Sexuality Policy Watch. Available online at www.sxpolitics.org/frontlines/home/index.php (accessed 22 November 2007).

Ilkkaracan, P. and Jolly, S. (2007) 'Gender and sexuality: overview report', BRIDGE/Development, Institute of Development Studies, Brighton. Available online at www.bridge.ids.ac.uk/reports/CEP-Sexuality-OR.pdf (accessed 22 November 2007).

Ilkkaracan, P. and Seral, G. (2000) 'Sexual pleasure as a human right', in P. Ilkkaracan (ed.) *Women and Sexuality in Muslim Societies*, Istanbul: Women for Women's Human Rights – New Ways.

Imam, A. (2000) 'The Muslim right ("fundamentalists")', in P. Ilkkaracan (ed.) *Women and Sexuality in Muslim Societies*, Istanbul: Women for Women's Rights – New Ways.

—— (2005) 'Women's reproductive and sexual rights and the offence of Zina in Muslim laws in Nigeria', in W. Chavkin and E. Chesler (eds) *Where Human Rights Begin – Health, Sexuality, and Women in the New Millennium*, New Brunswick: Rutgers University Press.

Institute of Medicine/National Academy of Sciences (1986) *Confronting AIDS: Directions for Public Health, Health Care, and Research*, Washington, DC: Institute of Medicine/National Academy of Sciences.

Iraq Body Count (2007) Available online at www.iraqbodycount.org/ (accessed 17 November 2007).

Irvine, J. (ed.) (1994) *Sexual Cultures and the Construction of Adolescent Identities*, Philadelphia: Temple University Press.

Jackson, P. (1989) *Dear Uncle Go: Male Homosexuality in Thailand*, Bangkok: Bua Luang Publishing.

—— (1997) '*Kathoey* – gay – man: the historical emergence of gay male identity in Thailand', in L. Manderson and M. Jolly (eds) *Sites of Desire/Economies of Pleasure: Sexualities in Asia and the Pacific*, Chicago: University of Chicago Press.

—— (2007) 'An explosion of Thai identities: global queering and re-imagining queer theory', in R. Parker and P. Aggleton (eds) *Culture Society and Sexuality: A Reader*, London: Routledge.

Jacobs, H. (1987) 'Incidents in the life of a slave girl', in H.L. Gates, Jr. (ed.) *The Classic Slave Narratives*, New York: New American Library.

Jacobson, J. (2006) 'Analysis of the Uganda political situation', paper presented to a Sexuality Policy Watch research meeting in Toronto, August.

Jagose, A. (1996) *Queer Theory*, Melbourne: University of Melbourne Press.

Jakobsen, J.R. and Pellegrini, A. (2003) *Love the Sin: Sexual Regulation and the Limits of Religious Tolerance*, New York: New York University Press.

Jantzen, G.M. (1995) *Power, Gender and Christian Mysticism*, Cambridge: Cambridge University Press.

—— (2000) 'Good sex', in P.B. Jung, M.E. Hunt, and R. Balakrishna (eds) *Good Sex: Feminist Perspectives from the World's Religions*, New Brunswick: Rutgers University Press.

Jayasree, A.K. (2004) 'Searching for justice for body and self in a coercive environment: sex work in Kerala, India', *Reproductive Health Matters*, 12(23): 58–67.

Jelen, T.G. and Wilcox, C. (eds) (2002) *Religion and Politics in Comparative Perspective: The One, The Few, and The Many*, Cambridge: Cambridge University Press.

John, M. and Nair, J. (1998) *A Question of Silence: The Sexual Economies of Modern India*, New Delhi: Kali for Women.

Johnson, A., Field, J., Wadsworth, J., and Wellings, K. (1994) *Sexual Attitudes and Lifestyles*, London: Blackwell Scientific.

Johnson, C. (2004) *The Sorrows of Empire: Militarism, Secrecy, and the End of the Republic*, New York: Metropolitan Books.

Jones, E. (1961) *Life and Work of Sigmund Freud*, New York: Basic Books.

Jones, J.H. (1997) *Alfred C. Kinsey: A Public/Private Life*, New York: Norton.

Jordan, W.D. (1968) *White Over Black: American Attitudes Towards the Negro, 1550–1812*, New York and London: W.W. Norton.

Jung, P.B., Hunt, M.E., and Balakrishna, R. (eds) (2001) *Good Sex: Feminist Perspectives from the World Religions*, New Brunswick: Rutgers University Press.

Kahn, S. (1996) 'Under the blanket: bisexualities and AIDS in India', in P. Aggleton (ed.) *Bisexualities and AIDS: International Perspectives*, London: Taylor & Francis.

Kammerer, C.A., Hutheesing, O.K., Maneeprasert, R., and Symonds, P.V. (1995) 'Vulnerability to HIV infection among three hill tribes in northern Thailand', in H. Brummelhuis and G. Herdt (eds) *Culture and Sexual Risk: Anthropological Perspectives on AIDS*, New York: Gordon & Breach.

Kapur, R. (2002) 'The tragedy of victimization rhetoric: resurrecting the "native" subject in international/post-colonial feminist legal politics', *Harvard Human Rights Journal*, 15: 1–37.

—— (2005) *Erotic Justice: Law and the New Politics of Post-colonialism*, London: Glasshouse Press.

Katz, J. (1976) *Gay American History: Lesbians and Gay Men in the USA*, New York: Avon Books.

—— (1995) *The Invention of Heterosexuality*, New York: Dutton.

Kaul, I., Grunberg, I., and Stern, M.A. (1999) *Global Public Goods: International Cooperation in the 21st Century*, New York: UNDP/Oxford University Press.

Kelves, D.J. (1985) *In the Name of Eugenics: Genetics and the Uses of Human Heredity*, New York: Knopf.

Kempadoo, K. (1998) 'Globalizing sex workers' rights', in K. Kempadoo and J. Doezema (eds) *Global Sex Workers: Rights, Resistance, and Redefinition*, New York and London: Routledge.

—— (ed.) (1999) *Sun, Sex, and Gold: Tourism and Sex Work in the Caribbean*, Lanham, MD: Rowman & Littlefield.

—— (2005) 'Shifting the debate on the traffic of women', *Cadernos Pagu*, 25: 55–78. Available online at www.scielo.br/scielo.php?script=sci_arttext& pid=S0104–83332005000200003&lng=en&nrm=iso (accessed 4 September 2007).

Kempadoo, K. and Doezema, J. (1998) *Global Sex Workers: Rights, Resistance, and Redefinition*, New York and London: Routledge.

Kendall, K. (1998) ' "When a woman loves a woman" in Lesotho: love, sex and the (Western) construction of homophobia', in S.O. Murray and W. Roscoe (eds) *Boy-wives and Female Husbands: Studies in African Homosexualities*, New York: Palgrave.

Kennedy, M.D. and Davis, E.L. (1993) *Boots of Leather, Slipper of Gold: The History of A Lesbian Community*, Harmondsworth: Penguin.

Kessler, S. and McKenna, W. (1978) *Gender: An Ethnomethodological Approach*, Chicago: University of Chicago Press.

Khalidi, R. (2004) *Resurrecting Empire: Western Footprints and America's Perilous Path in the Middle East*, Boston: Beacon Press.

Kheshwa, B. and Wieringa, S. (2005) ' "My attitude is manly … a girl needs to walk on the aisle": butch-femme subculture in Johannesburg, South Africa', in R. Morgan and S. Wieringa (eds) *Tommy Boys, Lesbian Men and Ancestral Wives: Female Same-sex Practices in Africa*, Johannesburg: Jacana.

Kinsey, A., Martin, C.E., and Pomeroy, W. (1948) *Sexual Behavior in the Human Male*, Philadelphia: Saunders.

Kinsey, A., Martin, C.E., Gebhard, R.H., and Pomeroy, W. (1953) *Sexual Behavior in the Human Female*, Philadelphia: Saunders.

Kippax, S., Connell, R., Crawford, J., and Dowsett, G. (1993) *Sustaining Safer Sex: Gay Communities Respond to AIDS*, London: Falmer Press.

Kirp, D.L. and Bayer, R. (1992) *AIDS in the Industrialized Democracies: Passions, Politics, and Policies*, New Brunswick: Rutgers University Press.

Kissling, F. (1999) 'Roman Catholic fundamentalism: what's sex (and power) got to do with it?', in C.W. Howland (ed.) *Religious Fundamentalisms and the Human Rights of Women*, New York: St Martin's Press.

—— (2003) 'Dancing against the Vatican', in R. Morgan (ed.) *Sisterhood is Forever: The Women's Anthology for a New Millennium*, New York: Washington Square Press.

Klassen, A.D., Levitt, E.E., and Williams, C.J. (1989) *Sex and Morality in the U.S.: An Empirical Enquiry Under the Auspices of the Kinsey Institute*, Middleton, CT: Wesleyan University Press.

Kligman, G. (1998) *The Politics of Duplicity: Controlling Reproduction in Ceau{s}escu's Romania*, Berkeley: University of California Press.

Klugman, B. (2000) 'Sexual rights in Southern Africa: a Beijing discourse or strategic necessity?', *Health and Human Rights*, 4(2): 144–173.

Knerr, W. and Philpott, A. (2006) 'Putting the sexy back into safer sex: the pleasure project', *IDS Bulletin*, 37(5): 105–109.

Kontula, O. and Haavio-Mannila, E. (1995) *Sexual Pleasures: Enhancement of Sex Life in Finland 1971–1992*, Aldershot: Dartmouth.

Kordela, A.K. (2005) 'A grammar of sensual and visceral reason', *Parallax*, 11(3): 55–71.

Kothari, S. and Sethi, H. (eds) (1991) *Rethinking Human Rights: Challenges for Theory and Action*, New York/Lokayan, Delhi: New Horizons Press.

Kotiswaran, P. (2001) 'Preparing for civil disobedience: Indian sex workers and the law', *Boston College Third World Law Journal*, 21(2). Available online at www.bc.edu/bc_org/avp/law/lwsch/journals/bctwj/21_2/01_FMS.htm (accessed 4 September 2007).

Krafft-Ebing, R. (1939 [orig. 1886]) *Psychopathia Sexualis*, 12th edn, New York: Pioneer Press.

Kulick, D. (1998) *Travesti: Sex, Gender and Culture among Brazilian Transgendered Prostitutes*, Chicago: University of Chicago Press.

Lacan, J. (1968) *The Language of the Self: The Function of Language in Psychoanalysis*, Baltimore: Johns Hopkins University Press.

—— (1977) *Écrits: A Selection*, New York: W.W. Norton.

—— (1981) *Speech and Language in Psychoanalysis*, Baltimore: Johns Hopkins University Press.

Lamberts-Bendroth, M. (1999) 'Fundamentalism and the family: gender, culture, and the American Pro-family Movement', *Journal of Women's History*, 10: 35–54.

Lancaster, R.N. (1992) *Life is Hard: Machismo, Danger, and the Intimacy of Power in Nicaragua*, Berkeley and Los Angeles: University of California Press.

—— (1995) ' "That we should all turn queer?": homosexual stigma in the making of manhood and the breaking of a revolution in Nicaragua', in R. Parker and J.H. Gagnon (eds) *Conceiving Sexuality: Approaches to Sex Research in a Postmodern World*, New York and London: Routledge.

Lancaster, R.N. and di Leonardo, M. (eds) (1997) *The Gender/Sexuality Reader: Culture, History, Political Economy*, New York and London: Routledge.

Landesman, P.A. (2002) 'Woman's work', *New York Times Magazine*, 15 September.

Lasky, M.P. (2006) *Iraqi Women Under Siege*. Report by CODEPINK: Women for Peace and Global Exchange. Available online at www.codepink4peace.org (accessed 27 September 2007).

Laumann, E. and Gagnon, J. (1995) 'A sociological perspective on sexual action', in R. Parker and J. Gagnon (eds) *Conceiving Sexuality: Approaches to Sex Research in a Postmodern World*, New York and London: Routledge.

Laumann, E., Ellingson, S., Mahay, J., Paik, A., and Youm, Y. (eds) (2004) *The*

Sexual Organization of the City, Chicago and London: University of Chicago Press.

Laumann, E.O., Gagnon, J.H., and Michael, R.T. (1994a) 'A political history of the national sex survey of adults', *Family Planning Perspectives*, 26(1): 34–38.

Laumann, E.O., Gagnon, J.H., Michael, R.T., and Michaels, S. (1994b) *The Social Organization of Sexuality: Sexual Practices in the United States*, Chicago: University of Chicago Press.

Laurie, M. and Petchesky, R. (2008) 'Gender, health, and human rights in sites of political exclusion', *Global Public Health*, 3(1): 25–41.

Laws, J. and Schwartz, P. (1977) *Sexual Scripts: The Social Construction of Female Sexuality*, Hinsdale, IL: Dryden Press.

Lawyers Collective (2001) Writ Petition in Delhi High Court (mimeo).

Leap, W. (ed.) (1999) *Public Sex, Gay Space*, New York: Columbia University Press.

Lederer, E.M. (2006) 'Women under attack in Iraq, Afghanistan', *Boston Globe*, 27 October.

Le Minh, G. and Nguyen, T.M.H. (2007) 'From family planning to HIV/AIDS in Vietnam: shifting priorities, remaining gaps', in R. Parker, R. Petchesky, and R. Sember (eds) *SexPolitics: Reports from the Frontlines*. Sexuality Policy Watch. Available online at www.sxpolitics.org/frontlines/home/index.php (accessed 22 November 2007).

Levinas, E. (2003) *Humanism of the Other*. Urbana and Chicago: University of Illinois Press.

Levine, M.P., Gagnon, J.H., and Nardi, P.M. (eds) (1997) *In Changing Times: Gay Men and Lesbians Encounter HIV/AIDS*, Chicago: University of Chicago Press.

Lewis, J. and Gordon, G. (2006) 'Terms of contact and touching change: investigating pleasure in an HIV epidemic', *Sexuality Matters, IDS Bulletin*, 37(5): 110–116.

Long, S. (2004) 'When doctors torture; the anus and the State in Egypt and beyond', *Health and Human Rights, Special Focus Sexuality*, 7(2): 114–140.

—— (2006) 'Violence erupts'. Available online at http://washingtonblade.com/2006/redpride/index.cfm (accessed 28 August 2007).

Longmore, M.A. (1998) 'Symbolic interactionism and the study of sexuality', *Journal of Sex Research*, 35(1): 44–57.

Lorde, A. (1984) *Sister Outsider: Essays and Speeches*, Trumansberg, NY: The Crossing Press.

Lorway, R. (2006) 'Dispelling "heterosexual African AIDS" in Namibia: same-sex sexuality in the township of Katutura', *Culture, Health and Sexuality*, 8(5): 435–449.

Lotringer, S. (1996) *Foucault Live: Interviews, 1961–1984*, Cambridge, MA: MIT Press.

Luibhéid, E. (2002) *Entry Denied: Controlling Sexuality at the Border*, Minneapolis: University of Minnesota Press.

Luibhéid, E. and Cantú, L. (2005) *Queer Migrations: Sexuality, US Citizenship and Border Crossings*, Minneapolis: University of Minnesota Press.

Lurie, P., Hintzen, P., and Lowe, R.A. (1995) 'Socioeconomic obstacles to HIV prevention and treatment in developing countries: the roles of the International Monetary Fund and the World Bank', *AIDS*, 9: 539–546.

Lützen, K. (1995) '*La mise en discours* and silences in research on the history of sexuality', in R. Parker and J. Gagnon (eds) *Conceiving Sexuality: Approaches to Sex Research in a Postmodern World*, New York and London: Routledge.

MacCormack, C. and Strathern, M. (eds) (1980) *Nature, Culture and Gender*, Cambridge: Cambridge University Press.

Macklin, A. (2004) 'Like oil and water, with a match: militarized commerce, armed conflict, and human security in Sudan', in W. Gyles and J. Hyndman (eds) *Sites of Violence: Gender and Conflict Zones*, Berkeley: University of California Press.

MADRE (2006) War on civilians: a MADRE guide to the Middle East Crisis. Available online at http://madre.org/articles/me/waroncivilians.html (accessed 19 July 2007).

Mahmood, S. (2005) *Politics of Piety*, Princeton and Oxford: Princeton University Press.

Malinowski, B. (1927) *Sex and Repression in Savage Society*, New York: Harcourt, Brace & Company.

—— (1929) *The Sexual Life of Savages in North-western Melanesia*, London: Routledge.

—— (1944) *A Scientific Theory of Culture and Other Essays*, Chapel Hill: University of North Carolina Press.

Maluwa, M., Aggleton, P., and Parker, R. (2002) 'HIV and AIDS-related stigma, discrimination, and human rights', *Health and Human Rights*, 6(1): 1–18.

Mama, A., Pereira, C., and Manuh, T. (2005) 'Editorial: sexual cultures', *Feminist Africa*, 5. Available online at www.feministafrica.org/05-2005/editorial.html (accessed 22 November 2007).

Manalansan, M. (2003) *Global Divas: Filipino Gay Men in the Diaspora*, Durham, NC: Duke University Press.

Manderson, L. (1992) 'Public sex performances in Patpong and explorations of the edges of imagination', *Journal of Sex Research*, 29: 451–475.

Manderson, L. and Jolly, M. (eds) (1997) *Sites of Desire/Economies of Pleasure: Sexualities in Asia and the Pacific*, Chicago: University of Chicago Press.

Mannoni, O. (1971) *Freud*, New York: Pantheon Books.

Marcuse, H. (1966) *Eros and Civilization: A Philosophical Inquiry on Freud*, 2nd edn, Boston: Beacon Press.

Marsh, M., Navani, S., and Purdin, S. (2006) 'Addressing sexual violence in humanitarian emergencies', *Global Public Health*, 1(2): 133–146.

Martinot, S. and James, J. (eds) (2001) *The Problems of Resistance: Studies in Alternate Political Cultures*, Amherst, NY: Prometheus Books.

Masike, L. (2007) 'Tensions as 18 homosexuals appear in court', *Behind the Mask*. Available online at www.mask.org.za/article.php?cat=nigeria&id=1675 (accessed 4 September 2007).

Mayer, J. (2005) 'The experiment', *New Yorker*, 11 and 18 July.

—— (2006) 'The hidden power', *New Yorker*, 3 July.

—— (2007) 'The black sites', *New Yorker*, 13 August.

McFadden, P. (2003) 'Sexual pleasure as feminist choice', *Feminist Africa*, 2: 50–60.

McGinn, T. and Purdin, S. (2004) 'Reproductive health and conflict: looking back and moving ahead', *Disasters*, 28(3): 235–238.

McKenna, N. (1996) *On the Margins: MSM and HIV in the Developing World*, London: The Panos Institute.

Mead, G.H. (1934) *Mind, Self, and Society*, Chicago: Chicago University Press.

Mead, M. (1928) *Coming of Age in Samoa*, Chicago: Morrow.

—— (1935) *Sex and Temperament in Three Primitive Societies*, New York: Morrow.

—— (1949) *Male and Female: A Study of the Sexes in a Changing World*, London: Gollancz.

Meekers, D. and Calves, A.E. (1997) '"Main" girlfriends, girlfriends, marriage, and money: the social context of HIV risk behaviour in sub-Saharan Africa', *Health Transition Review*, 7: 361–375.

Menon, N. (1999) 'Introduction', in N. Menon (ed.) *Gender and Politics in India*, New Delhi: Oxford University Press.

Mernissi, F. (2000) 'The Muslim concept of active women's sexuality', in P. Ilkkaracan (ed.) *Women and Sexuality in Muslim Societies*, Istanbul: Women for Women's Human Rights.

Michaels, S. and Giami, A. (1999) 'Sexual acts and sexual relationships: asking about sex in surveys', *Public Opinion Quarterly*, 63: 401–420.

Miller, A.M. (2000) 'Sexual but not reproductive: exploring the junctions and disjunctions of sexual and reproductive rights', *Health and Human Rights*, 4(2): 68–109.

—— (2004) 'Sexuality, violence against women, and human rights: women make demands and ladies get protection', *Health and Human Rights*, 7(2): 16–47.

—— (2006) 'Sexual rights words and their meanings: the gateway to effective human rights work on sexual and gender diversity', paper presented at the International Commission of Jurists and International Services on Human Rights Expert Meeting on Human Rights, Sexual Orientation and Gender Identity, Yogyakarta, Indonesia, November.

Miller, N. (1995) *Out of the Past: Gay and Lesbian History from 1869 to the Present*, New York: Vintage Books.

Millet, K. (1979) *Sexual Revolution*, London: Virago Press.

Minter, S.P. (2006) 'Do transsexuals dream of gay rights? Getting real about transgender inclusion', in P. Currah, R.M. Juang, and S.P. Minter (eds) *Transgender Rights*, Minneapolis: University of Minnesota Press.

Misra, G. and Chandiramani, R. (2005) *Sexuality, Gender and Rights: Exploring Theory and Practice in South and Southeast Asia*, New Delhi: Sage.

Mitchell, J. (1974) *Psychoanalysis and Feminism: Freud, Reich, Laing and Women*, New York: Vintage Books.

Mohanty, C.T. (2003) *Feminism without Borders: Decolonizing Theory, Practicing Solidarity*, Durham, NC, and London: Duke University Press.

Moodie, T.D., Ndatsche, V., and Sibuyi, B. (1988) 'Migrancy and male sexuality in the South African gold mines', *Journal of Southern African Studies*, 14(2): 228–256.

Morgan, R. and Wieringa, S. (eds) (2005) *Tommy Boys, Lesbian Men and Ancestral Wives: Female Same-sex Practices in Africa*, Johannesburg: Jacana Media.

MSF/DND (Médecins Sans Frontière/Drugs for Neglected Diseases Working Group) (2002) *The Crisis of Neglected Diseases: Developing Treatments and Ensuring Access*, Working Group Expert Papers, New York: MSF/DND.

Mujica, J. (2007) *Economía Política del Cuerpo: La Reestructuración de los Grupos Conservadores y el Biopoder*, Lima: PROMSEX.

Mukerjee, M. (2006) 'The Prostitutes' Union', *ScientificAmerican.com*. Available online at www.sciam.com/article.cfm?articleID=00034A71-B1CD-1419-ABA683414B7F0101&sc=I100322 (accessed 17 November 2007).

Mukherjee, V.N. (2002) 'Gender matters', *Beyond Numbers Seminar* 511. Available online at www.india-seminar.com/2002/511/511%20vanita%20nayak%20mukherjee.htm (accessed 22 November 2007).

Muñoz-Laboy, M. (2004) 'Beyond "MSM": sexual desire among bisexually active Latino men in New York City', *Sexualities*, 7(1): 55–80.

Murdock, G.P. (1949) 'The social regulation of sexual behavior', in P.H. Hoch and J. Zubin (eds) *Psychosexual Development in Health and Disease*, New York: Grune & Stanton.

Murray, S. (1992) 'Components of gay community in San Francisco', in G. Herdt (ed.) *Gay Culture in America: Essays from the Field*, Boston: Beacon Press.

Mydans, S. (2007) 'Thais to vote on a constitution that would restore civilian rule in diluted form', *New York Times*, 18 August.

Myre, G. (2006) 'Under heavy police guard, gay rights advocates rally in Jerusalem', *New York Times*, 11 November.

Najmabadi, A. (2005) *Women with Mustaches and Men without Beards: Gender and Sexual Anxieties of Iranian Modernity*, Berkeley, Los Angeles and London: University of California Press.

Nanda, S. (1990) *Neither Man nor Woman: The Hijras of India*, Belmont: Wadsworth Publishing.

—— (1994) 'Hijras: an alternative sex and gender role in India', in G. Herdt (ed.) *Third Sex, Third Gender: Beyond Sexual Dimorphism in Culture and History*, New York: Zone Books.

—— (2007) 'The Hijras of India: cultural and individual dimensions of an institutionalized third gender role', in R. Parker and P. Aggleton (eds) *Culture, Society and Sexuality: A Reader*, London and New York: Routledge.

Narrain, A. (2001) 'Human rights and sexual minorities: global and local contexts', *Law, Social Justice and Global Development*, 2: 1–19.

—— (2004) 'The articulation of rights around sexuality and health: subaltern queer cultures in India in the era of Hindutva', *Health and Human Rights*, 7(2): 142–164.

Newton, E. (1972) *Mother Camp: Female Impersonators in America*, Englewood Cliffs, NJ: Prentice-Hall.

New York Times (2006a) 'Rushing off a cliff', editorial, 28 September.

—— (2006b) 'Turning back the clock on rape', editorial, 23 September.

—— (2007) 'Abu Ghraib swept under the carpet', editorial, 30 August.

Ng, V. (1990) 'Homosexuality and the state in late Imperial China', in M. Duberman, G. Chauncey, Jr., and M. Vicinus (eds) *Hidden From History: Reclaiming the Gay and Lesbian Past*, New York: Meridian.

NHRC (National Human Rights Commission) (2002) 'Final order on Gujarat', Delhi, 31 May. Available online at http://nhrc.nic.in/guj_finalorder.htm (accessed 23 November 2007).

Nowicka (2007) 'The struggle for abortion rights in Poland', in R. Parker, R. Petchesky, and R. Sember (eds) *SexPolitics: Reports From the Frontlines*. Sexuality Policy Watch. Available online at www.sxpolitics.org/frontlines/home/index.php (accessed 22 November 2007).

NRC (Norwegian Refugee Council) (2006) *Internal Displacement: Global Overview of Trends and Developments in 2005*, Geneva: Internal Displacement Monitoring Center.

Nussbaum, M.C. (1999) *Sex and Social Justice*, New York: Oxford University Press.

—— (2006) *Frontiers of Justice: Disability, Nationality, Species Membership*, Cambridge, MA: Harvard University Press.

Nussbaum, M.C. and Glover, J. (eds) (1995) *Women, Culture, and Development: A Study of Human Capabilities*, WIDER Studies in Development Economics, Oxford: Clarendon Press; New York: Oxford University Press.

Nuwayhid, I., Cortas, C.S., and Zurayk, H. (2006) 'Resilience during war and its implications for public health interventions, education, and training', paper presented at the Global Forum for Health Research Annual Meeting, Cairo, Egypt, 29 October to 2 November.

Okidi, J.A. and Mugambe, G.K. (2002) *An Overview of Chronic Poverty and Development Policy in Uganda*, Working Paper 11, Kampala: Chronic Poverty Research Center.

Okin, S.M. (1979) *Women in Western Political Thought*, Princeton: Princeton University Press.

Ortiz-Ortega, A. (2005) 'The politics of abortion in Mexico: the paradox of doble discurso', in W. Chavkin and E. Chesler (eds) *Where Human Rights Begin: Health, Sexuality, and Women in the New Millennium*, New Brunswick: Rutgers University Press.

Ortner, S.B. and Whitehead, H. (eds) (1981) *Sexual Meanings: The Cultural Construction of Gender and Sexuality*, New York: Cambridge University Press.

Osakue, G. and Martin-Hilber, A. (1998) 'Women's sexuality and fertility in Nigeria: breaking the culture of silence', in R. Petchesky and K. Judd (eds) *Negotiating Reproductive Rights*, International Reproductive Rights Research Action Group (IRRRAG), London and New York: Zed Books.

OSI (Open Society Institute) (2007) 'Anti-Prostitution Pledge' Materials. Available online at www.soros.org/initiatives/health/focus/sharp/articles_publications/publications/ pledge_20070612 (accessed 1 November 2007).

Ottosson, D. (2007) 'State homophobia: a world survey of laws prohibiting same sex activity between consenting adults', ILGA Report. Available online at www.ilga.org/news_results.asp?LanguageID=1&FileID=769&ZoneID=7&FileCategory=1 (accessed 18 August 2007).

Oxfam (2006a) 'Public health at risk', Oxfam Briefing Paper, Oxfam International. Available online at www.oxfam.org/en/policy/briefingpapers/bp86_thailand_publichealth (accessed 27 September 2007).

—— (2006b) 'Patents vs. patients: five years after the Doha Declaration', Oxfam International. Available online at www.oxfam.org/en/policy/briefingpapers/bp95_patentsvspatients_061114 (accessed 27 September 2007).

—— (2007) 'Indian ruling against pharmaceutical giant Novartis a victory for public health, say leading aid and advocacy agencies', Oxfam International. Available online at www.oxfam.org/en/news/2007/pr070806_india_ruling_against_novartis (accessed 27 September 2007).

Padgug, R.A. (1979) 'Sexual matters: on conceptualizing sexuality in history', *Radical History Review*, 20: 3–23.

Padilla, M. (2007) *Caribbean Pleasure Industry: Tourism, Sexuality, and AIDS in the Dominican Republic*, Chicago: University of Chicago Press.

Padilla, M., Hirsch, J.S., Muñoz-Laboy, M., Sember, R.E., and Parker, R.G. (eds) (2007) *Love and Globalization: Transformations of Intimacy in the Contemporary World*, Nashville: Vanderbilt University Press.

Paiva, V. (2000) 'Gendered scripts and the sexual scene: promoting sexual subjects among Brazilian teenagers', in R. Parker, P. Aggleton, and R.M. Barbosa (eds) *Framing the Sexual Subject: The Politics of Gender, Sexuality, and Power*, Berkeley, Los Angeles, and London: University of California Press.

—— (2003) 'Beyond magical solutions: prevention of HIV and AIDS as a process of psychosocial emancipation', *Divulgacao em Saúde para Debate*, 27: 192–203.

Pankurst, J.O. (2002) 'The Ugandan success story? Evidence and claims of HIV-1 prevention', *Lancet*, 360: 78.

Parker, R. (1987) 'Acquired immunodeficiency syndrome in urban Brazil', *Medical Anthropology Quarterly*, 1: 155–172.

—— (1991) *Bodies, Pleasures and Passions: Sexual Culture in Contemporary Brazil*, Boston: Beacon Press.

—— (1999) *Beneath the Equator: Cultures of Desire, Male Homosexuality and Emerging Gay Communities in Brazil*, New York and London: Routledge.

—— (2001) 'Sexuality, culture and power in HIV/AIDS research', *Annual Review of Anthropology*, 30: 163–179.

—— (2007) 'Sexuality, health, and human rights', *American Journal of Public Health*, 97(6): 972–973.

Parker, R. and Aggleton, P. (1999) 'Introduction', in R. Parker and P. Aggleton (eds) *Culture, Society and Sexuality: A Reader*, London: University College London Press.

—— (eds) (2007) *Culture, Society and Sexuality: A Reader*, 2nd edn, London and New York: Routledge.

Parker, R. and Corrêa, S. (eds.) (2003) *Sexualidade e Política na América Latina*, Rio de Janeiro: ABIA.

Parker, R. and Gagnon, J. (1995) *Conceiving Sexuality: Approaches to Sex Research in a Post-modern World*, New York and London: Routledge.

Parker, R., Aggleton, P., and Barbosa, R.M. (eds) (2000a) *Framing the Sexual Subject: The Politics of Gender, Sexuality, and Power*, Berkeley, Los Angeles, and London: University of California Press.

Parker, R., Aggleton, P., and Khan, S. (1998) 'Conspicuous by their absence? Men who have sex with men (MSM) in developing countries: implications for HIV prevention', *Critical Public Health*, 8(4): 329–346

Parker, R., Easton, D., and Klein, C. (2000b) 'Structural barriers and facilitators in HIV prevention: a review of international research', *AIDS*, 14 (suppl. 1): S2–S32.

Parker, R., Guimarães, K., Mota, M., Quemmel, R., and Terto, V. (1995) 'AIDS prevention and gay community mobilization in Brazil', *Development*, 2: 49–53.

Parker, R., Petchesky, R., and Sember, R. (eds) (2007) *SexPolitics: Reports from the Front Lines*. Sexuality Policy Watch. Available online at www.sxpolitics. org/frontlines/home/index.php (accessed 22 November 2007).

Pateman, C. (1988) *The Sexual Contract*, Stanford: Stanford University Press.

Patrick, E. (2007) 'Sexual violence and firewood collection in Darfur', *Forced Migration Review*, 27: 40–41.

Patton, C. (1990) *Inventing AIDS*, New York and London: Routledge.

Pazello, M. (2005) 'Sexual rights and trade', *Peace Review: A Journal of Social Justice*, 17: 155–162.

Peacock, B., Eyre, S., Kegeles, S., and Quinn, S.C. (2001) 'Delineating differences: sub-communities in the San Francisco gay community', *Culture, Health and Sexuality*, 3: 183–201.

People's Union of Civil Liberties – Karnataka (2003) *Human Rights Violations against the Transgender Community: A Study of Kothi and Hijra Sex Workers in Bangalore, India*, Bangalore: People's Union of Civil Liberties.

Petchesky, R. (1990) *Abortion and Women's Choice: The State, Sexuality and Reproductive Freedom*, Boston: Northeastern University Press.

—— (2000) 'Sexual rights: inventing a concept, mapping an international practice', in R. Parker, P. Aggleton, and R.M. Barbosa (eds) *Framing the Sexual Subject: The Politics of Gender, Sexuality and Power*, Berkeley, Los Angeles and London: University of California Press.

—— (2003) *Global Prescriptions: Gendering Health and Human Rights*, London and New York: Zed Books.

—— (2005) 'Rights of the body and perversions of war: sexual rights and wrongs ten years past Beijing', *International Social Science Journal*, 57(2): 301–318.

Petchesky, R. and Judd, K. (eds) (1998) *Negotiating Reproductive Rights*, International Reproductive Rights Research Action Group (IRRRAG), London and New York: Zed Books.

Petchesky, R. and Laurie, M. (2007) 'Gender, health and human rights in sites of political exclusion', Report for World Health Organization, Commission on the Social Determinants of Health (Women and Gender Knowledge Network).

Peteet, J. (2002) 'Male gender and rituals of resistance in the Palestinian Intifada', in R. Adams and D. Savran (eds) *The Masculinity Studies Reader*, Malden, MA, and Oxford: Blackwell.

Phillips, A. (2002) 'Multiculturalism, universalism, and the claims of democracy', in M. Molyneux and S. Razavi (eds) *Gender Justice, Development and Rights*, Oxford: Oxford University Press.

Phillips, K. (2002) *Wealth and Democracy: A Political History of the American Rich*, New York: Broadway Books.

Phillips, O. (2001) 'Conscripts in camp: making military men', *African Gender Institute Newsletter*, 8. Available online at http://web.uct.ac.za/org/agi/pubs/newsletters/vol8/camp.htm (accessed 27 September 2007).

Philpott, A., Knerr, W., and Boydell, V. (2006) 'Pleasure and prevention: when good sex is safer sex', *Reproductive Health Matters*, 14(28): 23–31.

Platform for Action (1995) 'Fourth World Conference on Women, Beijing'. Available online at www.un.org/womenwatch/daw/beijing/platform/ (accessed 28 September 2007).

Plummer, K. (1975) *Sexual Stigma*, London: Routledge & Kegan Paul.

—— (1982) 'Symbolic interactionism and sexual conduct: an emergent perspective', in M. Brake (ed.) *Human Sexual Relations: Toward a Redefinition of Sexual Politics*, New York: Pantheon.

—— (1995) *Telling Sexual Stories: Power Change and Social Worlds*, London and New York: Routledge.

—— (2003) *Intimate Citizenship: Private Decisions and Public Dialogues*, Seattle and London: University of Washington Press.

Pomeroy, W.B. (1972) *Dr. Kinsey and the Institute for Sex Research*, New York: Harper & Row.

Presser, H. and Sen, G. (2000) 'Women's empowerment and demographic processes: laying the groundwork', in H. Presser and G. Sen (eds) *Women's Empowerment and Demographic Processes: Moving Beyond Cairo*, Oxford: Oxford University Press.

Preston-Whyte, E.M. (1995) 'Half-way there: anthropology and intervention oriented AIDS research in KwaZulu/Natal, South Africa', in H. ten Brummelhuis and G. Herdt (eds) *Culture and Sexual Risk: Anthropological Perspectives on AIDS*, New York: Gordon & Breach.

Preston-Whyte, E., Blose, F., Oosthuizen, H., Roberts, R., and Varga, C. (2000) 'Survival sex and HIV/AIDS in an African city', in R.G. Parker, P. Aggleton, and R.M. Barbosa (eds) *Framing the Sexual Subject: The Politics of Gender, Sexuality, and Power*, Berkeley: University of California Press.

Prieur, A. (1998) *Mema's House, Mexico City: On Transvestites, Queens, and Machos*, Chicago: University of Chicago Press.

Programme of Action (1994) United Nations International Conference on Population and Development, Cairo. Available online at www.un.org/ecosocdev/geninfo/populatin/icpd.htm (accessed 7 September 2007).

Puar, J.K. (2004) 'Abu Ghraib: arguing against exceptionalism', *Feminist Studies*, 30(2): 1–14.

Quine, M.S. (1996) *Population Politics in Twentieth Century Europe*, London and New York: Routledge.

Radosh, D. (2004) 'The culture wars: why know?', *New Yorker*, 6 December.

Ramasubban, R. (1995) 'Patriarchy and the risks of STD and HIV transmission to women', in M. das Gupta, L.C. Chen, and T.N. Krishnan (eds) *Women's Health in India: Risk and Vulnerability*, Bombay: Oxford University Press.

—— (2007) 'Culture, politics, and discourses on sexuality: a history of resistance to the anti-sodomy law in India', in R. Parker, R. Petchesky, and R. Sember (eds) *SexPolitics: Reports From the Frontlines*. Sexuality Policy Watch. Available online at www.sxpolitics.org/frontlines/home/index.php (accessed 22 November 2007).

Ramdas, K.N. (2006) 'Women's rights another victim of the Iraq catastrophe', *Baltimore Sun*, 22 December.

Ramonet, I. (2007) 'Polish witch hunt'. Available online at http://mondediplo.com/2007/04/01poland (accessed 4 September 2007).

Ramsden, E. (2003) 'Social demography and eugenics in the interwar United States', *Population and Development Review*, 29(4): 547–593.

Rashid, A. (2000) *Taliban*, New Haven and London: Yale University Press.

Reddy, G. (2005) *With Respect to Sex: Negotiating Hijra Identity in South India*, Chicago: University of Chicago Press.

Reich, W. (1971) *The Sexual Revolution: Toward a Self-governing Character Structure*, New York: Farrar, Straus & Giroux.

—— (1973a) *Selected Sex-pol Essays, 1934–37*, London: Socialist Reproduction.

—— (1973b) *The Function of the Orgasm: Discovery of the Orgone*, New York: Farrar, Straus & Giroux.

Reisman, J. (1998) *Kinsey, Crimes and Consequences*, Crestwood, KY: The Institute for Media Education.

Reiter, R. (ed.) (1975) *Toward an Anthropology of Women*, New York: Monthly Review Press.

Reuters (2005) 'Polish PM candidate says homosexuality unnatural'. Available online at www.redorbit.com/news/international/ (accessed 4 September 2007).

Rhode, D. and Sanger, D. (2007) 'How the "Good War" in Afghanistan went bad', *New York Times*, 12 August.

Rich, A. (2007) 'Compulsory heterosexuality and lesbian existence', in R. Parker and P. Aggleton (eds) *Culture, Society and Sexuality: A Reader*, 2nd edn, London and New York: Routledge.

Richardson, D. (2000) 'Claiming citizenship?: sexuality, citizenship and lesbian/feminist theory', *Sexualities*, 3(2): 255–272.

Richey, L.A. (2005) 'Uganda: HIV/AIDS and reproductive health', in W. Chavkin and E. Chesler (eds) *Where Human Rights Begin – Health, Sexuality, and Women in the New Millennium*, New Brunswick: Rutgers University Press.

Riley, D. (1988) *Am I That Name? Feminism and the Category of 'Women' in History*, Minneapolis: University of Minnesota Press.

Rios, R.R. (2006) 'Para um direito democrático da sexualidade', *Horizontes Antroplóógicos*, 12(26): 71–100.

Risen, J. (2006) *State of War: The Secret History of the CIA and the Bush Administration*, New York: Simon & Schuster; Free Press.

Risen, J. and Golden, T. (2006) 'Three prisoners commit suicide at Guantanamo', *New York Times*, 11 June.

Robinson, P. (1976) *The Modernization of Sex*, New York: Harper.

Rodrik, D. (2000) 'Global governance of trade: as if development really mattered', background paper for the 2002 *Human Development Report*, 'Making Trade Work for People', New York: UNDP.

Rofel, L. (2007) *Desiring China: Experiments in Neoliberalism, Sexuality, and Public Culture*, Durham, NC: Duke University Press.

Rojas, L. (2001) *El Debate sobre los Derechos Sexuales en México*, Mexico City: Programa de Salud Reproductiva y Sociedad, Colégio de México.

Rosaldo, M.Z. and Lamphere, L. (eds) (1974) *Woman, Culture, and Society*, Stanford: Stanford University Press.

Rosenberg, T. (2001) 'The Brazilian solution', *New York Times Magazine*, 28 June.

Ross, E. and Rapp, R. (1983) 'Sex and society: a research note from social history and anthropology', in A. Snitow, C. Stansell, and S. Thompson (eds) *Powers of Desire: The Politics of Sexuality*, New York: Monthly Review Press.

Ross, E.B. (1998) *The Malthus Factor: Poverty, Politics and Population in Capitalist Development*, London and New York: Zed Books.

Roubus, K. (2007) 'Rally denounces homosexuality', *Behind the Mask*. Available online at www.mask.org.za/article.php?cat=uganda&id=1671 (accessed 31 August 2007).

Rubin, G. (1975) 'The traffic in women: notes on the "political economy" of sex', in R. Reiter (ed.) *Toward an Anthropology of Women*, New York: Monthly Review Press.

—— (1982) 'The leather menace', *Body Politic*, 82(34).

—— (1984) 'Thinking sex: notes for a radical theory of the politics of sexuality', in C. Vance (ed.) *Pleasure and Danger: Exploring Female Sexuality*, Boston: Routledge & Kegan Paul.

—— (1991) 'The Catacombs: a temple of the butthole', in M. Thompson (ed.) *Leatherfolk: Radical Sex, People, Politics, and Practice*, Boston: Alyson Publications.

—— (1996) 'The outcasts: a social history', in P. Califia and R. Sweeney (eds) *The Second Coming: A Leatherdyke Reader*, Los Angeles: Alyson Publications.

—— (1997) 'Elegy for the Valley of the Kings: AIDS and the leather community in San Francisco, 1981–1996', in M.P. Levine, P.M. Nardi, and J.H. Gagnon (eds) *In Changing Times: Gay Men and Lesbians Encounter HIV/AIDS*, Chicago: University of Chicago Press.

—— (2000) 'Sites, settlements, and urban sex: archaeology and the study of gay leathermen in San Francisco 1955–1995', in R. Schmidt and B. Voss (eds) *Archaeologies of Sexuality*, London and New York: Routledge.

—— (2002) 'Studying sexual subcultures: the ethnography of gay communities in urban North America', in E. Lewin and W. Leap (eds) *Out in Theory: The Emergence of Lesbian and Gay Anthropology*, Urbana: University of Illinois Press.

—— (2003) 'Samois', in M. Stein (ed.) *Encyclopedia of Lesbian, Gay, Bisexual, and Transgender History in America*, New York: Charles Scribner's Sons.

Saad-Filho, A. and Johnston, D. (eds) (2005) *Neoliberalism: A Critical Reader*, London and Ann Arbor: Pluto Press.

Sabrang and The South Asian Citizens Web (2003) 'Appendix', in *The Foreign Exchange of Hate*, Mumbai: Sabrang Communications.

Saghal, G. and Yuval-Davis, N. (1992) *Refusing Holy Orders: Women and Fundamentalism in Britain*, London: Verso.

Saiz, I. (2004) 'Bracketing sexuality: human rights and sexual orientation – a decade of development and denial at the United Nations', *Health and Human Rights*, 7: 48–81.

Sambanis, N. (2006) 'It's official: there is now a civil war in Iraq', *New York Times*, Op-Ed, 23 July.

Sangini (India) Trust (2005) 'List of LGBT groups in India', unpublished mimeo.

Sangram (2005) 'Of veshyas, vamps, whores and women', November, Sangli: Sangram. Available online at www.sangram.org/vampnews/index.html (accessed 4 September 2007).

Sarkar, S. (2002) 'Hindutva and history', in S. Sarkar, *Beyond Nationalist Frames: Relocating Postmodernism, Hindutva and History*, Delhi: Permanent Black.

Saunders, P. (2004) 'Prohibiting sex work projects, restricting women's rights: the international impact of the 2003 U.S. global AIDS act', *Health and Human Rights*, 7(2): 179–192.

Schiebinger, L. (1993) *Nature's Body: Gender in the Making of Modern Science*, Boston: Beacon Press.

Schoepf, B. (1992) 'Women at risk: case studies from Zaire', in G. Herdt and S. Lindenbaum (eds) *The Time of AIDS: Social Analysis, Theory, and Method*, Newbury Park, CA: Sage.

Schrecker, T. (1998) 'Private health care for Canada: north of the border, an idea whose time shouldn't come?', *Journal of Law, Medicine and Ethics*, 26(2): 138–148.

Schutz, A. (1967) *The Phenomenology of the Social Word*, Evanston: Northwest University Press.

Sedgwick, E. (1990) *Epistemology of the Closet*, Berkeley and Los Angeles: University of California Press.

—— (1993) *Tendencies*, Durham, NC: Duke University Press.

Seidman, S. (1996) *Queer Theory/Sociology*, Cambridge: Blackwell.

—— (1998) 'Are we all in the closet? Notes towards a sociological and cultural turn to queer theory', *European Journal of Cultural Studies*, 1: 177–192.

Semple, K. (2006) 'Kidnapped in Iraq: victim's tale of clockwork death and ransom', *New York Times*, 7 May.

Sen, A. (1995) Population Policy: Authoritarianism versus Cooperation, International Lecture Series on Population Issues, 17 August, New Delhi, The John D. and Catherine T. MacArthur Foundation. Available online at www.abep. nepo.unicamp.br/docs/PopPobreza/AmartyaSen.pdf (accessed 22 November 2007).

—— (1999) *Development as Freedom*, New York: Alfred A. Knopf.

Sen, G. (2005) 'Neolibs, neocons and gender justice: lessons from global negotiations', United Nations Research Institute for Social Development Occasional Paper 9, September, Geneva: UNRISD.

Sen, G. and Corrêa, S. (2000) 'Gender justice and economic justice: reflections on the five year reviews of the UN Conferences of the 1990s', *DAWN Informs*, January, Suva, Fiji.

Seshu, M. (2005) 'Organizing women in prostitution: the case of SANGRAM', in R. Ramasubban and B. Rishyasringa (eds) *AIDS and Civil Society: India's Learning Curve*, Jaipur and New Delhi: Rawat Publications.

Sex Workers Project (2007) 'Critique of the anti-prostitution pledge and its global impact'. Available online at www.sexworkersproject.org/working-group/downloads/20070330-BriefingPaperOnAnti-ProstitutionPledge.pdf (accessed 30 August 2007).

Shane, S. and Mazzetti, M. (2007) 'Advisers fault harsh methods in interrogation', *New York Times*, 30 May.

Sharma, J. (2006) 'Reflections on the language of rights from a queer perspective', *IDS Bulletin*, 37(5): 52–57.

Shepherd, G. (1987) 'Rank, genders and homosexuality: Mombassa as a key to understanding sexual options', in P. Caplan (ed.) *The Cultural Construction of Sexuality*, London: Tavistock Publications.

Simms, C. (2004) *Low Credit: A Report on the World Bank's Response to HIV/AIDS in Developing Countries*, Action Aid International. Available online at www.actionaid.org.uk/doc_lib/85_1_low_credit.pdf (accessed 24 October 2007).

Simon, W. (1996) *Postmodern Sexualities*, New York and London: Routledge.

Simon, W. and Gagnon, J.H. (1984) 'Sexual scripts', *Society*, 23(1): 53–60.

—— (1986) 'Sexual scripts: permanence and change', *Archives of Sexual Behavior*, 15: 97–120.

—— (1987) 'A sexual scripts approach', in J.H. Geer and P. Donohue (eds) *Theories of Human Sexualities*, New York: Plenum.

—— (1999) 'Sexual scripts', in R. Parker and P. Aggleton (eds) *Culture, Society and Sexuality: A Reader*, London: University College London Press.

Simon, P., Dourlen-Rollier, A.-M., Gondonneau, J., and Mironer, L. (1972) *Rapport sur le comportement sexual des français*, Paris: Julliard, Charron.

Singer, M. (ed.) (1998) *The Political Economy of AIDS*, Amityville, NY: Baywood Publishing.

Smith-Rosenberg, C. (1985) *Disorderly Conduct: Visions of Gender in Victorian America*, New York: Alfred A. Knopf.

Sobo, E.J. (1995) *Choosing Unsafe Sex: AIDS Risk Denial among Disadvantaged Women*, Philadelphia: University of Pennsylvania Press.

Sow, F., Mukherjee, V., and Pazello, M. (2007) 'The remaking of a secular social contract', unpublished paper.

Spade, D. (2006) 'Compliance is gendered: struggling for gender self-determination in a hostile economy', in P. Currah, R.M. Juang, and S.P. Minter (eds) *Transgender Rights*, Minneapolis: University of Minnesota Press.

Spees, P. (2003) 'Women's advocacy in the creation of the International Criminal Court: changing the landscapes of justice and power', *SIGNS*, 28(4): 1233–1254.

Spiegel, P. (2004) 'HIV/AIDS among conflict-affected and displaced populations: dispelling myths and taking action', paper presented at 20th meeting of the Inter-Agency Advisory Group on AIDS, United Nations High Commission on Refugees, 9–10 February, Geneva, Switzerland. Available online at http://intranet.theirc.org/docs/Dispelling%20Myths%20and%20Taking%20Action%20-%20IAAG.pdf (accessed 29 October 2007).

Spira, A., Bajos, N., and ACSF Group (1994) *Sexual Behaviour and AIDS*, Aldershot: Avebury.

Srinivasan, B. (2004) 'Falling through the cracks', *Scripts*, 4, April: 36–7, Mumbai: Labia.

Standing, H. (1999) *Framework for Understanding Gender Inequities and Health Sector Reforms: An Analysis and Review of Policy Issues*, Working Paper Series, No. 99.06, Cambridge, MA: Harvard Center for Population and Development Studies.

Stein, A. and Plummer, P. (1994) ' "I can't even think straight": "queer" theory and the missing sexual revolution in sociology', *Sociological Theory*, 12(2): 178–187.

Steiner, G. (2005) *Anthropocentrism and Its Discontents: The Moral Status of Animals in the History of Western Philosophy*, Pittsburgh: University of Pittsburgh Press.

Stiglitz, J. (2002) *Globalization and its Discontents*, New York: W.W. Norton.

Stiglitz, J., Ocampo, J.A., Spiegel, S., French-Davis, R., and Nayyar, D. (2006) *Stability with Growth: Macroeconomics, Liberalization, and Development*, Oxford: Oxford University Press.

Stoler, A.L. (1997) 'Carnal knowledge and imperial power', in R.N. Lancaster and M. di Leonardo (eds) *The Gender/Sexuality Reader: Culture, History, Political Economy*, New York and London: Routledge.

Stout, D. (2007) 'Bush seeks to double spending for AIDS program', *New York Times*, 30 May. Available online at www.nytimes.com/2007/05/30/washington/30cnd-prexy.html?_r=1&hp&oref=slogin (accessed on 19 December 2007).

Strathern, M. (1972) *Women in Between*, London: Academic Press.

Stryker, S. (1994) 'My words to Victor Frankenstein above the village of Chamounix – performing transgender rage', *GLQ*, 1(3): 277–254.

Susskind, Y. (2007) *Promising Democracy, Imposing Theocracy: Gender Based Violence and the US War on Iraq*, New York: MADRE.

Swamy, A.R. (2003) *Hindu Nationalism – What's Religion Got to Do with It?* Asia-Pacific Center for Security Studies, Occasional Paper Series, Honolulu, March.

Symonds, P.V. (1998) 'Political economy and cultural logics of HIV/AIDS among the Hmong in Northern Thailand', in M. Singer (ed.) *The Political Economy of AIDS*, Amityville, NY: Baywood Publishing.

Tamale, S. (2006) 'Eroticism, sensuality and "women's secrets" among the Baganda', *IDS Bulletin*, 37(5): 89–97.

Taminnen, T. (1996) 'Hindu revivalism and the Hindutva movement', *Temenos*, 32: 221–238.

Tan, M. (1996) 'Silahis: looking for the missing Filipino bisexual male', in P. Aggleton (ed.) *Bisexualities and AIDS: International Perspectives*, London: Taylor & Francis.

—— (1999) 'Walking the tightrope: sexual risk and male sex work in the Philippines', in P. Aggleton (ed.) *Men Who Sell Sex: International Perspectives on Male Prostitution and HIV/AIDS*, London: University College London Press.

Taylor, C.L. (1985) 'Ethnographic materials on Mexican male homosexual transvestites', *Journal of Homosexuality*, 11(3): 117–136.

Terto Jr., V. (1989) *No Escurinho do Cinema: Sociabilidade Orgiástica nas Tardes Cariocas*, unpublished Master's thesis in psychology, Rio de Janeiro: PUC.

—— (2000) 'Male homosexuality and seropositivity: the construction of social identities in Brazil', in R. Parker, P. Aggleton, and R.M. Barbosa (eds) *Framing the Sexual Subject: The Politics of Gender, Sexuality, and Power*, Berkeley, Los Angeles, and London: University of California Press.

The Pleasure Project (2007). Available online at www.thepleasureproject.org (accessed 29 September 2007).

The Times of India (2005) 'Anti-prostitution law for drastic revamp', 1 October. Available online at http://timesofindia.indiatimes.com/articleshow/msid-1248700, prtpage-1.cms (accessed 15 May 2005).

Thomas, K. (2006) 'Afterword: are transgender rights inhuman rights?', in P. Currah, R.M. Juang, and S.P. Minter (eds) *Transgender Rights*, Minneapolis: University of Minnesota Press.

Touraine, A. (1997) *Pourrons nous vivres ensemble, egaux et difference?*, Paris: Fayard.

Touraine, A. and Khosrohavar, F. (1999) *La recherché de Soi*, Paris: Fayard.

Treichler, P. (1988) 'AIDS, homophobia and biomedical discourse: an epidemic of signification', in D. Crimp (ed.) *AIDS: Cultural Analysis and Cultural Activism*, Cambridge, MA: MIT Press.

—— (1999) *How to Have Theory in an Epidemic: Cultural Chronicles of AIDS*, Durham, NC: Duke University Press.

Trejos, N. (2007) 'Iraq's woes are adding major risks to childbirth', *Washington Post*, 4 January.

Trías, E. (1998) 'Thinking religion', in J. Derrida and G. Vattimo (eds) *Religion*, Stanford: Stanford University Press.

Trumbach, R. (1977) 'London's sodomites: homosexual behaviour and Western culture in the eighteenth century', *Journal of Social History*, 11: 1–33.

Truong, T.D. (1990) *Sex, Money and Morality: Prostitution and Tourism in South East Asia*, London: Zed Books.

Tully, M. and Masani, Z. (1988) *From Raj to Rajiv: 40 Years of Indian Independence*, London: BBC.

Turkle, S. (1981) *Psychoanalytic Politics: Freud's French Revolution*, New York: Basic Books.

Turner, C.F., Miller, H.G., and Moses, L.E. (eds) (1989) *AIDS: Sexual Behavior and Intravenous Drug Use*, Washington, DC: National Academy Press.

Turshen, M. (1995) 'Response: societal instability in international perspective: relevance to HIV/AIDS prevention', in *Assessing the Social and Behavioral Science Base for HIV/AIDS Prevention and Intervention*, Washington, DC: National Academy Press.

—— (1998) 'The political economy of AIDS', in M. Singer (ed.) *The Political Economy of AIDS*, Amityville: Baywood Publishing.

Tushnet, M. (1984) 'An essay on rights', *Texas Law Review*, 62: 1363–1403.

UN (United Nations) (2007) Application of General Assembly Resolution 60/25 of March 15th 2006 entitled 'Human Rights Council'. Report from Special Rapporteur on Freedom of Religion and Conviction (Ms Asma Jahangir). Geneva. A/HRC/4/21.

UNAIDS (United Nations Programme on HIV/AIDS) (2006) *Report on the Global AIDS Epide*mic, Geneva: UNAIDS.

—— (2004) 'Democracy in Latin America: towards a citizenship democracy'. Available online at www.democracia.undp.org/Informe/Default.asp?Menu=15&Idioma=1 (accessed 28 August 2007).

—— (2005) International Cooperation at a Crossroads: Aid, Trade and Security in an Unequal World (Human Development Report 2005), New York: Oxford University Press.

UNFPA (United Nations Population Fund) (2003) 'Study finds maternal deaths have tripled in Iraq', Communications Consortium Media Center. Available online at msnmagazine.com/news/uswirestory.asp?id=8155 (accessed 5 November 2003).

UNFPA (2006) *State of World Population 2006: A Passage to Hope – Women and International Migration*, New York: UNFPA.

UNHCR (United Nations High Commission on Refugees) (2005) *Global Refugee Trends*, Geneva: UNHCR.

—— (2007a) The Iraq Situation. Available online at www.unhcr.org/iraq.html (accessed 29 September 2007).

—— (2007b) *2006 Global Trends: Refugees, Asylum-Seekers, Returnees, Internally Displaced and Stateless Persons*, Geneva: UNHCR, Division of Operational Services, June, revised 16 July.

—— (2007c) 'Press release – independent experts express serious concerns over draft Nigerian bill outlawing same-sex relations'. Available online at www.unhchr.ch/huricane/huricane.nsf/view01/A8F5CC6EAC2D6C52C125728B0054CD9B?opendocument (accessed 15 May 2007).

United States 108th Congress (2003) 'United States Leadership against HIV/AIDS, Tuberculosis, and Malaria Act of 2003', Title III, Sec. 104A, e & f, Washington, DC: United States Congress.

United States Supreme Court (1986) *Bowers v. Hardwick*, 478 U.S. 186 (1986). Available online at http://supreme.justia.com/us/478/186/case.html (accessed 25 November 2007).

—— (2003) *Lawrence* v. *Texas*, 539 U.S. 558 (2003). Available online at http://supreme.justia.com/us/539/558/case.html (accessed 25 November 2007).

USAID (2003) 'Male circumcision and HIV prevention', U.S. Agency for International Development, Bureau for Global Health, August. Available online at www.hawaii.edu/hivandaids/Male_Circumcision_and_HIV_Prevention.pdf (accessed 23 November 2007).

US Committee for Refugees and Immigrants (USCRI) (2006) 'World Refugee Survey 2006'. Available online at www.refugees.org/article.aspx?id=1565& subm=19&ssm=29&area=Investigate& (accessed 22 November 2007).

US Congress (2002) 'Hearing on Communal Violence in Gujarat, India', U.S. Congress Commission on International Religious Freedom, Washington, DC, 10 June.

Vance, C.S. (1984) 'Pleasure and danger: toward a politics of sexuality', in C. Vance (ed.) *Pleasure and Danger: Exploring Female Sexuality*, Boston: Routledge & Kegan Paul.

—— (1989) 'Social construction theory: problems in the history of sexuality', in A. van Kooten Niekerk and T. van der Meer (eds) *Homosexuality, Which Homosexuality?*, Amsterdam: An Dekker, Imprint Schorer.

—— (1999) 'Anthropology rediscovers sexuality: a theoretical comment', in R. Parker and P. Aggleton (eds) *Culture, Society and Sexuality: A Reader*, London: University College London Press.

Vatican (2004) 'Catechism of the Catholic Church', Part Three, Section Two, Chapter 2, Article 6, Para. 2357. Available online at www.usccb.org/catechism/text/pt3sect2chpt2art6.htm (accessed 23 November 2007).

—— (2005a) 'Instruction Concerning the Criteria for the Discernment of Vocations with regard to Persons with Homosexual Tendencies in view of their Admission to the Seminary and to Holy Orders', *Congregation for Catholic Education*, 4 November. Available online at www.papalencyclicals.net/Ben16/Instructions.htm (accessed 23 November 2007).

—— (2005b) 'Deus Caritas Est', The first Encyclical by Pope Benedict XVI. Available online at www.vatican.va/holy_father/benedict_xvi/encyclicals/documents/-hf_ben-xvi_enc_20051225_deus-caritas-est_en.html (accessed 23 November 2007).

—— (2006) 'Discorso di Sua Santità Benedetto XVI in Occasione del XXV Anniversario Dalla Fondazione del Pontificio Istituto Giovanni Paolo II per Studi su Matrimonio e Famiglia'. Available online at www.vatican.va/holy_father/benedict_xvi/speeches/2006/may/documents/hf_ben-xvi_spe_20060511_istituto-gp-ii_it.html (accessed 23 November 2007).

Vattimo, G. (1998) 'The trace of the trace', in J. Derrida and G. Vattimo (eds) *Religion*, Stanford: Stanford University Press.

—— (2006) *O amor é fraco*. Suplemento Mais, Folha de São Paulo, 2 July. Available online at www.fsp/indices/inde02072006.htm (accessed 3 January 2007).

Vianna, A.R.B. and Carrara, S. (2007) 'Sexual politics in Brazil: a case study', in R. Parker, R. Petchesky, and R. Sember (eds) *SexPolitics: Reports from the Front Line*, Sexuality Policy Watch. Available online at www.sxpolitics.org/frontlines/book/pdf/capitulo1_brazil.pdf (accessed 23 November 2007).

Vicinus, M. (1985) 'Distance and desire: English boarding-school friendships', in E.B. Freedman, B.C. Gelpi, S.L. Johnson, and K.M Weston (eds) *The Lesbian Issue: Essays from SIGNS*, London: University of Chicago Press.

Voices Against 377 (2004) 'Rights for all: ending discrimination against queer desire under Section 377'. Available online at www.voicesagainst377.org/images/voices_report.pdf (accessed 22 November 2007).

von Zielbauer, P. (2007a) 'Army Colonel acquitted in Abu Ghraib abuse case', *New York Times*, 29 August.

—— (2007b) 'General and two colonels censured for poor investigation into Haditha killings', *New York Times*, 6 September.

Wallace, R., Fullilove, M.T., Fullilove, R., Gould, P., and Wallace, D. (1994) 'Will AIDS be contained within the U.S. minority urban populations?', *Social Science and Medicine*, 39: 1051–1062.

Warner, M. (1991) 'Introduction: fear of a queer planet', *Social Text*, 9(4): 3–17.

—— (1993) *Fear of a Queer Planet; Queer Politics and Social Theory*, Minneapolis: University of Minnesota Press.

—— (2000) *The Trouble With Normal: Sex, Politics, and the Ethics of Queer Life*, Cambridge, MA: Harvard University Press.

Watney, S. (1987) *Policing Desire: Pornography, AIDS and the Media*, Minneapolis: University of Minnesota Press.

WCC (World Council of Churches) (2006) 'HIV prevention: current issues and new technologies', *Contact Magazine*, 182 (August).

Webb, D. (1997) *HIV and AIDS in Africa*, London and Chicago: Pluto Press.

Weber, M. (1993) *Sociology of Religion*, Boston: Beacon Press.

Weeks, J. (1977) *Coming Out: Homosexual Politics in Britain from the Nineteenth Century to the Present*, London and New York: Quartet Books.

—— (1979) 'Movements of affirmation: sexual meaning and homosexual identities', *Radical History Review*, 20: 164–180.

—— (1981) *Sex, Politics, and Society: The Regulation of Sexuality Since 1800*, New York: Longman.

—— (1985) *Sexuality and its Discontents: Meanings, Myths and Modern Sexualities*, London: Routledge & Kegan Paul.

—— (1986) *Sexuality*, London: Horwood and Tavistock.

—— (1991) *Against Nature: Essays on History, Sexuality and Identity*, London: Rivers Oram Press.

—— (1999a) 'Discourse, desire and sexual deviance: some problems in a history of homosexuality', in R. Parker and P. Aggleton (eds) *Culture, Society and Sexuality: A Reader*, London: University College London Press.

—— (1999b) 'The sexual citizen', in M. Featherstone (ed.) *Love and Eroticism*, London: Sage.

—— (2000) *Making Sexual History*, Cambridge: Polity Press.

—— (2003) *Sexuality*, 2nd edn, London and New York: Routledge.

—— (2005) 'Remembering Foucault', *Journal of the History of Sexuality*, 14(1/2): 186–201.

Weeks, J. and Holland, J. (eds) (1996) *Sexual Cultures: Communities, Values and Intimacy*, New York: St Martins Press.

Weiss, T.G. and Korn, D.A. (2006) *Internal Displacement: Conceptualization and Its Consequences*, London and New York: Routledge.

Wellings, K., Bajos, N., Collumbien, M., Hodges, H., Singh, S., Slaymaker, E., and Patel, D. (2006) 'Sexual behaviour in context: a global perspective', *The Lancet*, 368: 1706–1728.

West, D. and Zimmerman, C. (1991) 'Doing gender', in J. Lorber and S. Farrell (eds) *The Social Construction of Gender*, Newbury Park, CA: Sage.

Whitehead, T. (1997) 'Urban low-income African American men, HIV/AIDS, and gender identity', *Medical Anthropology Quarterly*, 11: 411–447.

WHO (World Health Organization) (2002) 'Technical consultation on sexual health, working definitions', Geneva. Available online at www.who.int/-reproductive-health/gender/sexual_health.html#2 (accessed 25 February 2007).

Wieringa, S., Bhaiya, A., and Blackwood, E. (eds) (2007) *Women's Sexualities and Masculinities in a Globalizing Asia*, New York: Palgrave Macmillan.

Williams, W. (1986) *The Spirit and the Flesh: Sexual Diversity in American Indian Culture*, Boston: Beacon Press.

Wintemute, R. (2007) 'Comments on "X vs. Colombia" – Ramifications on Gay Rights Internationally, e-mail to sogi@list.arc-international.net, 7 August.

WLUML (Women Living under Muslim Laws) (1997) *Plan of Action*, Dhaka. Available online at www.wluml.org/english/pubs/rtf/poa/dhakapoa.rtf (accessed 29 November 2007).

Wojcicki, J. (2002) 'Commercial sex work or Ukuphanda?: sex-for-money exchange in Soweto and Hammskraal area, South Africa', *Culture, Medicine, and Psychiatry*, 26: 339–370.

Wong, E. (2006) 'G.I.s investigated in slayings of four and rape in Iraq', *New York Times*, 1 July.

Woolf, V. (1983 [orig. 1933]) *Flush*, San Diego, New York and London: Harcourt.

World Bank (2006) 'Male circumcision: evidence and implications', World Bank Global HIV/AIDS Program Monitoring and Evaluation Team, March.

Yogyakarta Principles (2007) Available online at www.yogyakartaprinciples.org/index.php?item=25 (accessed 9 September 2007).

Young, I.M. (1990) *Justice and the Politics of Difference*, Princeton: Princeton University Press.

Zangana, H. (2006) 'All Iraq is Abu Ghraib', *Guardian*. Available online at http://commentisfree/guardian.co.uk/haifa_zangana/2006/07 (accessed 5 July 2006).

Zarkov, D. (2001) 'The body of the other man: sexual violence and the construction of masculinity, sexuality and ethnicity in Croatian media', in C.O.N. Moser and F.C. Clark (eds) *Victims, Perpetrators, or Actors? Gender, Armed Conflict, and Political Violence*, London: Zed Books.

Zernike, K. (2006) 'Senate approves broad new rules to try detainees', *New York Times*, 29 September.

Zinn, E.F. (1924) 'History, purpose and policy of the National Research Council's Committee for Research on Sex Problems', *Mental Hygiene*, 8: 94–105.

Zinn, M.B. and Dill, B.T. (1996) 'Theorizing difference from multiracial feminism', *Feminist Studies*, 22: 321–331.

Žižek, S. (2002) *Welcome to the Desert of the Real*, London and New York: Verso.

Zoepf, K. (2007) 'Iraqi refugees, in desperation, turn to the sex trade in Syria', *New York Times*, 29 May.

Index

D30852

CPSIA information can be obtained at www.ICGtesting.com
Printed in the USA
BVOW02s2159080114

341268BV00003B/42/P

9 780415 351188